Basic immunology and its medical application

Basic immunology and its medical application

James T. Barrett

Professor of Microbiology, University of Missouri,
Columbia, Missouri

with 122 illustrations

Saint Louis

The C. V. Mosby Company

1976

Printed in the United States of America

Distributed in Great Britain by Henry Kimpton, London

Library of Congress Cataloging in Publication Data

Barrett, James T 1927-
Basic immunology and its medical application.

Bibliography: p.
Includes index.
1. Immunology. 2. Immunopathology. I. Title.
[DNLM: 1. Immunity. 2. Immunochemistry.
3. Serology. QW504 B274b]
RC584.B35 616.07'9 75-42465
ISBN 0-8016-0496-6

VH/VH/VH 9 8 7 6 5 4 3 2 1

To my parents

Preface

The emphasis on immunology in medical, dental, and other health science curricula is not surprising. Immunology has been the scene of many significant discoveries in the past few decades. Those discoveries of medical importance have quite naturally been incorporated into the clinical practice of pediatrics, medicine, obstetrics, surgery, and others. However, this period of expansion in immunology has not been restricted to its human and medical applications; the entire subject of immunology has grown dramatically. This has required more extensive discussions of immunochemistry, immunopharmacology, immunopathology, and immunity in such fields as biochemistry, anatomy, pathology, pharmacology, and microbiology. For the most part, these changes have been all to the good, but it is clear that instruction in immunology has fallen into the classic pattern in which the fundamental features of the subject are presented in the first and second years of an educational program, followed by a consideration of its applications at some later time.

It is obvious that there are many applied aspects of immunology that can be presented successfully to students in the preclinical years. A student need not have training in obstetrics and gynecology to understand the practical aspects of hemolytic disease of the newborn and Rh problems any more than he is required to study pediatrics and medicine to appreciate the importance of prophylactic immunizations in the control of infectious disease. In fact, the description of these professional applications of immunologic knowledge whets the appetite for further understanding of immunology in both its basic and applied form. The advice "Teach by example" can be interpreted appropriately either to present or be the example.

This book was written with two goals in mind: to present the basic subject matter of immunology to the reader in a condensed form and to illustrate by case histories and clinical correlations how this information is applied to the solution of medical problems. The title of the text was chosen to indicate this emphasis. Since it was expected that the primary users of this text would be preclinical students, the case histories have not included the entire clinical laboratory "printout" of all the data often assembled by these laboratories. Much of this data would be superfluous to the case histories presented and, by forcing the student to refer constantly to a table of normal values, would detract from the primary immunologic message. Examples of exotic conditions are few in number and, when included, are designed to emphasize some basic immunologic tenet rather than to represent a regular encounter in medical practice. Instead, a genuine effort has been made to include and discuss everyday immunologic problems—penicillin and ragweed allergy, myeloma, serologic tests for syphilis, immunization schedules, and the like, since these are the problems the student is most likely to face later in the "real world."

James T. Barrett

Contents

Basic immunology and its medical application

chapter 1

Scope of medical immunology

HISTORICAL BACKGROUND

There is no disputing the fact that immunology originated from the study of immunity. The study of immunity itself had little scientific basis until the investigations of Louis Pasteur in the second half of the 19th century. It was at approximately this time that techniques were being developed to recognize, cultivate, and attenuate the microbes that caused certain infectious diseases. Pasteur's genius allowed him to capitalize on these developments, to add to them his own knowledge from his background in chemistry and biology, and to emerge as the father of immunology.

The groundwork of immunity as a science probably originated in ancient China, where the inhalation of dried smallpox crusts was practiced as a preventive of this disease. Presumably the viral agent of this disfiguring and lethal disease lost some of its infectivity in drying, so that it was a mixture of inactivated and active viral particles that was actually inhaled. Because of the long incubation period for smallpox, some immunity could be developed during the period in which the few active viral particles generated a sufficient number of its kind to produce disease. Consequently, the disease was milder than "wild" smallpox, and this form of immunization was perpetuated.

In Turkey a different form of variolation (smallpox was then known as variola) was observed by Lady Montagu, wife of the British Ambassador. There, pustular material was taken from the lesions of a person with a mild case of smallpox and transferred by a common needle into a vein or tissue of the person desiring the immunization. Hopefully, a mild form of smallpox would develop and apparently did with sufficient regularity for Lady Montagu to have her own children vaccinated in this manner. In 1718 she introduced this procedure in England, and she is credited with introducing the method to the western world.

Obviously these earlier methods of immunization had inescapable risks—there was no assurance that variolation would result in only a mild case of smallpox, and there was also a possibility of transferring syphilis, leprosy, hepatitis, or most any other disease of the donor. Jenner's system of smallpox vaccination, advanced by him in 1798 as a result of his study of cowpox and smallpox in English milkmaids, avoided these problems and began to place immunity on a firm scientific footing. Jenner observed simply that milkmaids who contracted cowpox were thereafter immune to smallpox. Cowpox is a mild pox of cattle that causes pustule formation on the teats of the cow. Milkers are inescapably exposed to the disease and develop cowpox lesions on their hands. These heal and disappear with little outward noticeable change in the individual. However, Edward Jenner, an English countryside physician, noted that such persons never contracted smallpox, and he set up an experiment to test this more critically. Jenner took pustular material from a cowpox lesion on the thumb of a milkmaid named Sarah Nelmes and used it to inoculate a farm boy named James Phipps. Surely enough young Phipps developed cowpox. Then Jenner performed the critical part of the experiment. After Phipps had recovered from cowpox, Jenner inoculated him with smallpox and demonstrated his immunity to this disease as well. Like so many remarkable advances, this lifesaving discovery was mocked and not widely adopted until well into the 19th century. Admittedly, Jenner had capitalized on a rare occurrence—the creation of a permanent immunity to one disease on recovery from another. This phenomenon is known as cross-immunity, and Jenner had witnessed it in its most perfect form. We now recognize that the cowpox and smallpox viruses are nearly identical twins, and because of their close relationship, immunity to one is immunity to the other. There is, in fact, only one other example of good cross protective immunity of this sort practiced in human medicine and that is the use of the bovine strain of the tubercle bacillus to immunize against the human form of tuberculosis.

Pasteur's fame and status as the father of immunology also stems in part from an unusual circumstance. Of course, Pasteur made many famous discoveries, including the relationship of crystal structure to optical isomerism, the process of pasteurization, the attenuation of virulence of infectious agents, and his rabies vaccine (Fig. 1-1). Prior to his study of rabies but eventually to be closely linked to it was Pasteur's recognition that the virulence of the anthrax bacillus and that of the bacterium

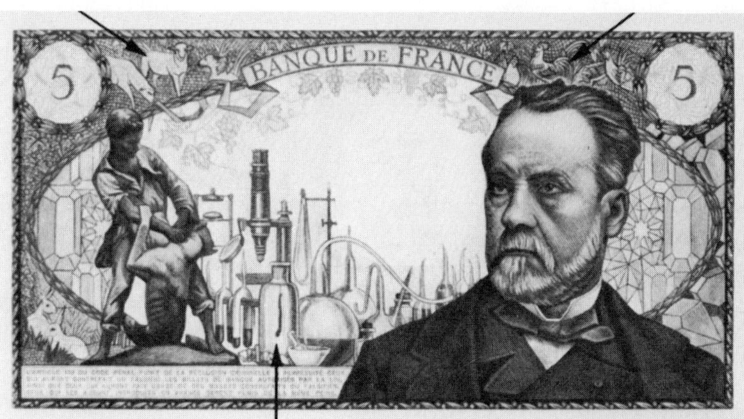

Fig. 1-1. **French five franc notes illustrate many of Pasteur's scientific accomplishments** in a true art form. Upper left and upper right arrows point to sheep and chickens that commemorate development of attenuated vaccines for anthrax and chicken cholera. Lower arrow indicates rabid rabbit spinal cord in a drying jar first used to treat Joseph Meister, the young boy shown battling a rabid dog. Rabbits in lower left corner possibly portray Pasteur's entry into bacterial warfare and his deliberate infection of rabbits who were burrowing into a friend's wine cellar and dislodging the masonry with disastrous results. Crystals at left and right center illustrate relationships of crystal structure to optical rotation, grape clusters refer to Pasteur's study of diseases of wine and discovery of pasteurization, and swan-necked flask near Pasteur's portrait is a reminder of his disputation of the theory of spontaneous generation. Flagellated bacilli surrounding number 5 in each upper corner of note refer to his discovery of anaerobic life. The reverse side of the bill is also beautiful and illustrates fungi, mulberry, and grapes with the portrait of Pasteur.

that causes chicken cholera could be reduced by manipulation of the age or growth temperature of cultures of these bacteria. Both of these discoveries were serendipitous—the first from an effort to use cultures that had been placed in a faulty incubator and the second from a similar use of cultures that had set for several days on a laboratory bench. When Pasteur observed that dried spinal cords of rabbits dead from experimental rabies could not transmit the disease although fresh spinal cord material from these rabbits would, he correctly reasoned that, as in the experiments with chicken cholera and anthrax, the noninfective material might make a good vaccine. Laboratory studies confirmed this, and eventually he was prevailed on to try his Pasteur treatment on a young boy, Joseph Meister, who had been bitten many times by a rabid dog. The Pasteur treatment consisted of a series of inoculations beginning with aged and ending with fresh spinal cord from a rabid rabbit. This method protected Joseph Meister and thousands like him from rabies and led to the great popular fame of Pasteur and the construction of Pasteur Institutes throughout the world dedicated to him and his discovery.

In the case of rabies a second unique situation exists—an exceptionally long incubation time of the disease. As a consequence of this, immunization with rabies vaccine after exposure to the virus has time to generate sufficient immunity to resist the disease. For practically all other diseases except smallpox, which also has a long incubation time, vaccination must be performed prior to exposure. The word "vaccination" (from the Latin *vacca,* meaning cow) was used by Pasteur to honor Jenner's contribution and the use of microorganisms to prevent the very diseases they cause.

Another successful form of immunization, and one in which the use of the term "vaccination" is generally considered less appropriate, is the use of bacterial toxoids. It is surprising that toxoids were not used for prophylactic immunization against human diseases until 1923, since Behring and Kitasato had recognized as early as 1890 that certain bacteria, of which diphtheria and tetanus are examples, cause disease almost entirely by virtue of the potent exotoxins they excrete. Moreover, complete immunity against these diseases is based on the presence of special toxin-neutralizing antibodies, or antitoxins, present in the blood of individuals who have recovered from these diseases. Such antibodies can be formed by a person who is injected with tiny doses of these toxins, but this is obviously a dangerous undertaking. Nontoxic, neutral mixtures of toxin and antitoxin (taken from an immune laboratory animal) were used for immunization instead, that is, until 1923 when Ramon found that treatment of these exotoxins with formaldehyde would convert them to harmless molecules called toxoids. These toxoids would generate the same degree of immunity as the toxins without their obvious drawback, and toxoids have been used for immunizations ever since. Unfortunately there are few diseases caused by exotoxins, but diphtheria and tetanus are such widespread and serious diseases that toxoid-induced immunity is still considered an important development in preventive medicine.

Emil von Behring received a Nobel Prize in 1901, the first ever offered in medicine and physiology, for his studies with antitoxins. However, immunity is not entirely founded on the ability of an animal to respond to vaccines or toxoids of pathogenic organisms by the formation of antibodies. Metchnikoff, the volatile Russian, was one of the first to recognize this when he noticed that the cell-eating behavior of certain cells, the circulatory and tissue phagocytes, resulted in the death of the foreign cells they ate. Presently there is a resurgence of interest in phagocytic cells as the key to tumor immunity. Other recent studies of human patients with functionally inept phagocytes, who consequently suffer from a continuous stream of bacterial infections, are beginning to unravel the means these cells use to destroy their phagocytic victims. For his discovery of phagocytic cells, Metchnikoff received a Nobel Prize in 1908.

In the three quarters of a century that have passed since these early awards to immunologists for their contributions in the realm of immunity, immunology has taken new directions in chemistry, genetics, medicine, and surgery. Immunologists are concerned with the chemistry of blood proteins, of histocompatibility antigens, of the red blood cell membrane, of mast cell degranulation, and of other biochemical problems. Problems of tissue transplantation, hemolytic disease of the newborn, the inheritance of allergies, the functions of lymphocytes, and other topics outside the realm of immunity as such dominate much of modern-day immunology. At the same time diseases, not necessarily infectious in nature, such as tumor immunity and the autoimmune diseases are under investigation by immunologists. The expanding interest in and information about the subdivisions of immunology have been so great that special methods and a special jargon for each has emerged. Old terms are being used in new ways and new terms are being originated. Unfortunately this has resulted in duplicate definitions and vague or imprecise descriptions. Normally a vocabulary for a science develops gradually as knowledge of the science itself grows, but wherever uncertainty exists, reference to a dictionary or glossary becomes inevitable. Such a glossary is presented at the end of this book. Although it might be possible to memorize a brief glossary, a better appreciation of the manner in which immunologic terms are used may be conceived from the following condensed introductory sketch of medical immunology.

IMMUNOLOGIC REAGENTS

The science of immunology is dynamic in the sense that it analyzes the response of the body to substances that are foreign to the body. Often the first foreign substances that come to mind are bacteria, viruses, or other infectious agents that the immunologist calls *antigens*. Actually, cells are composed of many complex macromolecules that are antigenic, and this includes such molecules in red blood cells, grafted tissues, and other noninfectious as well as infectious cells. The body can also respond to many nonantigenic substances, *haptens*, when these are linked into hapten-antigen conjugates, but not to the hapten alone. Haptens are customarily of lower molecular weight or simpler structure than antigens, so it can be seen that the animal body has evolved a method of reacting to simple as well as complex molecules. This response can be magnified if the antigen or *neoantigen* is presented to the animal with an *adjuvant*.

Adjuvants improve the immune response (immune response is the term used even though the antigen or hapten has no connection with an infectious agent) by influencing the behavior of host cells. Tissue *macrophages*, a type of *phagocyte*, engulf and partially degrade the antigen, passing on *antigenic determinants* to *B* and *T lymphocytes*. The B lymphocytes in birds are easily recognized because they pass through and are altered by a cloacal gland called the *bursa of Fabricius*. This alteration allows them to respond to antigenic determinants with a reproductive burst that terminates in the *plasma cell* as the product of *lymphocyte transformation*. The plasma cell excretes *antibodies (immunoglobulins)* that are found in the gamma globulin fraction of the blood. These antibodies are synthesized in such a way that they can combine with that specific antigen (and certain *cross-reactive* antigens) that stimulated its formation. Several different molecular classes of these immunoglobulins are formed. This includes IgG, IgM, IgA, IgD, and IgE plus several subclasses, or *allotypes*. Oncogenesis of plasma cells results in an excessive synthesis of the immunoglobulins or their structural parts as seen in *multiple myeloma, Waldenström's macroglobulinemia,* or other *immunoproliferative diseases*. Since this may create an imbalance in the defensive armory, plasma cell proliferation, just as a genetic absence of plasma cells, may produce an *immunodeficiency disease*. Immunodeficiency due to *hypogammaglobulinemia* may be either genetic or acquired.

Simultaneous with these events, the antigen-exposed T lymphocyte has emitted a message that results in the appearance of a more actively phagocytic and a more powerfully digestive macrophage known as the *activated macrophage,* which is consequently more active in modifying the antigen. The T lymphocyte progresses through a proliferative phase and becomes concentrated with macrophages in cell packets termed *germinal centers*. Proliferating B cells also create germinal centers. The T lymphocyte, so named because it is modified by the thymus, may stimulate the B cell in its immunoglobulin response *(helper T cell)* or restrict B cell activities *(suppressor T cell)*. Perhaps more important is the T cell production of *lymphokines* that alter host cells to make them refractory to intracellular parasites *(interferon)*, attract macrophages *(chemotaxin)*, arrest macrophage migration *(macrophage migration inhibitor factor)*, or attack foreign cells directly *(lymphotoxin)*. Other lymphokines may function in *cell-mediated immune* reactions or *cell-mediated (delayed) hypersensitivity. Humoral immunity* and the *immediate hypersensitivities* are dependent on antibodies.

To these adaptive responses or reactants must be added those of the *complement* system that participate in antigen-antibody reactions to stimulate phagocytosis by generating *opsonins* and *chemotaxins* and encouraging *immune adherence*. Other undesirable complement-related activities include those associated with *anaphylatoxin* and *kinin* formation. Complement activation can also be initiated by the antibody-independent *properdin* pathway.

IMMUNOLOGIC REACTIONS

The union of an antigen with its antibody with or without the participation of complement or other accessory factors is the subject matter for serology. When the antigen is soluble, the reaction is described as a *precipitation* reaction. Serologic precipitates can also form when the reagents diffuse through gels and combine with each other. There are many variations to such *immunodiffusion* tests—*radial (Mancini) immunodiffusion,* double diffusion of the *Ouchterlony type, immunoelectrophoresis, crossed immunoelectrophoresis, counterimmunoelectrophoresis,* etc. When the antigen is cellular or particulate, the serologic reaction is an *agglutination* reaction or, as in the case of erythrocyte antigens, *hemagglutination*. Fluid antigens can be absorbed to cells to convert precipitation tests to *passive agglutination* tests. When complement is present, it is fixed in the serologic reaction *(complement fixation)*, and this may be measured as a cytolytic reaction *(bacteriolysis* or *hemolysis)*. When phagocytic cells are present, the serologic reaction may be seen to favor phagocytosis of the antigen. Occasionally no outward sign of an antigen- or hapten-antibody reaction may be noted. This may demand the use of *fluorescent antibody* procedures, *radioimmunoassay,* or *antiglobulin* (double antibody) techniques.

The result of immunologic reactions in vivo that destroy or resist foreign cells or their products is usually classified as immunity. This explains the origin of the terms "transplantation immunity" and "tumor immunity," since tumors usually have a new set of antigens that makes them foreign. When the immune response is directed against self-antigens, an *autoimmune disease* is often the result. This may take the form of an *autoimmune hemolytic disease* or *immune complex disease* involving antigens of thrombocytes, kidney, or other cells. Autoimmune diseases associated with misdirected T cell activities as in postinfectious encephalomyelitis are also known. When disease results from immune responses to external antigens, these diseases are usually labeled *allergies*. The *immediate* or *immunoglobulin-dependent allergies* rely on the attachment of *reagin (cytotropic IgE)* to the surface of *mast cells*. Combination of this IgE with antigen initiates *mast cell degranulation* with the liberation of *vasoactive amines* such as *histamine* and *serotonin*. The antigen-antibody reaction may trigger the *Hageman pathway* and the eventual release of *bradykinin* and other *kinins*. White blood cells may also release pharmacologically active substances. *Antihistamines* and *β-adrenergic drugs* such as adrenaline modify these toxic reactions. In their milder forms these reactions are associated with the *atopic illnesses,* hay fever or other *respiratory allergies,* and *food allergies*. In their more severe form these are seen as life-threatening *anaphylactic reactions*.

T cell activities may also be expressed as allergies and *contact dermatitis,* including reactions to cosmetics, dyes, animal products, and *poison ivy,* and other sources of haptenic compounds have much in common with *tuberculin reactions* and other *allergies of infection*.

From this compact overview of immunology it is apparent that the behavior of the involved cells is complex, and this will be treated in the following chapter on immunocytology. The chemicals these cells respond to and the cell products they respond with are considered in the chapter on immunobiochemistry. Serologic reactions and immunity are discussed in separate chapters, as is immunohematology. Thereafter separate chapters will fill in the details of B and T cell–mediated allergies, autoimmunity, transplantation, and tissue immunity. It can be seen that the first chapters are devoted to basic immunology, whereas the latter are devoted to its medical applications.

BIBLIOGRAPHY

Textbooks on general immunology

Abramoff, P., and La Via, M.: Biology of the immune response, New York, 1970, McGraw-Hill Book Co.

Barrett, J. T.: Textbook of immunology, ed. 2, St. Louis, 1974, The C. V. Mosby Co.

Bigley, N. J.: Immunologic fundamentals, Chicago, 1975, Year Book Medical Publishers, Inc.

Eisen, H. N.: Immunology, Hagerstown, Md., 1974, Medical Department, Harper & Row, Publishers, Inc.

Gold, E. R., and Peacock, D. B.: Basic immunology, Bristol, 1970, John Wright & Sons, Ltd.

Henriksen, S. D.: Immunology, Baltimore, 1970, The Williams & Wilkins Co.
Roitt, I. M.: Essential immunology, ed. 2, Oxford, 1974, Blackwell Scientific Publications, Ltd.

Textbooks and monographs on medical immunology

Alexander, J. W., and Good, R. A.: Immunobiology for surgeons, Philadelphia, 1970, W. B. Saunders Co.
Bellanti, J. A.: Immunology, Philadelphia, 1971, W. B. Saunders Co.
Gell, P. G. H., Coombs, R. R. A., and Lachmann, P. J., eds.: Clinical aspects of immunology, ed. 13, Oxford, 1975, Blackwell Scientific Publications, Ltd.
Good, R. A., and Fisher, D. W., eds.: Immunobiology, Stamford, Conn., 1971, Sinauer Associates.
Humphrey, J. H., and White, R. G.: Immunology for students of medicine, ed. 3, Philadelphia, 1970, F. A. Davis Co.
Park, B. H., and Good, R. A.: Principles of modern immunobiology: basic and clinical, Philadelphia, 1974, Lea & Febiger.
Sell, S.: Immunology, immunopathology, and immunity, ed. 2, Hagerstown, Md., 1975, Medical Department, Harper & Row, Publishers, Inc.
Turk, J. L.: Immunology in clinical medicine, ed. 2, New York, 1972, Appleton-Century-Crofts.
Weiser, R., Myrvik, Q., and Pearsall, N.: Fundamentals of immunology for students of medicine and related sciences, Philadelphia, 1969, Lea & Febiger.

chapter 2

Immunocytology

The cells of the body that respond to antigens are variously categorized as belonging to the hematopoietic system, the reticuloendothelial system, or lymphoid system. The organs and tissues comprising these systems are not as well defined as those of the nervous system, endocrine system, etc., which tend to exist as distinct structural organs and have a clear, often singular, physiologic role. The cells of the immune system originate from hematopoietic tissue, and after leaving this they acquire or express functions that place them in the reticuloendothelial or lymphoid system (Fig. 2-1).

HEMATOPOIETIC SYSTEM

The cells of the reticuloendothelial and lymphoid systems and those of the recently delineated mononuclear phagocytic system arise from the bone marrow. The average adult has about 3 kg of bone marrow, making it the largest organ of the body. In addition to the vascular and adipose tissue of marrow that represent about one half of the tissue, about one half of the tissue in bone marrow is dedicated to hematopoiesis or blood cell formation. The development of blood cells arises from a primitive, undifferentiated stem cell, the reticulum cell, and diverges into several distinct lines. Of these, only the cells of the granulocytic, lymphocytic, and monocytic series are of fundamental importance in the immunologic response, although cells of the erythroid and megakaryocytic series are often important as targets of the immune response.

RETICULOENDOTHELIAL SYSTEM

The so-called reticuloendothelial system (RES) is a collection of cells of diverse morphology and tissue residence united by the sole property of an ambitious phagocytic behavior. Classically the RES has been divided into tissue and blood phagocytes of large size, macrophages, and those of lesser size, microphages. The macrophages have now been united and elevated to the status of a system by a WHO expert committee and called the mononuclear phagocytic system. The characteristics of the cells in the new system include a pronounced phagocytic ability, a cell diameter of 10 to 25 μ, a nucleus-cytoplasm ratio of about 1:1 or somewhat less, a relatively large oval or kidney-shaped nucleus, a granular texture in their cytoplasm due to its content of lysosomal granules, and numerous cytoplasmic vacuoles. These cells arise from the monocytic series of the hematopoietic system and are represented in blood by circulating monocytes. The peripheral blood monocytes serve as the source of the free and fixed tissue macrophages. Tissue macrophages have specific names according to their anatomic location; thus histiocytes are found in connective tissue, Kupffer's cells in liver, alveolar macrophages in lung, microglial cells in the neural system, and free and fixed macrophages in spleen, lymph nodes, and other organs (Fig. 2-2).

The mononuclear phagocytes have surface receptors for immunoglobulins and complement that may assist in the attachment of antigens to these cells. Other blood

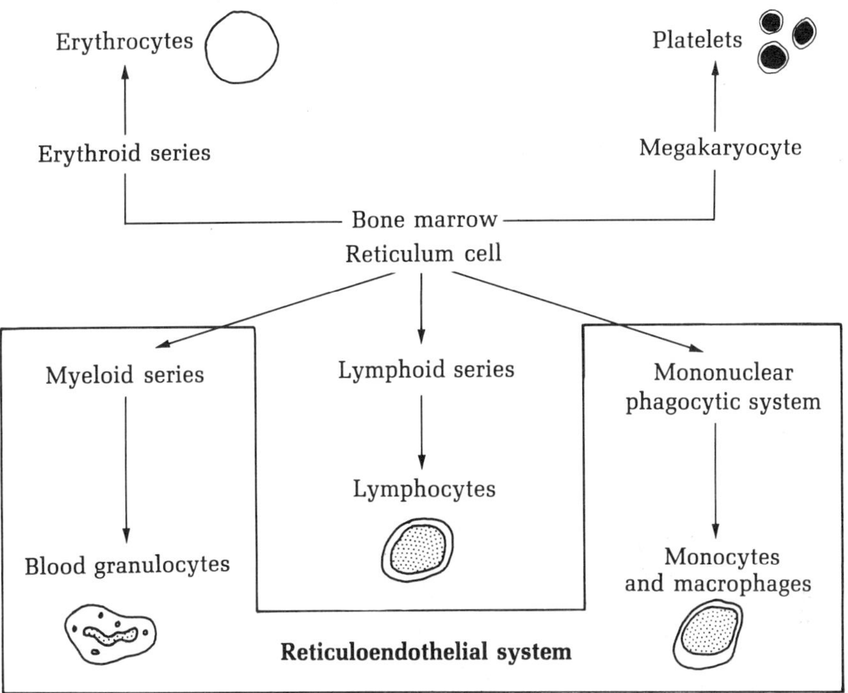

Fig. 2-1. Origin of immunologically vital cells from bone marrow. Granulocytes and monocytes have traditionally been considered as the two halves of the reticuloendothelial system, but the latter are now being treated as a separate unit. The lymphoid system represents the third important cell line. Cells of the erythroid series and megakaryocytes are important as antigens.

proteins (opsonins—to prepare for eating) may assist in phagocytosis. Once the engulfed particle is taken internally, it eventually contacts a lysosomal granule. When this occurs, the lysosome disgorges an array of hydrolytic enzymes into the phagocytic vacuole. This now becomes the phagolysosome, a structure in which a combination of forces seeks to reduce bacteria, viruses, other pathogens, or antigens into their smaller constituents. These forces include an acid pH resulting from the intracellular accumulation of lactic acid arising from glycolysis. Antibody and complement, which may also utilize the enzyme lysozyme, are lytic for certain cells. Oxidative halogenation and hydrolytic degradation also destroy antigens. Among the lysosomal hydrolases known to be released during phagocytosis are phosphatases, ribonucleases, deoxyribonucleases, proteases, lipases, glycosidases, and esterases. Certain lysosomal proteins may contribute to the destruction of engulfed cells by nonenzymatic processes, for example, phagocytin.

The polymorphonuclear neutrophilic (PMN) leukocytes, the neutrophilic granulocytes of blood, represent about 60% of all blood leukocytes. The eosinophils and basophils, the other granulocytes, represent only 1% each. These two latter cell types are important in allergic reactions but have feeble phagocytic powers compared to the PMNs. The granulocytes are about 12 μ in diameter (Fig. 2-3) and have a granulated cytoplasm that has an affinity for either basic dyes (basophils), acid dyes such as eosin (eosinophils), or both (neutrophils). The neutrophils are easily recognized by their neutrophilic granula-

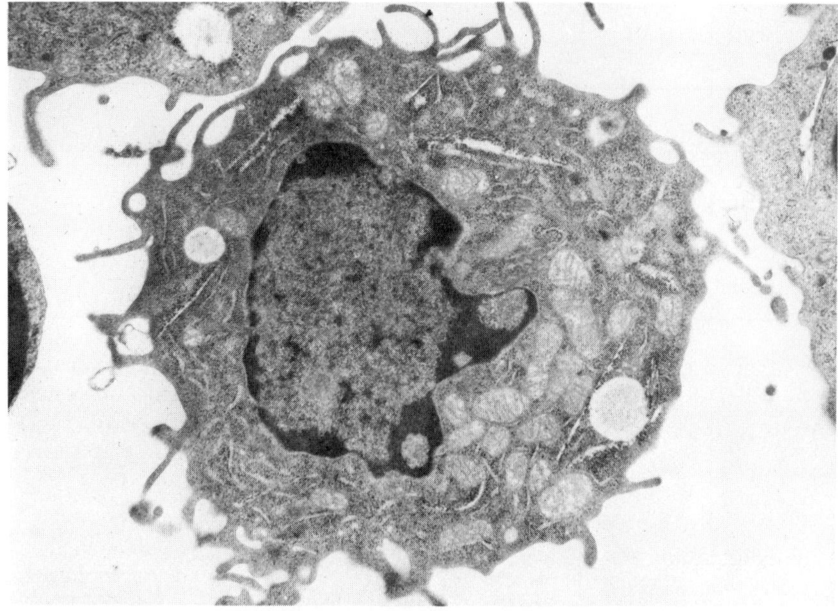

Fig. 2-2. This macrophage, seen as it appears under the electron microscope, is not necessarily typical of all macrophages. They differ slightly from organ to organ, except for their large cytoplasmic volume and numerous inclusions and granules. The numerous extensions from its cytoplasmic membranes are an indication of its extensive membrane activity, which is helpful for both motility and phagocytosis. (Courtesy Dr. E. Adelstein.)

tion and their tri- or multilobed nucleus. Their granules apparently do not differ from the lysosomal granules of tissue macrophages, but the granules of eosinophils and basophils are not lysosomal. Thus the result of phagocytosis by PMNs and macrophages is essentially the same, the enclosure of the engulfed object into a phagocytic vacuole, coalescence of the phagocytic vacuole and lysosome to form a phagolysosome, and the death and digestion of the cell.

Although enzymes derived from lysosomes are undoubtedly important in the degradation of ingested pathogenic bacteria or other cells, it is no longer believed that these enzymes are directly responsible for the death of such bacterial cells. Examination of leukocytes with impaired bactericidal activity from patients with chronic granulomatous disease and similar disorders reveals that inept phagocytes lack the ability to form singlet oxygen ($^1O_2$). Singlet oxygen is believed to be the ultimate bactericidal weapon of the phagocyte. Singlet oxygen might be provided by the decomposition of the superoxide radical (O_2^-) formed during oxidation of reduced pyridine nucleotides. The feasibility of this hypothesis is strengthened by the knowledge that phagocytic cells exhibit a respiratory burst during phagocytosis and have the possibility to involve nicotinamide adenine dinucleotide (NAD or NADP) extensively in oxidation-reduction reactions. Alternatively an excited singlet oxygen could arise from the interaction of the myeloperoxidase–hydrogen peroxide–halide system in which hypochlorite or other halides could interact with myeloperoxidase and H_2O_2 as indicated in Fig. 2-4. Absolute proof that granulocytes form singlet oxygen is not available; however, they can form the superoxide ion, and since they lack the enzyme superoxide dismutase that decomposes the superoxide ion, singlet oxygen

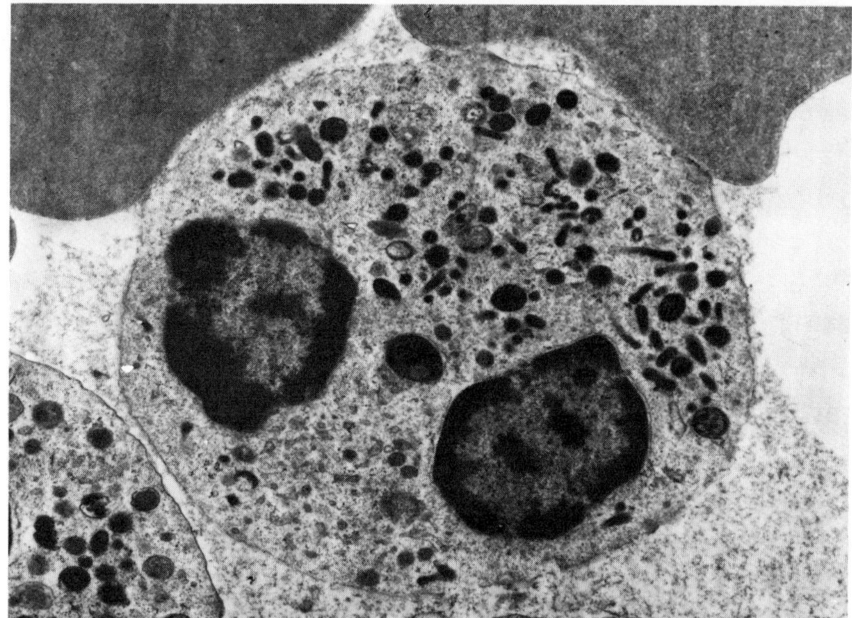

Fig. 2-3. Electron microscopic appearance of polymorphonuclear leukocyte (PMN or neutrophil). Section through the cell gives the illusion that its trilobed nucleus exists as three separate nuclei. Many of the dark granules in the upper portion of the cell are lysosomes. Phagolysosomes are not in evidence. (Courtesy Dr. E. Adelstein.)

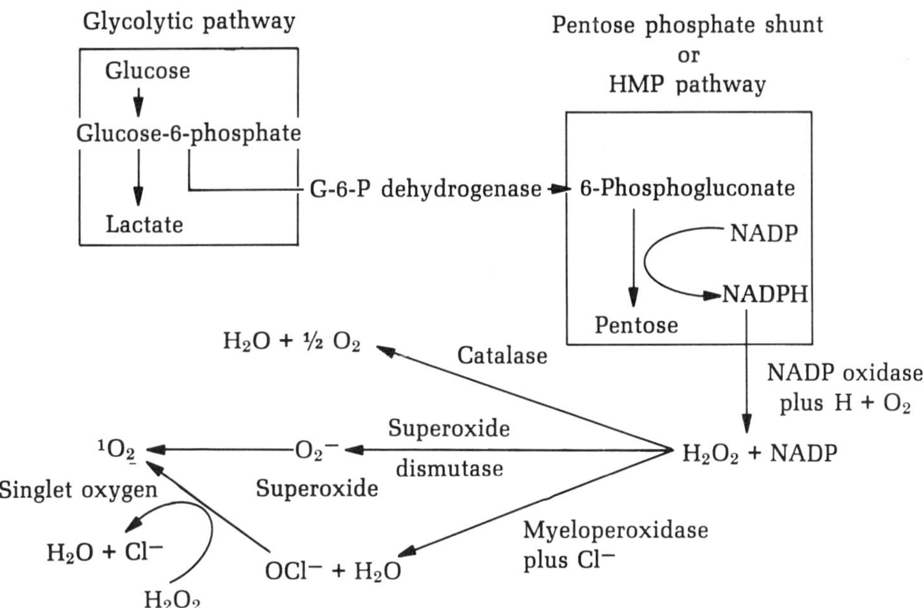

Fig. 2-4. Metabolism by normal phagocytes in glycolytic and pentose phosphate shunt leads to formation of H_2O_2. Then the microbicidal singlet oxygen is formed by alternate pathways, two of which are shown. Phagocytic defects at the level of G-6-P dehydrogenase, NADP oxidase, myeloperoxidase, and superoxide dismutase would obviously impair intracellular killing by the phagocyte.

formation by the spontaneous dismutation of superoxide ion would be expected to occur. Carotenoid pigments of bacteria protect them against intraphagocytic killing and are known to quench singlet oxygen, a finding that strongly incriminates this form of oxygen as the bactericidal substance.

LYMPHOID SYSTEM

The lymphocyte is the dominant cell of the lymphoid system, which is generally discussed in terms of the central and peripheral lymphoid tissues. Included among the central lymphoid tissues are bone marrow and thymus. Lymph nodes, spleen, tonsils, intestinal lymphoid tissue (Peyer's patches), and others constitute the peripheral lymphoid tissues. Fowl have a second central lymphoid organ, the bursa of Fabricius, that is critical to the development of immunoglobulin-producing cells.

Central lymphoid organs

Bone marrow. The structure of bone marrow was described in the preceding section on the hematopoietic system.

Thymus. The mammalian thymus is a flat, bilobed organ situated below the thyroid gland along the neck and extending into the thoracic cage. In the chicken the thymus is a multilobed structure rarely extending into the thoracic cavity and usually lying along the neck. The thymus emerges from the third and fourth branchial pouches during embryonic development and is a fully developed organ at birth, when it weighs 15 to 20 gm. By puberty it will reach 40 gm, after which it will atrophy, becoming less significant structurally and functionally.

The thymus exists as an epithelial pouch filled with lymphocytes, occasionally called thymocytes. The epithelial cells and connective tissue subdivide the thymus gland into a series of lobes, each of which is filled with lymphocytes. The outer portion of each lobule, the thymic cortex, has the greatest density of lymphocytes, and the central or medullary portion of the gland is relatively free of these cells. In the medulla the lobes blend into a common field of reticulum cells, a few lymphocytes, and structures known as Hassall's corpuscles—concentric rings of hyaline epithelial cells of uncertain origin or function.

Bursa of Fabricius. Situated near the cloaca of fowl is a lymphoid organ not possessed by mammals known as the bursa of Fabricius. It is a saclike structure, about 3 cm in diameter at the time of its maximal development, that is very much like the thymus in structure. It is subdivided into lobes or follicles by epithelial cells and connective tissue. At the external margin of these follicles (in the cortical region of the gland), as in the thymus, the lymphocytes are gathered. In the more central portions of the gland (its medulla), lymphocytes are less prominent.

Interest in the bursa as a lymphoid organ resulted from the discovery that the surgical removal of the gland from young chicks restricted their antibody response to bacterial vaccines. The treatment of developing chick embryos with 19-nortestosterone prevents the development of the bursa, and the hatching chicks are even more severely penalized in terms of immunoglobulin production than are surgically bursectomized birds. The greater residuum of antibody-synthesizing ability in surgically as compared to hormonally bursectomized birds can be related to the fact that surgical bursectomy is performed later, after potential antibody-forming cells have been dispersed to the peripheral lymphoid organs.

Because of the morphologic similarities of thymus and bursal tissues, the effects of thymectomy were also examined. In this case it was found that certain immune reactions dependent on lymphocytes, such as graft rejection, and certain hypersensitive reactions of the delayed or cell-mediated type were lost. These reactions were known to be dependent on lymphocytes, and because of the experiments with bursectomy, it was now concluded that there were two major classes of lymphocytes, the thymic or T lymphocytes and the bursal or B lymphocytes. The T lymphocytes, although only partially related to the antibody-forming arm of the immune system, come from the bone marrow, probably as predestined T cells, and are imprinted with T cell characteristics in the thymus. Likewise the B lymphocytes, probably predestined to be such, are imprinted in the bursa to serve as the key cells in the immunoglobulin response. Since mammals have no bursa, an intense but largely disappointing search for a bursal equivalent has been conducted. Unlike chickens, mammals have apparently not placed all their immunoglobulin-forming cells in one basket, but have distributed them among several lymphoid organs. Bone marrow is used as the source of B cells in mammalian experiments.

Lymphocytes imprinted in the bursa, or its equivalent, and thymus are distributed from these organs through the blood to the peripheral lymphoid organs.

Peripheral lymphoid organs

The lymph nodes are situated along the lymphatic vessels that drain the solid tissues and are the first of the organized lymphoid tissues to encounter most antigens, except those entering through the cardiovascular system. Lymph nodes tend to be clustered near the ankle, knee, wrist, elbow, and at the juncture of the extremities with the torso. The internal structure of lymph nodes can be described as a spongelike meshwork through which macrophages, granulocytes, and lymphocytes course on their return to the blood. The lymphocytes are assembled in greatest density near the perimeter of the gland, which is divided into lobules or follicles. The bursal-derived or B lymphocytes are more prominent in the far cortical region of the gland and along the medullary cords leading from its center, whereas the thymus-derived or T lymphocytes tend to have a paracortical and more medullary location. This semisegregated distribution is readily discerned in thymectomized animals or those genetically deficient in thymus, having few lymphocytes in the paracortical region of their lymph nodes. Bursectomized birds and mammals with agammaglobulinemia have few lymphocytes in the far cortical region of their lymph nodes.

The tonsils are lymphoid tissues that, like the thymus, are rather large in childhood and tend to diminish in size with age. The internal structure of tonsils is very reminiscent of the thymus, bursa, and lymph nodes, being divided into follicles that are more lymphoid in nature near their outer, cortical perimeter.

The spleen is an important responder to blood-borne antigens. This response occurs in the white pulp of the organ, which is its lymphoid portion; the red pulp is reserved for the removal of aged or damaged erythrocytes. As with the other lymphoid organs, the lymphoid sections of the spleen are segregated into pockets of lymphocytes, which are dominantly of the bursal type. The abundance of splenic macrophages and B lymphocytes is evidence that the gland is well suited for immunoglobulin formation. The spleen is a vital organ in youth, but splenectomy in adulthood has no serious influence on resistance to infectious disease or life expectancy.

Other potentially important collections of lymphoid tissue exist in the appendix, Peyer's patches, and the lamina propria of the intestine.

Lymphocytes

The important cell common to all lymphoid tissue is the lymphocyte. Lymphocytes are derived from lymphoblasts in bone marrow and are dispersed into the

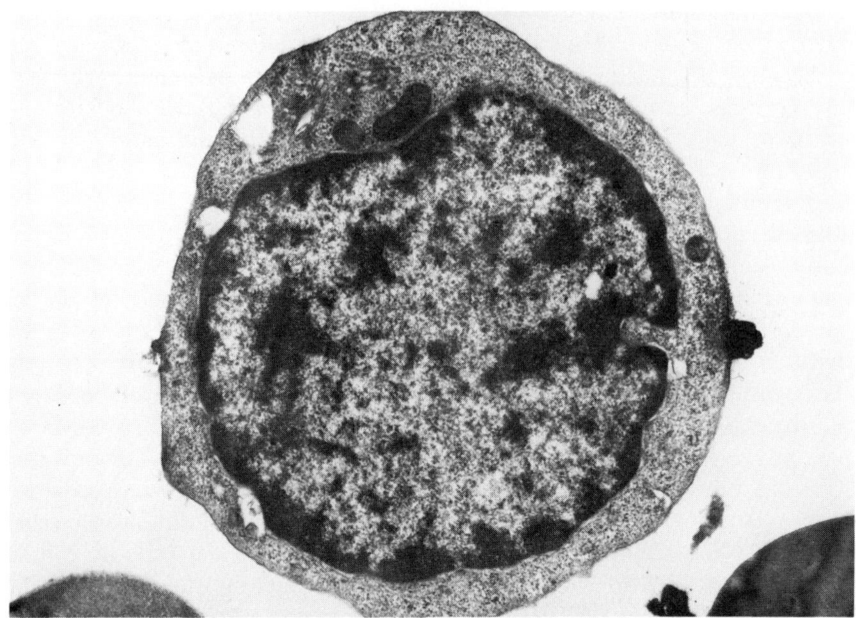

Fig. 2-5. Electron microscopic view of a lymphocyte in which no cytoplasmic endoplasmic reticulum can be seen. Scant margin of cytoplasm, isolated mitochondria, and diffuse nuclear chromatin assist in its identification as a lymphocyte. (Courtesy Dr. E. Adelstein.)

blood where they represent about 30% of the circulating leukocytes. Lymphocytes carried by the blood course through many organs, but important events take place in the thymus and bursa of Fabricius (or its mammalian equivalent) that regulate the response of these lymphocytes to antigens. Many more lymphocytes are present in tissues than in blood. Lymphocytes are collected from tissues and drawn into the lymphatic system, passing through lymph nodes and finally being returned to the blood from the thoracic lymph duct. Lymphocytes average about 7 μ in diameter and have a large, rounded nucleus surrounded by a small fringe of cytoplasm. The nucleus, which may have a single indentation, displays an irregular distribution or clumping of its chromatin. The cytoplasm has a faint granular texture, but these granules stain lightly, are small, and do not resemble lysosomal granules. When seen under an electron microscope, the cytoplasm appears clear (Fig. 2-5).

T versus B lymphocytes. Two major classes of lymphocytes, the T and B lymphocytes, are known, and there may be several subdivisions of each. The characteristics that distinguish T and B cells from each other are numerous, although they share a common origin (Table 2-1). When the T cells are modified in the thymus, they acquire a distinguishing surface antigen, the T or theta (θ) antigen. Lymphocytes bearing the T antigen are involved in cell-mediated immune and cell-mediated hypersensitivity reactions. Although these immune reactions appear to require a direct or nearly direct contact of the T cell with the foreign cell, these protective functions are mediated by lymphokines. T lymphocytes represent approximately 85% of all blood lymphocytes and are the dominant type of lymphocyte in thoracic duct lymph. These cells are present in peripheral lymphoid tissue, and when stimulated by antigens or certain mitogens, undergo cell growth and division, a process

Table 2-1. Differences of T and B lymphocytes

Characteristic	*T lymphocyte*	*B lymphocyte*
Tissue where modified	Thymus	Bursa of Fabricius or bursal equivalent
Unique surface antigen	T or θ-antigen	B or β-antigen
Surface immunoglobulin	Absent or masked	Readily detectable
Phytoagglutinin receptors	Yes, especially concanavalin A	Yes, especially phytohemagglutinin
Complement receptors	No	Yes, for C3
Antigen receptors	Yes, but mechanism unknown	Yes, through surface immunoglobulin
Tissue distribution	High in thoracic duct, lymph, and blood	High in spleen, low in blood
Lymphocyte transformation	Yes, to small lymphocytes	Yes, to plasma cells
Cell product	Lymphokines	Immunoglobulins
Germinal center location	Paracortical and medullary regions of lymph nodes	Far cortical regions of lymph nodes
Sensitivity to immunosuppression	Less than B cells	Greater than T cells
Response to conjugated antigens	Mostly to carrier	Good hapten response
Immune tolerance	Occurs early and persists, low-antigen doses are effective	Less sensitive than T cells

called lymphocyte transformation. Concanavalin A is a highly specific T cell mitogen. T lymphocyte replication in peripheral lymphoid tissue as a result of repeated antigenic stimulation results in the creation of distinct germinal (growth) centers. The germinal center consists of a well-defined oval structure (in cross section) containing a few centrally placed macrophages and lymphocytes. Larger lymphocytes undergoing nuclear and cytoplasmic growth can also be noted. Near the margin of the germinal center the smaller, mature lymphocytes are seen. Thymus and bursa, the central lymphoid organs, rarely have germinal centers. Germinal centers arising in peripheral lymphoid tissue from T lymphocytes can often be identified, at least in lymph nodes, by their tendency to form in the subcortical region, or more medullary area, of the gland. Although the location of germinal centers is not absolutely fixed, T cells tend not to be transported nor to initiate growth in the far cortical region of the lymph nodes.

The device used by T lymphocytes to recognize antigens or mitogens that launch the cell into a phase of growth and division is not clearly defined. It is apparently not a surface immunoglobulin of the usual type, although hypothetical immunoglobulins IgX or IgT have been postulated. T cells do have an unusual cell surface receptor for foreign erythrocytes, and sheep red blood cells are commonly used to identify these cells. A mixture of T lymphocytes from a nonimmune donor with sheep erythrocytes will result in a clumping of the erythrocytes around the T cell to form a rosette. Again the nature of the receptor responsible for rosette formation has not been identified, but it is one of the simplest tests for T cells.

Although lymphokine production wanes earlier than immunoglobulin production, it is believed that the T lymphocyte (or T memory cell) is longer lived than the B lymphocyte (or B memory cell). This belief is founded on the greater duration of T cell–mediated allergies than B cell–mediated allergies. Since several subpopulations of both B and T cells exist, some B cells conceivably could live longer than some forms of the T cells; thus the preceding is but a generalization. T cells are generally described as being more resistant to radiation, steroids, and several other chemical immunosuppressants such as cyclophosphamide than are B cells. Several adjuvants encourage T cell trapping in lymph nodes as the key to their mode of action, and T cells respond heavily to the carrier portion of hapten-antigen complexes with little in the way of a hapten-directed response. Specific immune tolerance of the low-dose type is believed due to the ease by which small quantities of antigen suppress T cell functions, much larger doses being required to inhibit B cells. Both T cells and B cells can be caused to transform by phytohemagglutinins that attach to specific cell receptors. Concanavalin A, an efficient stimulant of T cell transformation, attaches to α-D-glucosyl residues on the lymphocyte surface. Pokeweed mitogen and phytohemagglutinin are both more stimulatory of B lymphocytes.

For each of the features mentioned, the behavior of the B lymphocyte contrasts sharply with that of the T lymphocyte. The B lymphocyte has no T antigen, but it does have a unique surface antigen of its own, the B antigen, which is acquired in the bursa or bursa equivalent. The B lymphocyte is intimately involved in immunoglobulin formation, not that it is so generously endowed with this capacity itself but through B lymphocyte transformation to plasma cells. B lymphocyte transformation is initiated by antigens that attach to preformed antibody molecules on the surface of the lymphocyte. Cell growth and division of the B lymphocyte is presumed to pass through several stages, the first, perhaps, being the immunoblast. This cell is larger and has a more diffuse nuclear chromatin than the B cell. It is believed to be more sensitive to immunosuppressants than either

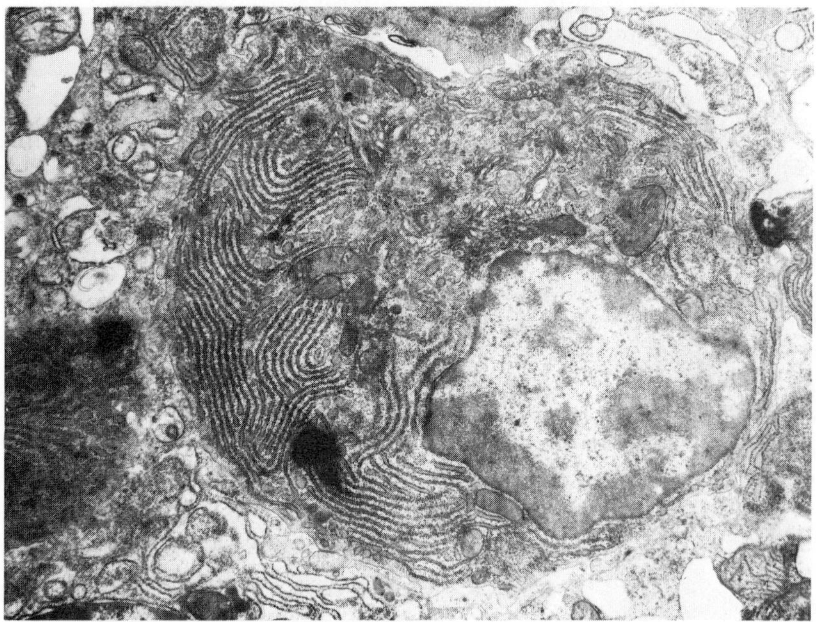

Fig. 2-6. Electron micrograph of a plasma cell in which the laminated, rough endoplasmic reticulum, where immunogloblulins are synthesized, is very apparent. The nucleus is eccentrically located. A few mitochondria are visible, and the Golgi apparatus extends from the upper left of the nucleus in an upward direction toward the outer cell membrane. (Courtesy Dr. E. Adelstein.)

the T or B lymphocytes. Another transitional cell on the path to the plasma cell is the "memory cell," a cell that has a long life expectancy and is responsible for the booster response to antigens, which can be triggered years after the first exposure to antigen. The memory cell may be a side product and not on the direct line to the plasma cell, but it must be convertible to the plasma or end cell in the immunoglobulin-producing line.

Plasma cells. The plasma cell is admirably equipped for its role in immunoglobulin production by virtue of a cytoplasm that is heavily endowed with rough endoplasmic reticulum. This serpentine system of parallel membranes is heavily laden with polysomes, the point of attachment for messenger RNA and the locus of protein synthesis. Few other structures can be seen in the cytoplasm of plasma cells when viewed by the electron microscope (Fig. 2-6). It is this endoplasmic reticulum that is responsible for the plasma cell being labeled as a pyroninophilic cell. Pyronine is a cationic (basic) dye that has a strong affinity for anionic molecules such as the nucleic acids, and staining of a plasma cell with pyronine results in an intense red cytoplasmic coloring.

Germinal centers

In the germinal centers that develop from transforming B cells the B lymphocytes and macrophages are centrally located and surrounded by a perimeter of immunoblasts and plasma cells in company with a few macrophages and other cells (Fig. 2-7). These germinal centers tend to be located at the perimeter of lymph nodes or along the medullary cords leading to the cortex of the gland. B lymphocytes represent only 15% of circulating lymphocytes in blood and are also dominated by T lymphocytes in lymphatic fluid and lymph nodes. The spleen and bone

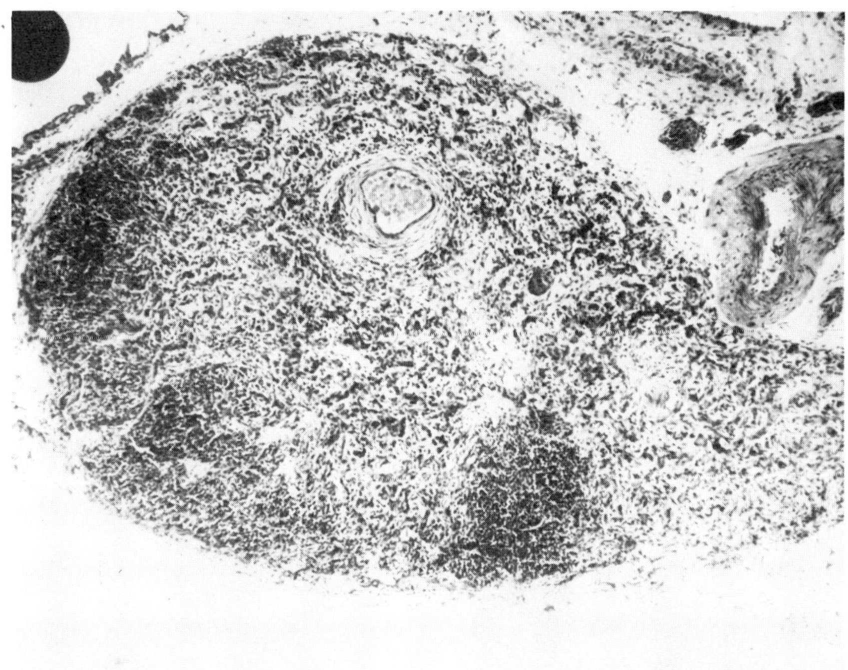

Fig. 2-7. Portion of spleen of hyperimmunized chicken. Dark area at left and two such areas at margin represent germinal centers, consisting of a collection of macrophages, lymphocytes, plasma cells, and antigen.

marrow are good sources of B lymphocytes. Plasma cells are extremely rare in peripheral blood and, since they arise from B lymphocytes, are found in spleen, bone marrow, lymph nodes, and other peripheral tissues.

The B lymphocyte is generally believed to be more sensitive to x-rays, steroids, and most other chemical immunosuppressants than T lymphocytes, but this sensitivity may be due more to immunoblasts than B cells per se. At least these treatments are often more effective when applied simultaneously with an antigen that stimulates the immediate transition of the B cell to the immunoblast stage. The hapten portion of hapten-antigen conjugates triggers B cells to respond with good levels of hapten-directed antibody, whereas the T cell response is more carrier oriented. B cells are more resistant than T cells to the induction of specific immune tolerance but are less responsive to adjuvants than T cells.

IMMUNOSUPPRESSANTS

Cells of the lymphoid and reticuloendothelial systems are more sensitive to several cytotoxic agents than are a number of other cell types. Although it is obvious that this is not likely to be of any natural survival benefit to the animal, it nevertheless has rendered the immune response susceptible to external manipulations. Just as it is possible to improve the immunologic response with adjuvants, the opposite action is possible with immunosuppressants. Since several autoimmune diseases and such alloimmune diseases as graft rejection and certain forms of hemolytic disease are dependent on antigen-reactive T and B cells, it is clear that immunosuppression provides a logical therapeutic avenue to minimize or prevent these diseases. Immunosuppression is an activity of cytotoxic chemicals, irradiation, and even immunoglobulins themselves.

CH_2OH / C=O / OH / O / O

Cortisone

CH_2OH / C=O / HO / OH / O

Hydrocortisone (cortisol)

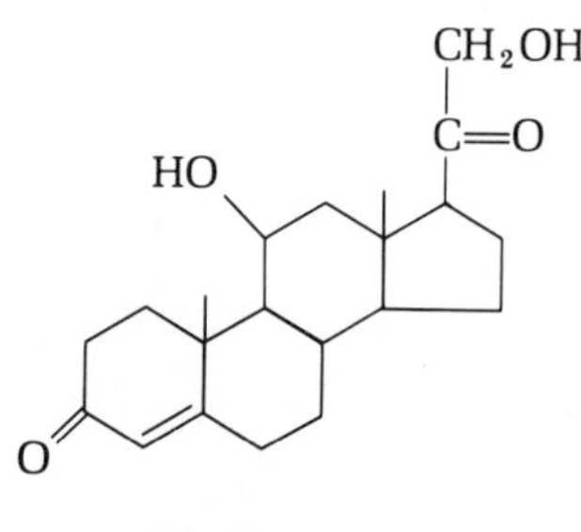

Corticosterone

Fig. 2-8. Steroidal structures represented here were among the first studied as immunosuppressants. Steroids in present use are structurally modified forms of these so as to reduce their undesirable side effects.

Chemical immunosuppressants

Chemicals with immunosuppressant activity can be placed in one of the following four groups: the corticosteroids, the alkylating agents, the antimetabolites, and a fourth group that appears to have no unifying feature.

The steroidal hormones produced in the adrenal glands contain a keto group in position 3 and a hydroxyl group in position 11 of the steroid ring (Fig. 2-8). The glucocorticoids, so named because of their ability to increase gluconeogenesis, are represented by cortisol, aldosterone, and corticosterone. Among the other important activities of the glucocorticoids is stimulation of protein catabolism, decrease in circulating lymphocytes and eosinophils, and an anti-inflammatory effect. The steroid level achieved in the blood during therapy is lympholytic, and this results in a lymphopenia that would have obvious effects on B and T cell responses. These drugs are also known to depress phagocytosis, and their suppressive effect on the inflammatory response, so useful in the treatment of rheumatoid arthritis, may endanger optimal antigen processing by macrophages.

A large number of synthetic steroid compounds have been prepared, and these

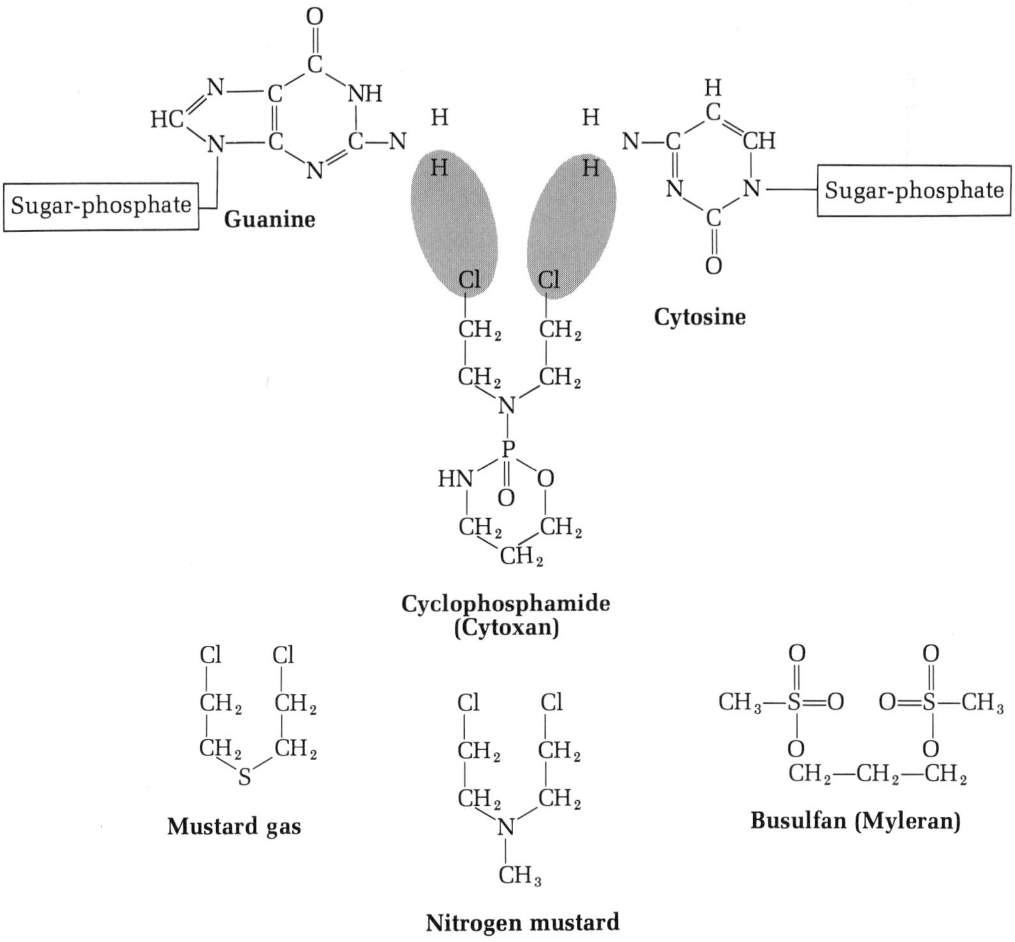

Guanine **Cytosine** **Cyclophosphamide (Cytoxan)** **Mustard gas** **Nitrogen mustard** **Busulfan (Myleran)**

Fig. 2-9. Structures of cyclophosphamide and busulfan, alkylating immunosuppressants, are clearly related to structure of mustard gas. Alkylating reaction of cyclophosphamide with nucleic acids is also illustrated.

have replaced the natural steroids in therapy since they have a higher specific activity and provoke less edema, an undesirable side effect of most steroidal drugs.

Alkylating agents have been patterned after the structure of mustard gas and have combined its basic cytotoxic activity with greater convenience and safety in handling (Fig. 2-9). Many of the original alkylating agents were sulfur-containing compounds that, by virtue of a pair of active halides, cross-linked nucleophilic zones between or within a single molecule. Nucleophilic centers are represented by amino, hydroxyl, and sulfhydryl groups, all of which exist in proteins and the first two of which are found in nucleic acids. Alkylation of two guanines in opposing strands of DNA would link them so that they could not separate during cell division. Such cells could continue to grow, and this probably accounts for the many large lymphoid cells observed in a premitotic phase following treatment with alkylating drugs. Alkylated DNA, as a first stage in protein synthesis, could be accompanied by alkylation of RNA and even of protein to create a complete interruption of the pathway to a functional immunoglobulin or lymphokine. The cytotoxic changes produced by cyclophosphamide, busulfan, phenylalanine mustard, and other alkylating compounds is so similar to that produced by x-irradiation that these drugs are often referred to as radiomimetic drugs.

Antimetabolites with immunosuppressive properties fall into two groups, those that are analogs of the purine and pyrimidine bases and those that are analogs of folic acid. Tetrahydrofolic acid, formed from dietary folic acid by dehydrofolate reductase, is an important coenzyme in

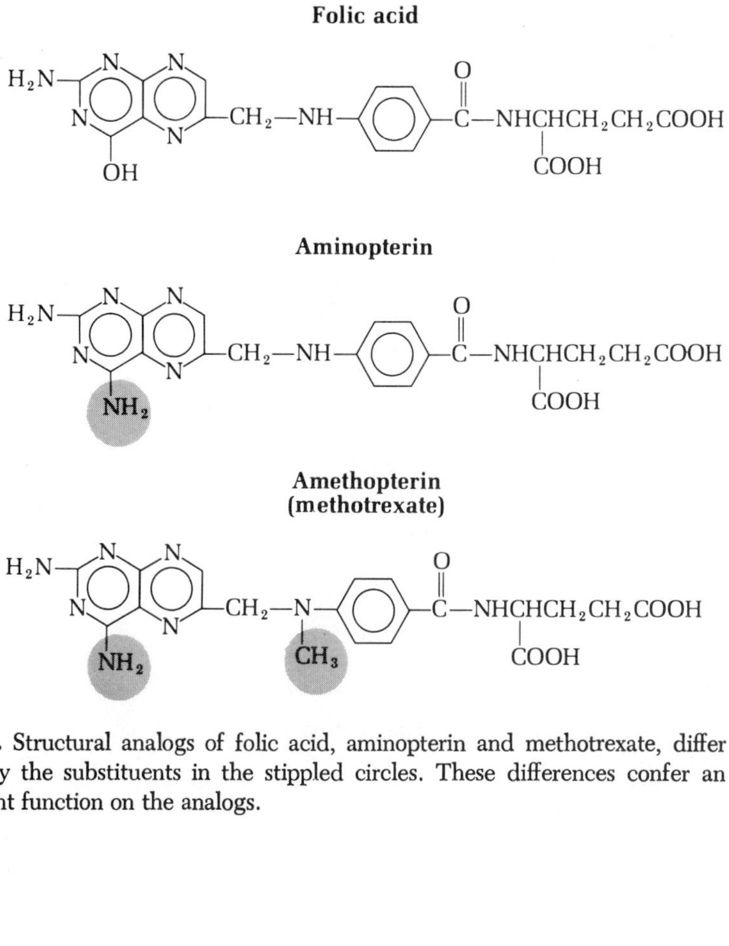

Folic acid

Aminopterin

Amethopterin (methotrexate)

Fig. 2-10. Structural analogs of folic acid, aminopterin and methotrexate, differ from the vitamin by the substituents in the stippled circles. These differences confer an immunosuppressant function on the analogs.

many one-carbon transfer reactions, including those involved in the synthesis of the amino acids methionine and serine and in the formation of the purines required in DNA and RNA. Aminopterin and methotrexate, which differ in structure only slightly from folic acid (Fig. 2-10), slow nucleic acid synthesis and protein synthesis in cells, arresting their development prior to the stage of cell division. Lymphocyte transformation and replication to form plasma cells is thus halted, suppressing the immunoglobulin response. T cell transformation is also interrupted with a consequent depression in lymphokine formation.

Purine and pyrimidine analogs are more direct antimetabolites of DNA and RNA formation (Fig. 2-11). Purine analogs such as 6-mercaptopurine, 6-thioguanine, and azathioprine are used as their free bases or can be converted to the nucleoside level and used as immunosuppressants. Use of the phosphate derivatives has not been practiced for the simple reason that they are not as active as the free bases or the ribose derivatives. This may be the result of a failure of phosphorylated derivatives to enter cells, and one reason afforded for the improved activity of azathioprine over 6-mercaptopurine is that blockage of the —SH group improves the cell permeability of the conjugated purine.

The activity of pyrimidine analogs as immune depressors is often based on the substitution of a fluorine or bromine atom for hydrogen as in 5-fluorouracil and 5-bromouracil. Substitution of a methyl group in the 5 position of cytosine or hydroxycytosine creates a cytotoxic compound. Several of the pyrimidine nucleosides are available, including 5-bromo-2-deoxyuridine (5-BUDR), 5-iodo-2-deoxyuridine, 5-iodo-2-deoxycytidine, 5-trifluoromethyl-2-deoxyuridine, and cytosine arabinoside. Some of these halogenated derivatives are incorporated into DNA, others such as cytosine arabinoside inhibit DNA polymerase and thus inhibit protein synthesis at its very origin.

Included in the miscellaneous group of

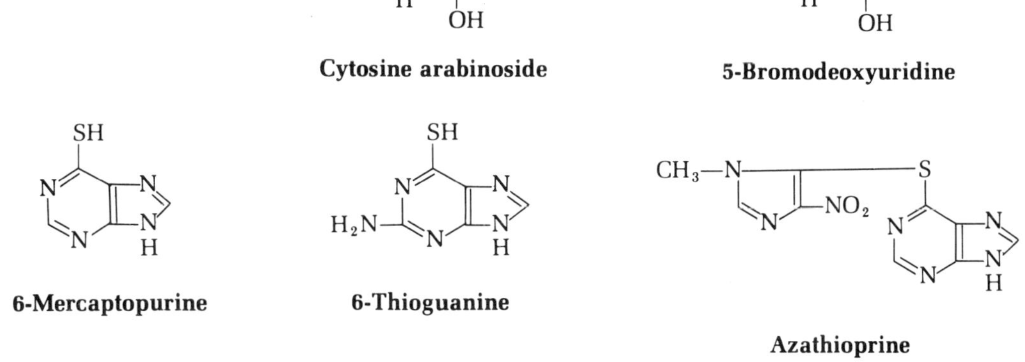

5-Fluorouracil

Cytosine arabinoside

5-Bromodeoxyuridine

6-Mercaptopurine

6-Thioguanine

Azathioprine

Fig. 2-11. Pyrimidine analogs (upper row) and purine analogs (lower row) with B and T cell–suppressing activity. A large number of similar compounds are available for human use.

immunosuppressant chemicals are the following antibiotics: mitomycin C, which behaves as an alkylating agent; puromycin, which inhibits at the RNA level; chloramphenicol, also an RNA inhibitor; and the highly toxic actinomycin D, which operates at the level of both DNA and RNA. Colchicine, vincristine, and vinblastine are plant alkaloids that halt cell division, a key activity of both T and B lymphocytes in their cellular transformation to functional immunocompetent cells. The enzymes ribonuclease and asparaginase diminish immune responses, possibly by interfering with nucleic acid functions.

Irradiation

Irradiation with x-rays (gamma rays) at sublethal doses is immunosuppressive. X-rays are highly cytotoxic for many cell types, but cells of the lymphoid system are especially sensitive. Irradiation blocks DNA synthesis and prevents the development of DNA polymerase needed in protein synthesis.

Immunoglobulins

Immunoglobulins of two different types can also be immunosuppressive. If human lymphocytes are used as antigens to immunize horses, the resulting antilymphocyte serum can be administered passively to human subjects with a resulting inhibition of lymphocyte functions. Since circulating lymphocytes, which are dominantly T-type cells, are used as the antigen, antilymphocyte serum (ALS) is generally a more effective inhibitor of T cells than of B cells. This is even more obviously the case when thymocytes are used to produce antithymocyte serum (ATS). Since extraneous serum proteins may produce undesirable reactions when ATS or ALS is used, the gamma globulin fraction of these antisera ATG or ALG are preferred for human use.

The treatments referred to previously are general immunosuppressants and reduce the capacity of the body to produce any or all antibodies or lymphokines. Prolonged treatment with these agents (or surgical removal of thymus or bursa early in life) will weaken the host's defense against infectious bacteria, their toxins, other pathogens, and tumor cells. Any patient on immunosuppressive regimens must be examined carefully and regularly for the emergence of these undesirable side effects. This handicap is eliminated in the second form of immunoglobulin suppression. It has been observed that if an antibody to a specific antigen is administered at about the same time as the antigen, the normal immunoglobulin response to that antigen is eliminated but the response to other antigens is unaffected. This has proved to be a completely effective and safe means of preventing hemolytic disease of the newborn and this procedure is described fully in Chapter 7.

Immunologic tolerance

Another antigen-specific form of suppression results when animals are pretreated with an antigen prior to the normal immunizing exposure to the antigen. Although this antigen-specific immune tolerance is more easily demonstrated when large first doses of the antigen are given, immune tolerance can also develop following the administration of minute doses of antigen. Immune tolerance is probably most easily demonstrated when antigen is given to fetal animals prior to the maturation of their immunologic system. In fact, prenatal exposure to antigens prior to the time the fetus has become immunocompetent is believed to be the basis for our failure to respond to self proteins and polysaccharides that otherwise meet all the criteria of antigens.

IMMUNOLOGIC MATURATION

After the peripheral lymphoid tissues are seeded with T and B cells, the primary lymphoid organs can be removed surgically or rendered inactive by radiation with a relatively slight effect on immune responsiveness. In old age, years after the atrophy of the central tissues, there is a gradual decline in the ability of an animal to respond to antigens. In prenatal life there is also an immune inadequacy until the lymphoid organs are developed and develop immunocompetency.

In the embryonic development of the human fetus, changes of immunologic importance are apparent by the fifth week of fetal life, when the spleen appears as a reticular structure even though it will have little in the way of lymphoid structure before the fifteenth week. The thymus emerges as a separate organ at 6 weeks and contains a few lymphocytes by the eighth week. At 10 weeks, when the thymus weighs only 20 mg, extensive lymphocytic development is noticeable in the cortex of the gland. By the twenty-sixth week the thymus weighs 4 gm, a 200-fold increase in weight in just 16 weeks. Lymph nodes do not become lymphoid until after the twentieth week of fetal life. Germinal centers and plasma cells are not normally seen until after birth. Lymphocytes appear in the blood between the seventh and eighth week of fetal existence but number only $1000/mm^3$ at 10 weeks, expanding to $10{,}000/mm^3$ at 20 to 25 weeks. At birth the infant may have twice the adult level (1 to 4.8×10^3) of lymphocytes. Primitive cells of the granulocytic series are detectable in the 8-week-old fetus, and cells at all levels of differentiation can be seen in bone marrow by the fifth month.

Although these tissues and cells are present anatomically, it is their physiologic activity that is critical to the immune system. Thymocytes taken from a 12-week-old fetus respond to phytohemagglutinin and pokeweed mitogen, although the percent of responding cells is much higher after 16 weeks. Mixed lymphocyte reactions have been noted between fetal lymphocytes taken from 12- to 14-week-old fetuses. After 13 weeks, flagellin binding to lymphocytes (a T cell function) is four to six times higher than the adult level, but by the twenty-fifth week this has fallen to the normal adult level (0.5% of lymphocytes). Similar data have been collected for β-galactosidase binding by cells, which is also a T cell function. T cell rosette formation with sheep red blood cells increases from 5% of blood lymphocytes at 13 weeks to 20% at 17 weeks. Fluorescent antibody studies have identified IgG in fetuses between 13 and 31 weeks of age, and incorporation of radiolabeled amino acids into IgM and IgG has been noted as early as 74 and 84 days, respectively. One report indicated that fetal synthesis of IgE could be detected by the seventeenth week and that cord blood contained about 15% of the adult level. Cord blood of the full-term infant contains tiny amounts of IgA. Traces of IgD can be found in approximately 18% of the infants. The IgG level of the sera of newborn infants is a reflection of the maternal IgG level, since it is the only immunoglobulin that easily transgresses the placental barrier. Congenital infection or other exposure to antigens, especially in the last trimester of pregnancy, stimulates the development of germinal centers and plasma cell formation with accompanying increases in the amounts of the immunoglobulins, particularly IgM.

Few detailed studies of the phagocytic capacity of fetuses are available, but the inability of tissues from young animals to synthesize antibody in vitro has been attributed to an immaturity of their macrophage population, which was reparable by the addition of macrophages from adult animals. Phagocytes of the newborn baby have a relatively normal phagocytic capacity but may have a low intracellular killing rate within the first 24 hours of life. This defect vanishes immediately thereafter.

These data reveal that the normal human infant is basically an immunologically complete individual at or shortly after birth. It has functional B and T cells and its phagocytic system is operative. The normal infant is well prepared to face the inevitable antigenic onslaught.

CELL INTERACTIONS IN THE IMMUNE RESPONSE

The direct influences of antigens and haptens on an animal are on the macrophages and the T and B lymphocytes. The origin, classification, maturation, and in part the functioning of these cells have already been discussed. In this section the function and the interaction of these cells will be considered further.

Macrophage to other cells

The first essential action on antigens is performed by the macrophages (Fig. 2-12). Lysosomal hydrolases released into the phagolysosome degrade the antigen but seem to preserve its antigenic determinants; that is, protein antigens are not necessarily reduced completely to their substituent amino acids. How antigenic determinant sites are preserved is enigmatic. It is known that these sites are not necessarily linear in peptide chains, and yet proteolysis would tend to eliminate tertiary aspects of molecular structure and destroy three-dimensional determinants. It is also unknown if certain macrophages are programmed or predestined to save a certain kind of determinant and leave other determinants for other cells. Antigen modification may not be required for all antigens—low molecular weight antigens may activate B and T cells directly.

However, there is evidence that macrophage extracts contain an RNA-antigen determinant linked complex that can be used to stimulate IgG synthesis by "virgin" lymphocytes in tissue cultures. This RNA

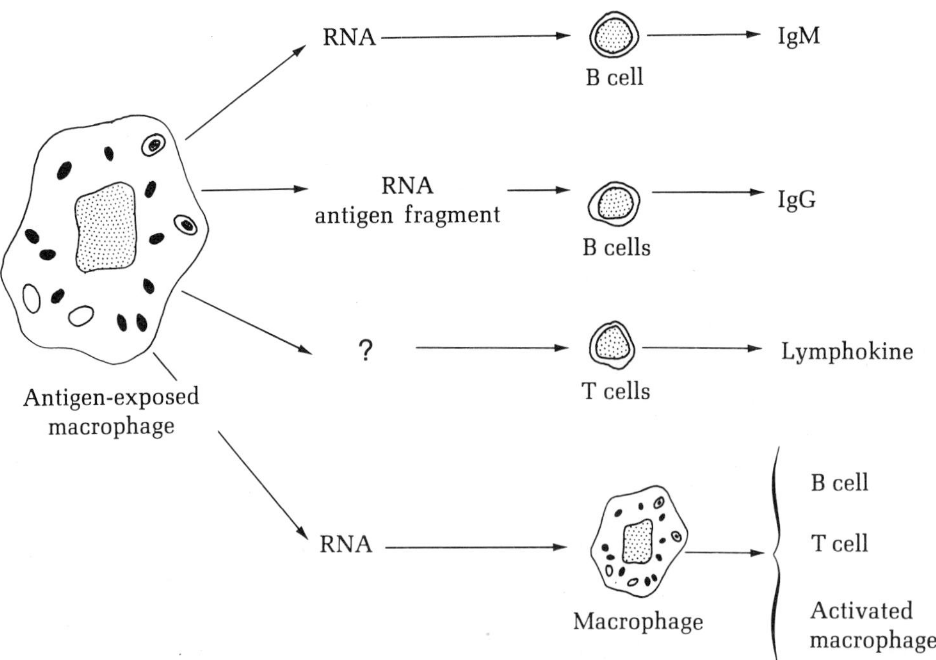

Fig. 2-12. One role of macrophages is to process antigens and send messages to B lymphocytes in the form of RNA or RNA-antigen fragments that inititate antibody synthesis. Similar molecules may stimulate T cells to produce lymphokines and to call forth activated macrophages, phagocytes with enhanced cytodestructive ability.

complex may contain as little as 15 amino acid residues and yet stimulate 400 to 1000 times the amount of antibody formation that the original antigen induces. A second RNA, free of antigenic determinants, is believed to be a specific spark for IgM synthesis. These RNA or RNA-antigen fragments must be considered informational RNA, since their activity is destroyed by RNAse and not by further proteolysis of the antigen fragment and because of genetic experiments. When RNA from an antigen-exposed rabbit of one allotype is transferred to a rabbit of a different allotype, the immunoglobulin formed is of the donor allotype.

Whether or not T cells receive RNA or other messages from macrophages is vaguely understood, but innocent macrophages do receive RNA messages and express this in terms of increased phagocytosis and intracellular destruction as activated macrophages.

T lymphocyte to other cells

The antigen-exposed T cell has two direct and opposite effects on B cells (Fig. 2-13). One of these, the helper cell effect of the T cell, has been extensively studied. The more recently discovered suppressor cell function of the T cell is, as a consequence, less well known.

The helper cell function of T lymphocytes on B lymphocytes has been studied in various animal models—the neonatal thymectomized animal; the nude mouse,

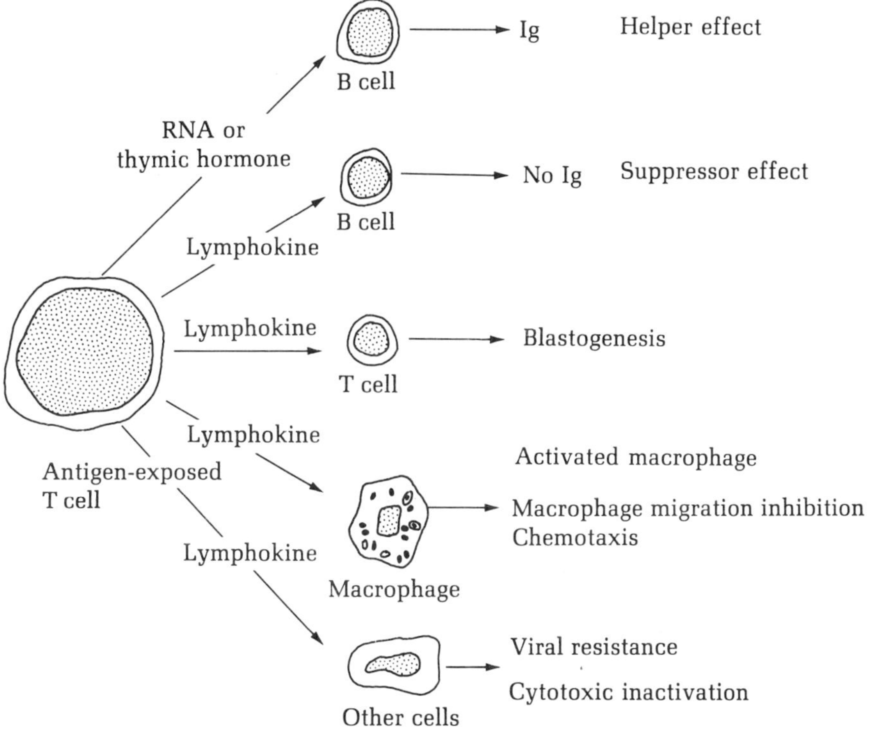

Fig. 2-13. Different lymphokines excreted by antigen-exposed T lymphocytes often function on other host cells rather than on the antigen. These lymphokines may either stimulate or inhibit B lymphocytes in the synthesis of immunoglobulins, attract macrophages, confer viral resistance on a cell, inactivate a tumor cell, etc. A distinct lymphokine is responsible for each activity.

which is congenitally deprived of a thymus; and animals treated with chemical immunosuppressants and irradiation and then reconstituted with B cells. In all of these systems it is possible to demonstrate that T cells, whether or not they are antigen exposed, assist the immunoglobulin response. This effect can be demonstrated more dramatically with certain antigens, termed the T cell–dependent antigens, than with others, the T cell–independent antigens. Antigens of the first class are often complex antigens or assortments of antigens as exist in bacteriophage, viruses, sheep red blood cells, large proteins, and other complex antigens. Simpler antigens such as the polyamino acids and pneumococcal polysaccharides stimulate the B lymphocyte without the mediation of the T cell. Of course, macrophages influence the B cell, especially when complex antigens are involved, by degrading the antigen and passing on its determinant groups and/or RNA.

The helper cell activity of the T lymphocyte may be expressed through some hormonelike substance. Immunologic reconstitution of thymus-deprived animals can be achieved by transplanting syngeneic thymus tissue into its normal anatomic location or by embedding the thymus tissue within semipermeable membranes that prevent emigration of thymus cells. Thymus gland extracts may also replace viable thymus tissue. These experiments demonstrate the possible cell-free nature of the thymus contribution. Many experimenters have attempted to define the biochemical nature of the "thymus hormone" responsible for the stimulation of B cells. One of these, thymosin, is a heat-stable, protease-sensitive peptide with a molecular weight near 10,000 or 12,000. Thymosin has a modest stimulating effect on B cells. A hormonelike peptide named lymphocyte-stimulating hormone has been partially purified and may be the B cell activator. Some evidence for an RNA from T cells as the responsible activator of the B cells also exists.

These thymus hormones may have an effect on T cells as well, and it is recognized that thymosin accelerates graft rejection and graft versus host immunity, which are both customarily cited as T cell activities. Another T cell–T cell interaction includes T lymphocyte transformation. The discovery that lymphocytes could produce a blastogenic or mitogenic agent that would act on other lymphocytes can be demonstrated rather simply in mixed lymphocyte culture (MLC). In this procedure, blood lymphocytes (85% T cells) from two antigenically distinct individuals are placed in a tissue culture environment. After several hours or a few days it will be possible to observe that many of the cells have undergone a morphologic transformation. Measurements of DNA or RNA synthesis or even of protein synthesis, through the use of radiolabeled nucleic acids or amino acids, are more sensitive indicators of lymphocyte transformation than observations of nuclear growth. The blastogenic factor responsible for this is an ill-defined lymphokine that is heat sensitive at 56° C for 30 minutes and is nondialyzable. Lymphokines are difficult to define exactly, but they are excretory products of T cells, most of which appear to be low molecular weight proteins that exhibit their activity on other cells.

T cells also elaborate lymphokines that operate on macrophages. One of these is a chemotactic factor that acts on free macrophages to attract them to areas where the T cell has come into contact with the antigen. If the antigen is a foreign invader, this would obviously contribute to cell-mediated immunity. T cells are also responsible for calling forth an activated macrophage that is more cell destructive than the ordinary macrophage. Once these macrophages are drawn to the T lymphocyte, a lymphokine called migration inhibition factor (MIF) prevents their egress from the T cell–antigen site. These macrophages may even be clumped by a factor called macrophage aggregation factor (MAF). The evidence now available indicates that MAF, MIF, and chemotactic activities are all exhibited by a single lymphokine.

Another lymphokine of T cells, interferon, acts on host cells to confer on them a resistance to infection by viruses and other intracellular parasites. The viruses invade the host cell but interferon has apparently adjusted the metabolism of the cell so that it will no longer accept foreign nucleic acid messages. Since most intracellular parasites instruct the host cell to synthesize structures of the parasite, interruption of that activity halts the intracellular infection. Lymphotoxin is also a highly protective substance produced by T lymphocytes. When a T cell is exposed to a tumor cell, allografted tissue, or possibly other cells, it becomes sensitized by that exposure so that on a second encounter with the cell it excretes the cytolytic lymphotoxin. Lymphotoxin causes the target cell to assume a spherical shape, lose its original cell shape, swell, cease its mobility, and rupture. A more rapid assay than cell destruction for lymphotoxin is designed about the use of ^{51}Cr-labeled cells. This isotope is released from cells at the first evidence of membrane damage or change in cell permeability—changes that preface death of the target cell.

B lymphocyte to other cells

It is surprising that there is so little known about the physiologic activities of B cells that influence macrophages and T cells. It is known that macrophages from nonimmune animals placed in antisera produced in other animals will absorb some of the antibodies on their surface (Fig. 2-14). Such cytophilic antibodies have been found on macrophages from immunized animals too, and the early, erroneous interpretation of this was that the macrophages were syn-

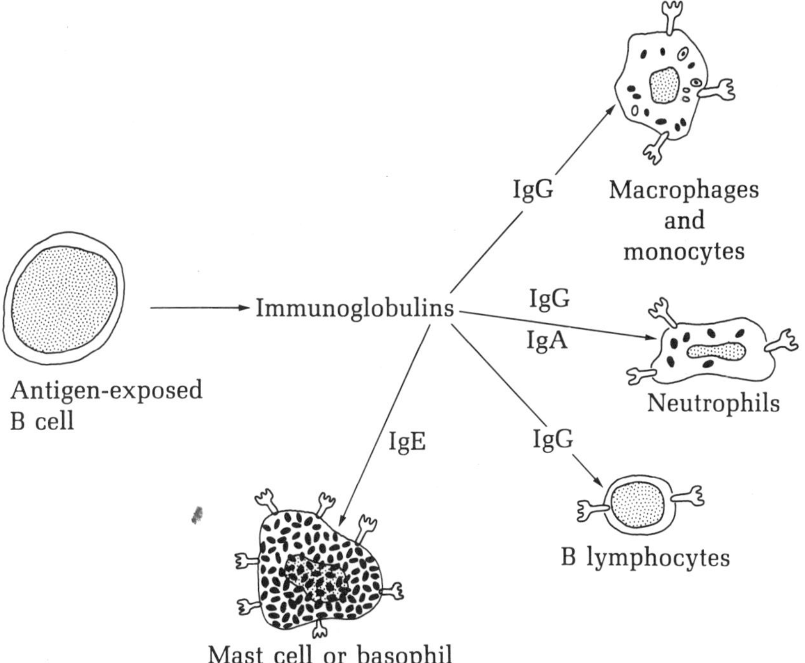

Fig. 2-14. Interaction of B lymphocytes with other cells of the immune system is based on the immunoglobulins released from plasma cells derived from B cells. Different classes of immunoglobulins interact with distinct cell types: cytotropic IgE with mast cells and basophils; cytophilic IgG with macrophages, neutrophils, and lymphocytes; etc.

thesizing antibodies. Now it is known that immunoglobulins will adhere to the surface of several cell types. Monocytes and macrophages of man adsorb IgGl, IgG3, and to a lesser extent IgG4. Neutrophils will also sponge these subclasses of IgG plus IgAl, IgA2, and secretory IgA. It is assumed that the presence of cytophilic antibodies on the surface of phagocytic cells enhances phagocytosis.

IgE is a well-known cytophilic antibody for which the term "cytotropic antibody" is sometimes reserved. IgE attaches primarily to the surface of mast cells and basophils. When the antigen combines with the cell-bound IgE, the mast cells degranulate, releasing histamine and heparin into the bloodstream. Heparin slows blood clotting, and histamine is a potent pharmacologic agent causing smooth muscle contraction and vasodilation. These activities are responsible for the major symptoms of the immediate type or immunoglobulin-mediated hypersensitivities.

CYTOKINETICS AND THE IMMUNE RESPONSE

Cytophilic antibodies on macrophages may serve as antigen receptors that facilitate antigen endocytosis by the cells as the first step in antigen processing. Some antigens may not require reduction to their antigen determinants and may stimulate the T and B lymphocytes directly, but RNA-antigen fragments or RNA alone from macrophages behaves as a superantigen. When the lymphocytes receive some form of the antigen, they are stimulated into a cycle of growth and division. Presumably this begins immediately and continues for variable periods of time, depending on the particular breed of lymphocyte that was stimulated. Lymphokines from the T lymphocytes can be detected in the blood of antigen-stimulated animals within a few hours; however, the level of these lymphokines diminishes quickly and they may be undetectable after 4 or 5 days. On the other hand, immunoglobulins, a reflection of B lymphocyte activation, are usually not detected in the blood until 5 to 10 days after antigen exposure. This may be in part due to the fact that B cell transformation progresses through several cell levels before terminating in the plasma cell, the dominant cell in immunoglobulin synthesis. The plasma cells destined to secrete IgM diminish in function in only a few days, just at the time that IgG-producing cells are reaching the peak of their activity. By this time only traces of antigen can be found in tissues. These traces of antigen are located in macrophages and lymphoid tissues in and around germinal centers. It is believed that the lymphocytes (and plasma cells) in a germinal center represent a clone of new cells originating from a single, stimulated cell. Only when this clone reaches a certain magnitude can its cellular product be detected in blood. Even in the case of B lymphocytes it has been shown with single-cell studies that antibody production begins within a few moments after antigen exposure; presumably these early antibody molecules are diluted too extensively in the body fluids to be measured in the blood until a few days have elapsed.

Primary immune response and secondary immune response

This initial burst of immunoglobulin and lymphokine production is referred to as the primary immune response (Fig. 2-15). It is quite different in respect to time from the secondary response that follows a second or subsequent exposure, provided this is after the primary immune response has been exhibited. Following this second exposure to antigen, referred to as the booster dose of antigen, there is a slight, immediate drop in the immunoglobulin content of blood as the newly inoculated antigen has combined with it and removed it from the circulation. The circulating level of the immunoglobulins quickly recovers as the

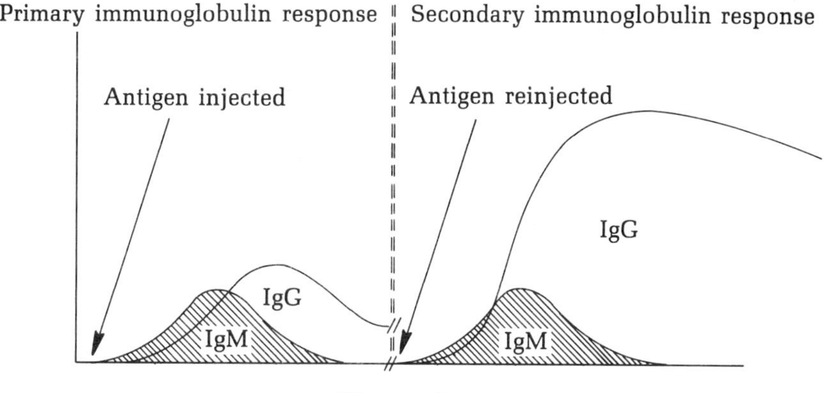

Fig. 2-15. Difference in IgG response to primary and secondary exposure to antigen indicates why it is termed the memory antibody. IgM, illustrated to exhibit no "memory," usually shows a slight anamnestic response.

cell population responsible for their production goes through a reproductive burst. The short time period required for this, as compared to the primary immune response, is believed due to the fact that the latter induced the formation of memory cells, which though not yet producing antibody were but a brief transitional stage away from plasma cells. Obviously IgM memory cells are more scant than IgG memory cells since the booster response of IgM is only 10-fold that of the primary response, whereas the booster response of IgG customarily results in a 100-fold or more increase. Other possibilities could account for this such as a greater rate of immunoglobulin synthesis by IgG plasma cells.

The anamnestic (without forgetting) or booster response is of considerable medical importance: it is dominated by the IgG response, which is one of the most important protective antibodies; it occurs within 2 or 3 days, so that the needed protection is almost immediately available; and the booster response can be repeated several times, a feature that permits the development of a truly hyperimmune serum. Also of importance is the observation that the booster response can be developed years after a prior antigen exposure, even at a time when the individual is presumably devoid of any immunoglobulin specific for that antigen. It should also be emphasized that since the anamnestic response is dominated by IgG, which has a longer half-life than any other immunoglobulin, the heightened antibody levels reached decay more slowly than after the primary response.

The primary and secondary responses can be modified if the antigen is injected with adjuvant. This extends the antigen elimination curve beyond that illustrated and blends the antibody responses of the primary and secondary types into a combined response. It should also be emphasized that although primary and booster responses are ordinarily discussed in terms of the antibody response, it is equally applicable to the lymphokine response. Repeated antigen exposures produce intensive germinal cell development of both B and T types of lymphocytes.

THEORIES OF ANTIBODY FORMATION

The presence of immunoglobulins on the surface of macrophages and B lymphocytes (but apparently not on T lymphocytes) taken from normal, newborn animals has provided considerable support for the clonal selection theory of antibody forwarded by Burnet, for which he and Peter B. Medawar won the Nobel Prize in Medicine and Physiology in 1960. The clonal selection theory of immunoglobulin formation surmises that lymphocytes are genetically endowed with the capacity to synthesize an immunoglobulin of a specific molecular class (IgG, IgM, etc.) or subclass to a specific antigenic determinant. The cell may be excreting trace amounts of these antibodies at all times, or its progeny, the plasma cell, may be formed in scant numbers, excreting faint amounts of the antibody. These few molecules become attached to the surfaces of macrophages and B lymphocytes and serve as the receptor for the antigen when it is eventually encountered. Surface changes caused by the combination of an antigen with its antibody provoke cell generation and maturation to produce clones of cells (germinal centers) producing antibody to that antigen. The consequence of this activity by many cells is the appearance of antibody in detectable quantities in the blood. A central key to this theory is that the cells are already capable of and probably are synthesizing minute quantities of antibody. The antigen "selects" that cell for proliferation. Note that the cell must be limited to the capacity to produce a single antibody or else there would be no specificity to the immune response. The cell could be pluripotent in its options, but once it opts to form one antibody this could block its capacity to respond to other antigens.

One objection to the clonal theory is that it supposes that the body contains cells that are potentially responsive to a myriad of antigenic determinants. Presumably this criticism would not apply to an instructive theory in which the antigenic determinant in some way directs the cell to form its corresponding antibody. However, there are drawbacks to the instructive theory also; for example, large doses of antigen would seem to provide a greater message and thus a greater antibody response, yet such doses often produce immunologic tolerance instead. Instructive theories seem to demand antigen retention for the whole time span that antibodies are being produced. Since this can encompass several years, it does not appear to harmonize with the basic dynamism of the immune as a special physiologic response. It is uncertain exactly what proofs are needed to convert the theories of antibody formation to facts, but the clonal selection theory is presently favored.

CLINICAL CORRELATION

A five-year study of human renal transplant success by two French surgeons included the use of antilymphocyte globulin (ALG) for each of the 126 patients.* Thoracic duct lymphocytes or human thymocytes recovered from children less than 3 years of age who died from traumatic incidents were used as the antigen and horse antisera were used. The globulin fraction of the serum was recovered by ammonium sulfate precipitation and tested in several ways for potency. No single potency test for ALG has been accepted as a standard. Transplant recipients were given 3 to 5 mg of ALG/kg intramuscularly or 8 to 20 mg/kg/day intravenously. After 10 to 60 days these injections were continued as intramuscular treatments of 3 to 5 mg/kg every second or third day.

An oral dose of 2.5 to 3 mg/kg/day of azathioprine was given. Prednisone and/or prednisolone were administered either orally or intravenously at a level of 0.2 mg/kg/day after ALG was started.

ALG was discontinued from the regimen of 19 patients in the first year and 9 in the second year due to allergic reactions. Forty-one patients were given immunosuppres-

*Touraine, J.-L., and Traeger, J.: Human renal allotransplantation and antilymphocyte globulin, Villeubanne, 1974, Foundation Merieux.

sants for as long as 2 years, and 31 of these received ALG. Some American surgeons have found it necessary to discontinue ALG for practically all transplant patients within 3 months. Variation in the tolerance to ALG is regulated in part by the dose, injection route, and purity of the product plus the influence of other suppressant treatments. Some of the patients in this study were subjected to thoracic duct drainage as an added suppressant, and this is an infrequent adjunct to therapy. Even so, two thirds of the patients in this study had some discomfort from ALG injection.

Azathioprine treatments can be continued almost indefinitely provided that the dosage is adjusted to maintain a leukocyte count near 5500/ml of blood with a granulocyte count over 3000/ml of blood. Corticosteroid treatments caused relatively few complications because the dosage used was less than that applied in many transplant centers; however, steroid treatment was deemed responsible for 16 incidents of gastrointestinal hemorrhage and transient psychiatric disturbances.

The most numerous complications were infectious in nature with the appearance of 26 cases of septicemia, 8 cases of bacterial pneumonia, and a case of purulent meningitis. Provisional pathogens accounted for many of these infections—*Pseudomonas, Klebsiella, Candida,* and *Escherichia* were involved in at least 15 of these cases. Viral infections were also frequent, with 14 cases of herpes simplex and 7 cases of extensive herpes zoster being observed. Liver disease of uncertain etiology was also common.

Transplant survival of 83.9% and 74.1% from sibling donors was noted at 1 and 3 years after transplantation; this fell to 48.4% and 39.1% for unrelated donors during the same time period.

BIBLIOGRAPHY

Abdou, N. I., and Richter, M.: The role of the bone marrow in the immune response, Adv. Immunol. **12**:202, 1970.

Aisenberg, A. C.: An introduction to immunosuppressants, Adv. Pharmacol. Chemother. **8**:31, 1970.

Allison, A. C.: Immunological tolerance, Clin. Immunobiol. **1**:113, 1972.

Carr, I.: The macrophage, New York, 1972, Academic Press, Inc.

Celada, F.: The cellular basis of immunologic memory, Prog. Allergy **15**:223, 1971.

Claman, H. N.: Corticosteroids and lymphoid cells, N. Engl. J. Med. **287**:388, 1972.

Claman, H. N., and Mosier, D. E.: Cell-cell interactions in antibody production, Prog. Allergy **16**:40, 1972.

Diener, E., and Langman, R. E.: Antigen recognition in induction of immunity, Prog. Allergy **18**:6, 1975.

Elves, M. W.: The lymphocytes, ed. 2, London, 1972, Lloyd-Luke (Medical Books), Ltd.

Gerebtzoff, A., Lambert, P. H. and Miescher, P. A.: Immunosuppressive agents, Annu. Rev. Pharmacol. **12**:287, 1972.

Good, R. A.: Structure-function relations in the lymphoid system, Clin. Immunobiol. **1**:1, 1972.

Greaves, M. F., Owen, J. J. T., and Raff, M. C.: T and B lymphocytes, Amsterdam, 1973, Excerpta Medica.

Howard, J. G., and Mitchison, N. A.: Immunological tolerance, Prog. Allergy, **18**:43, 1975.

Kaplan, S. R.: Immunosuppressive agents, N. Engl. J. Med. **289**:952, 1234, 1973.

Katz, D. H., and Benacerraf, B.: The regulatory influence of activated T cells on B cell responses to antigen, Adv. Immunol. **15**:1, 1972.

Lance, E. M., Medawar, P. B., and Taub, R. N.: Antilymphocyte serum, Adv. Immunol. **17**:1, 1973.

Luckey, T. D., ed.: Thymic hormones, Baltimore, 1973, University Park Press.

Mäkelä, O., and Cross, A. M.: The diversity and specialization of immunocytes, Prog. Allergy **14**:145, 1970.

Miller, J. F. A. P., Basten, A., Sprent, J., and Cheers, C.: Interactions between lymphocytes in immune responses, Cell. Immunol. **2**:469, 1971.

Pearsall, N. N., and Weiser, R. S.: The macrophage, Philadelphia, 1970, Lea & Febiger.

Schlesinger, M.: Antigens of the thymus, Prog. Allergy **16**:214, 1972.

Skinner, M. D., and Schwartz, R. S.: Immunosuppressive therapy, N. Engl. J. Med. **287**: 221, 281, 1972.

Unanue, E. R.: The regulatory role of macrophages in antigenic stimulation, Adv. Immunol. **15**:95, 1972.

Vernon-Roberts, R.: The macrophage, New York, 1972, Cambridge University Press.

Waksman, B. H.: Atlas of experimental immunology and immunopathology, New Haven, 1970, Yale University Press.

Warner, N. L.: Membrane immunoglobulins and antigen receptors on B and T lymphocytes, Adv. Immunol. **19**:67, 1974.

Weiss, L.: The cells and tissues of the immune system, Englewood Cliffs, N. J., 1972, Prentice-Hall, Inc.

Case histories

CASE 1. IMMUNOLOGIC PARALYSIS

Jeanette H., a slightly underweight 6-year-old girl, was taken to her pediatrician with what her mother recognized as bronchial pneumonia. Her mother was familiar with the symptoms of pneumonia because her daughter had contracted the disease six times within the past year and was believed to have had pneumonia 15 times in the past 3½ years. In those cases in which bacterial cultures had been made, *Streptococcus (Diplococcus) pneumoniae* type 3 had been isolated as the only pathogen, with occasional isolations of *Hemophilus influenzae.*

Questions

1. What is the antigenic composition of S. *pneumoniae* type 3, and how does this differ from that of other pneumococci?
2. What features of the pneumococci favor repeated infections rather than immunity?
3. What is immunologic paralysis? How does it differ, if at all, from immunologic tolerance?
4. Can immunologic paralysis be cured? Or is there a suitable vaccine for pneumococcal pneumonia?
5. What other medical situations involve immunologic paralysis?

Discussion

S. *pneumoniae* contains two major kinds of antigens, the somatic and the capsular antigens. The somatic antigens consist of a carbohydrate antigen or C substance that is specific to S. *pneumoniae* and is not antigenically the same as the C substances of other streptococci, a type-specific M protein, and an R protein antigen that has not yet been further characterized. The most important antigens of the pneumococci are the polysaccharide capsular antigens found on the smooth (S) but not rough (R) forms of the organism. Only the S forms are pathogenic for man, and only this form is isolated from human infections, as in the case under discussion. The rank of capsular types causing adult pneumococcal pneumonia is 1, 3, 2, 5, 8, and 7, with the first three of these causing 54% of all infections. For this reason it was believed that a vaccine containing the medically important types could be produced, or since type 3 causes the highest fatality rate, a vaccine of that type at least should be produced. This endeavor led to some interesting observations. One of these was that the purified pneumococcal capsule is either nonantigenic or a very impotent antigen for rabbits, although whole encapsulated bacteria induce suitable immunoglobulin formation. Thus for the rabbit, pure capsular substances appear to be haptenic rather than antigenic. This is not the case for mice and human subjects, who react to the pure capsular polysaccharide as to any other complete antigen.

But even in man and mice a failure to respond to pneumococcal polysaccharides can be observed as a dose-related phenomenon. Mice injected with only 0.01 μg of polysaccharide develop antibodies and resist infection by a pneumococcus of that polysaccharide type, but if the antigen dose were increased to 1000 μg, no protection could be demonstrated. This was described as immune paralysis. It is antigen specific and was at first thought to result from the large dose of antigen forming a depot that adsorbed the protective anticapsular antibodies thus reducing resistance to infection. This was an attractive hypothesis because it was known that pneumococcal polysaccharides tend to accumulate in the liver and are not hydrolyzed and removed as quickly as other antigens, but no corresponding accumulation of antibodies occurred in the liver of these animals.

Immune paralysis, immune unresponsiveness, and immune tolerance are now considered synonyms and known to relate to the specific antigenic suppression of T and B lymphocytes. T cells are easily suppressed by low doses of antigen, and this suppression persists relatively long compared to B cell suppression. However pneumococcal polysaccharides are T cell–independent antigens, which means T cells display no helper effect with this antigen. Consequently, tolerance to this antigen relies on suppression of B cells or high-dose tolerance. Patients with pneumococcal pneumonia often continue as carriers of the organism for weeks after their infection even in the presence of high blood levels of antibodies. During pneumococcal pneumonia the bacteria produce a large amount of their specific capsular substance. The polysaccharide substance can be recovered from tissues, sputum, urine, and, in cases of pneumococcal meningitis, from spinal fluid. Natural immune tolerance is a potential result of protracted exposure to this antigen. The more usual function of the pneumococcal polysaccharide is to function as a virulence factor. It has a pronounced antiphagocytic role that can easily be demonstrated in laboratory experiments to be the permissive factor in S. *pneumoniae* infections. Antibodies against the capsule are protective and R forms are not infective.

Variations in the chemical structure and the antigenic behavior of pneumococci have allowed their division into more than 80 serologic types. The exact structures of relatively few of these 80 capsular antigens are known, but all of them are polysaccharides. The composition of many of them is known, and type 3, for which the structure is also known, consists of repeating units of cellobiuronic acid linked by β-1,3-glycoside bonds. Cellobiuronic acid is a disaccharide of D-glucuronic acid and D-glucose joined by a β-1,4 bond. Some cross-reactions of these capsular antigens with polysaccharide antigens of other species do occur, and cross-reactions within the species of different serologic types are also known. For example, type 3 and type 8 polysaccharides each contain cellobiuronic acid (type 8 also includes D-galactose) and are cross-reactive.

In terms of frequency of pneumonia in children, type 3 ranks seventh; in incidence of pneumonia in all age groups, type 3 ranks second. Actually, Jeanette H. is an unusual case in that several of her repeated pneumonias were due to a pneumococcus of the same antigenic type. This may be due to incomplete cure of some chronic underlying infection or to her progression to a state of immune paralysis due to repeated or continual exposure to the antigen. This could be evaluated by determining if she has normal antipneumococcal antibody levels. If not, she is tolerant, and for this there is no reasonable cure.

Other human examples of naturally induced immune paralysis have been recognized to follow congenital infections such as rubella. Infection with the rubella virus in the first trimester of pregnancy leads to frequent abortion of the fetus, but when this does not occur and live births result, the rubella virus may establish a semi-chronic infection. Rubella virus is easily recovered from the blood and other tissues of the child for periods of several years following birth.

Congenital infections with rubella virus are known to produce nonprogressive defects in embryogenesis that include cataract formation, deafness, microcephaly, and arrested mental development. Recent descriptions of a delayed panencephalitis of progressive severity terminating in death have been attributed to fetal rubella infections. Rubella virus was not isolated from these patients who, in some cases, were not identified until they were 18 years of age. This syndrome was associated with high levels of antibody to the rubella virus in serum and spinal fluid, features not seen in normal children nor the usual child with congenital rubella. In at least one case assays of T cell function after exposure of the lymphocytes to rubella virus in culture indicated they were normal. It can be concluded that rubella infections in utero may lead to severe medical problems that are associated with viral persistence. Since the virus is an intracellular parasite, it can continue its reproductive cycle in an environment protected from antibodies and T cells.

REFERENCES

Felton, L. D., Kauffmann, G., Prescott, B., and Ottinger, B.: Studies on the mechanism of the immunological paralysis induced in mice by pneumococcal polysaccharides, J. Immunol. **74**:17, 1955.

Rawls, W. E.: Congenital rubella: the significance of virus persistence, Prog. Med. Virol. **10**:238, 1968.

Townsend, J. J., Baringer, J. R., Wolinsky, J. S., Malamud, N., Mednick, J. P., Panitch, H. S., Scott, R. A. T., Oshiro, L. S., and Cremer, N. E.: Progressive rubella panencephalitis, late onset after congenital rubella, N. Engl. J. Med. **292**:990, 1975.

Weil, M. L., Itabashi, H. H., Cremer, N. E., Oshiro, L. S., Lennette, E. H., and Carnay, L.: Chronic progressive panencephalitis due to rubella virus simulating subacute sclerosing panencephalitis, N. Engl. J. Med. **292**: 994, 1975.

CASE 2. LEUKOCYTE FUNCTION: CHRONIC GRANULOMATOUS DISEASE

Mark H., a 3-year-old boy, entered the hospital for the sixth time in the past 2½ years. His admission was for a fever of unknown origin. His white blood cell count was 18,500/mm^3, of which 46% were PMNs. His temperature was 101.8 and the liver and spleen were enlarged. Blood cultures were taken and reported to be positive for *E. coli*. On previous hospitalizations for septicemia, boils, cervical lymphadenopathy, and pneumonia, bacterial cultures had been positive for *E. coli* and/or *Klebsiella* and coagulase-positive staphylococci. A diagnosis of chronic granulomatous disease was considered and the following laboratory tests of interest were ordered: total gamma globulin, nitroblue tetrazolium (NBT) reductase test, and bactericidal killing test.

Questions

1. What is chronic granulomatous disease, and what are the hallmarks of leukocyte function in this disease?
2. What is the importance of the four special laboratory procedures, and what are the normal values of these tests?
3. How is chronic granulomatous disease treated?

Discussion

Chronic granulomatous disease is typified by repeated, slow-healing infections due to ordinarily feeble infectious organisms. The disease is seen only in young boys due to its sex-linked inheritance, although similar diseases are seen in female children. Granulomatous deposits in visceral organs, especially the lungs, facilitate a radiologic diagnosis; however, deficits in neutrophil function with normal T and B lymphocyte functions are instrumental in confirming the diagnosis.

Patients with chronic granulomatous disease, because of the frequent incidence of bacterial infections, have higher gamma globulin levels than normal, and this was seen in the case of Mark H., who had a total gamma globulin of 1400 mg/100 ml. The presence of such high levels of immunoglobulins promotes phagocytosis of bacteria but does not necessarily accelerate the intraphagocytic death rate of the ingested bacteria. For this reason a bactericidal killing test is performed. The buffy coat of heparinized blood from the patient is adjusted to a suitable neutrophil cell count rather than to some specific dilution. Cell counts are necessary due to the fluctuation in granulocyte counts in such patients. Generally 10^6 white blood cells/ml and 10^6 bacteria/ml are attained in the final mixture, which is contained in a tissue culture fluid supplemented with normal serum to the extent of 10%. After incubation of the mixture at 37° C for 30 minutes and at 30-minute intervals thereafter, penicillin and streptomycin are added to kill extracellular bacteria. (Penicillin-sensitive *Staphylococcus aureus* are used in the test.) The centrifuged pellet is subjected to total plate counts for surviving bacteria. The normal control utilizes white blood cells from a healthy subject.

Normal leukocytes kill staphylococci and most other bacteria rapidly, with a 1% viable remainder being typical after 2 hr of incubation. Patients with chronic granulomatous disease may have as much as 95% bacterial survival in the same test, although 70% survival would be more typical. PMNs from Mark H. reduced the staphylococcal population from 10^6 to only 8×10^5. Examination of white blood cell smears revealed that adequate ingestion had occurred.

Because the bactericidal killing test is cumbersome and time-consuming, the NBT reductase test is often used to evaluate neutrophil performance instead. The test is based on the knowledge that phagocytosis is accompanied by a burst in respiratory metabolism that can be detected by the ability of white blood cells to transfer hydrogen to the dye NBT. This reduces the dye and causes the appearance of dark blue dye granules inside the neutrophils. Neutrophils from patients with chronic granulomatous disease are genetically incapable of leaving their glycolytic energy-deriving system for the oxidative pathways associated with intraphagocytic killing. In the NBT reductase test, latex spherules are used as the phagocytic subject for white blood cells incubated with NBT. About 50% of the neutrophils will have phagocytosed at least five latex beads and be positive. Patients with chronic granulomatous disease will have decidedly lower scores, as will some other restricted patient categories and neonates. Mark H. had a score of 5%, definitely below the norm and compatible with the diagnosis.

There is no suitable therapy for chronic granulomatous disease other than treatment of the bacterial infections as they occur. For this reason the average life expectancy of such patients is only 10 years.

REFERENCES

Baehner, R. L., and Nathan, G.: Quantitative nitroblue tetrazolium test in chronic granulomatous disease, N. Engl. J. Med. **278**:971, 1968.

Holmes, B., Quie, P. G., Windhorst, D. B., and Good, R. A.: Fatal granulomatous disease of childhood. An inborn abnormality of phagocytic function, Lancet **1**:1225, 1966.

Park, B. H.: The use and limitations of the nitroblue tetrazolium test as a diagnostic aid, J. Pediatr. **78**:376, 1971.

Quie, P. G., and Hill, H. R.: Granulocytopathies, Disease-A-Month, p. 1, August, 1973.

chapter 3

Immunobiochemistry

On the chemical level immunology is dominated by macromolecules—the antigens, immunoglobulins, lymphokines, and proteins of the complement system nearly all exceed a molecular weight of 10,000. Molecules of low molecular weight such as the haptens, products of mast cells, antihistamines, and adrenergic drugs are also important in immunology. Because of their close relationship to antigens, only haptens will be considered in this chapter, and the complement system, because of its great importance to inflammation and immunity, will be discussed in a separate chapter.

ANTIGENS

Antigens defined

Antigens, once defined as substances that induce the formation of antibodies and react visibly with those antibodies, can no longer be defined in such simplistic terms if indeed they can be precisely defined at all. In terms of an operational definition, antigens can be defined as substances that catalyze B lymphocytes and T lymphocytes into specific adaptive responses to the antigen. For the B lymphocyte this response is a transformation into plasma cells that synthesize the antibodies (immunoglobulins) that react with the antigen. For the T lymphocyte this is the elaboration, also after cell transformation, of lymphokines that alter host cell behavior. Antigens may also activate macrophages directly or via lymphokine activities. These cellular interactions with antigens and each other were described in the preceding chapter. In this chapter the chemical nature of antigens will be emphasized.

Chemically, antigens are generally macromolecules that have a built-in chemical complexity; they are degradable by the animal exposed to them and can be considered as foreign to that animal. In terms of the first criterion, molecules greater than 10,000 daltons that possess antigenicity are legion—diphtheria toxin or toxoid, viral proteins, bacterial cell walls, hemoglobin, enzymes, high molecular weight dextrans, etc. are all antigenic. Although many molecules with a molecular weight of less than 10,000 can be antigenic (insulin, mol wt 6000; calcitonin, mol wt 3600; glucagon, mol wt 3485; and ACTH, mol wt 3900 are examples), as one progresses to lower and lower molecular weight molecules, fewer and fewer antigens are found. There is no specific lower molecular weight limit for antigenicity (Table 3-1). This is because the determination of antigenicity is regulated partially by the type of exposure the animal has to the antigen, the immunization dose and schedule, the health of the animal, its genetic capacity to respond to certain types of compounds, the sensitivity of the method used to measure the immunoglobulin or lymphokine response, and other structural features of the antigen other than size. For example, feeding a protein to an animal characteristically results in its digestion to low molecular weight peptides and amino acids, thus preventing an expression of an antigenicity that might have been demonstrated if the

Table 3-1. Selected low molecular weight antigens*

Antigen	*Molecular weight*
Oxytocin	1000
Vasopressin	1000
Dinitrophenylheptalysine	1080
Dinitrophenylbacitracin	1400
Gastrin	1800
Glucagon	3485
Thyrocalcitonin	3600
ACTH	3900
Ferredoxin	6000
Insulin	6000
Haptoglobin	9000

*These compounds have all demonstrated antigenicity, yet they have molecular weights (approximated here) of less than 10,000.

antigen were injected into the animal. Tiny doses of an antigen might be insufficient to trigger the immune response, and oddly enough, massive doses may result in a similar observation of antigenic tolerance.

Ir genes

Recent studies have demonstrated the existence of a genetic basis for the response to antigens, and this is located in the immune response (Ir) genes. Ir genes are more easily studied in laboratory animals with short gestation times and with molecules of low or feeble antigenicity that stimulate some but not all animals in a group. For example, the immunoglobulin response of C57 mice to a synthetic amino acid polymer composed of histidine, glutamic acid, alanine, and lysine is nil, whereas all CBA mice are good responders. C57 × CBA crossbreeding followed by antigen testing of the progeny revealed that the high response of CBA mice was dominant. Further breedings suggested that high responsiveness was under control of a single Ir gene, now identified as Ir-1. The immunoglobulin response of mice to other synthetic antigens is under the control of other genes —gene Ir-3 regulates the response to polymers of tyrosine, glutamic acid, proline, and lysine. Evidence concerning the inheritance of food allergies in man suggested half a century ago that human immunoglobulin responses to certain food antigens were under genetic control. It is now accepted that the antibody response in man to ragweed pollen antigens and the ABO and Rh blood group antigens is genetically controlled by Ir genes. A remarkable finding is that these Ir genes are transmitted with or are closely associated with the genes that regulate the synthesis of histocompatibility antigens found on the surface of tissue cells. This has been noticed in guinea pigs, mice, and rats and is not a unique finding in the human species. The meaning of this relationship has yet to be determined; however, the knowledge that genetic principles influence the immune response has been an exciting discovery for immunologists interested in tumor immunity, autoimmune disease, and tissue histocompatibility.

In returning to the chemistry of antigens a second quality expressed simply as molecular complexity is shared by most antigens. The synthetic amino acid polymers mentioned earlier have barely enough complexity to function as antigens. Complexity can be considered in terms of the primary structure of a molecule, including both the composition and sequence of its structural units. Proteins composed of 20 or more amino acids arranged in a variable, genetically regulated order generally achieve antigenicity when they reach a molecular weight of 10,000. Naturally occurring polysaccharides, since they are seldom composed of more than five different types of monosaccharide units, may not become antigenic until they reach a higher molecular weight. Proteins have a greater structural complexity at the primary level than most polysaccharides, and tertiary structural effects (coiling, branching, and folding) of very large molecules also contribute to antigenicity, as do quaternary structural (multichain) effects. Chemical complexity is not demonstrated by polymers of a single amino acid (homopolymers) or polymers of other repetitive types (for example, polystyrene), and these compounds are not antigenic. Protein and polysaccharide biopolymers are often antigens and demonstrate molecular complexity at several structural levels. Lipids and nucleic acids are structurally simpler and are not antigenic.

Antigenic tolerance

When antigens are injected into an animal, they are partially degraded by macrophages. Many synthetic polymers are not susceptible to hydrolysis by macrophage enzymes, and this is offered as a reason for their nonantigenicity. Nonantigenicity is also a characteristic of an animal's own proteins and polysaccharides. Human serum albumin meets all the above criteria for an antigen and is antigenic for fish, ducks, chickens, horses, cattle, rabbits, rats, mice, etc., but is not ordinarily antigenic for the person from whom the albumin was taken. The explanation offered for this is that the cells that might be expected to respond to self-antigens are still functionally immature cells when these antigens are first synthesized by the developing fetus. This premature contact of antigen and (ultimately) antigen-reactive cells suppresses the cells, creating a condition called antigen-specific immunologic tolerance. Such a hypothesis is obviously subject to experimental challenge—one simply injects a foreign antigen into a developing fetus, allows its birth and development, then reexposes it to the original plus a second antigen (Fig. 3-1). This type of experiment was conceived and conducted by Burnet and Medawar, and they received the Nobel Prize in Medicine and Physiology in 1960 when they demonstrated that an animal would respond to the second antigen that it had first encountered in adult life but not to the foreign antigen it met earlier in embryonic life.

Although Paul Ehrlich in the early 1900s stated that an animal does not ordinarily develop an immune response to its own normally circulating antigens and described this as the principle of *horror autotoxicus* (fear of self-poisoning), a self-directed immune response can nevertheless occur. Autoimmune diseases associated with the emergence of self- or autoantigens, discussed in Chapter 10, are an important type of human ailment. The terms "alloantigen" and "heteroantigen" must also be considered relative to autoantigen. An alloantigen is an antigen present in one member of a species but not in all other members of the species. Transplantation anti-

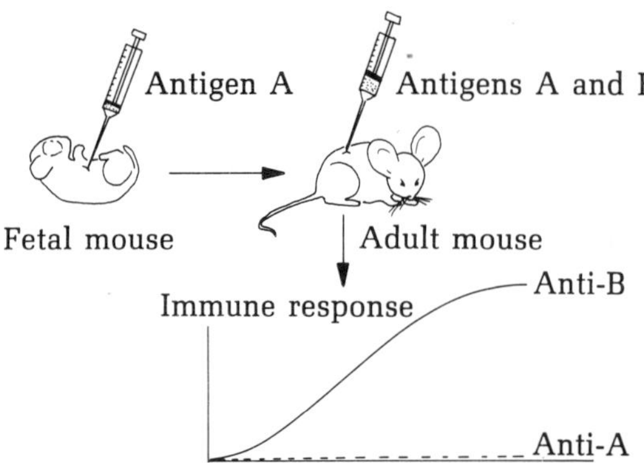

Fig. 3-1. Antigen-specific immune tolerance is easily demonstrated by exposing a fetal animal to an antigen. Later, in adult life, the animal does not respond to reexposure to that antigen but does to unrelated antigens.

gens and blood group antigens are examples. Heteroantigens are antigens of some species other than the species being immunized, and this applies to most of the antigens we contact—bacterial, viral, fungal, plant, and other antigens. A heterophil antigen is an antigen that is common or present in an assortment of diverse species (see case 1, p. 155).

Other uses of the word "antigen" that should be mentioned are homologous and heterologous antigen. Homologous antigen refers to the one used or previously associated with a situation, and heterologous refers to some other antigen. For example, if a vaccine of *Salmonella typhosa* were used to immunize a person and his blood later tested for its ability to react with *S. typhosa* and *S. paratyphi A,* then the former is the homologous antigen and the latter is the heterologous antigen. Actually, *S. typhosa* and *S. paratyphi A* are each composed of several antigens, but whenever a collection of antigens is present in a single structural unit—virus, bacterial cell, red blood cell, etc.—it is referred to in the singular.

The term "immunize" is also used in different ways. First, any antigenic exposure can be referred to as an immunization, even if the antigen is completely unrelated to any disease. This is simply the result of the historical development of immunology from the science of immunity. Active immunization means the individual under discussion received the antigen and the cells of his body were stimulated to respond with antibody and lymphokine synthesis. If the person received these antibodies and lymphokines from some other person, then the recipient is passively immunized. The use of the phrase adoptive immunization refers to the transfer of immunologically competent cells to an individual.

HAPTENS

Antigenic determinant sites

Although whole molecules are described as antigens, the immune response is ac-

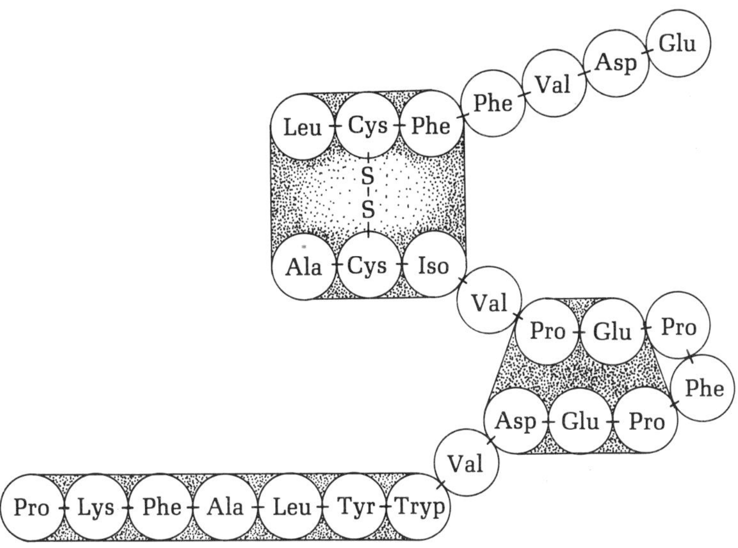

Fig. 3-2. Three antigenic determinant sites, represented by the stippled areas of five to seven amino acids in the peptide fragment shown, indicate that determinant sites may be either linear or nonlinear within a single peptide chain or across two peptide chains. Same features apply to polysaccharide antigens.

tually directed toward discrete portions of the antigen called antigenic determinant sites. Antigenic determinant sites are to antigens what catalytic sites are to enzymes, since they each represent the key functional unit. Antigenic determinant sites are equivalent in size to approximately six or eight amino acids in proteins and to six or eight monosaccharide units in polysaccharides, or roughly 25 to 50 Å (750 mol wt). The antigenic determinant sites in a molecule are not necessarily linear segments of a peptide or polysaccharide chain but consist instead of a geographic unit (Fig. 3-2). Thus an antigenic determinant could consist of three or four amino acids in one peptide chain plus three or four amino acids in a second peptide chain (in a protein with quaternary structure) if all these six or eight amino acids were proximal to each other in the natural, folded structure of the molecule. Antigens are believed to have two or more antigenic sites per molecule, roughly one to each 10,000 or 20,000 mol wt. These determinants are not necessarily of equal potency; it might be very easy to demonstrate an immune response to one, the immunodominant site, but not to others.

Much of our knowledge about antigenic determinants and antigenic specificity derives from the studies of haptens by Karl Landsteiner. Haptens are nonantigenic substances by definition, but they can modify existing antigens to create an antigenic determinant site that includes the attached hapten. These antigen-hapten complexes are described as conjugated antigens or neoantigens and are prepared by uniting a simple chemical grouping such as the dinitrophenyl radical to an antigen. This can be done by mixing dinitrochlorobenzene with a protein and performing a condensation reaction in which chlorine is lost from the hapten and hydrogen from the antigen as the dinitrophenyl antigen is formed. Injection of this conjugate into an animal will stimulate antibody formation against the new as well as the old determinant sites. This can be proved by various tests in which the animal's serum, now referred to as an antiserum since it contains antibodies, is mixed with the hapten or the hapten conjugated to a heterologous antigen. Radiolabeled or other tagged haptens are very useful in these tests, since hapten-antibody reactions take place without any visible change in the appearance of the reaction mixture. After the addition of the radiolabeled hapten to the antiserum, the antiserum will acquire radioactivity as the hapten attaches to it. It is usually

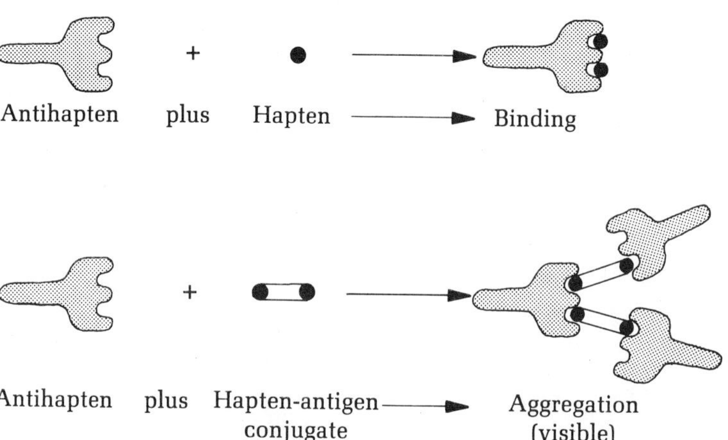

Fig. 3-3. An antibody directed to a hapten will bind to that hapten but cannot form large aggregates with it due to its monovalent nature. If more than one hapten moiety is present on a carrier antigen, then cross-linking and aggregate formation are possible.

necessary to separate the antibody-hapten complex from the unreacted hapten so that the amount of radiolabel actually bound to the antibody can be quantitated. Since the hapten is invariably smaller than the antibody-hapten complex, this can be accomplished by biochemical purification procedures based on size or weight differences such as ultrafiltration, molecular sieving, gradient density, and centrifugation. This use of sophisticated equipment and radiolabeled hapten can be avoided if the hapten is available in a conjugated form with a heterologous antigen. This form of the hapten will produce a visible reaction with the antiserum (Fig. 3-3). Any serologic reaction of the heterologous antigen-hapten conjugate with the antiserum to the original antigen-hapten complex can only be due to a specificity in the antiserum for the hapten. Thus haptens can react with antibodies directed against them, but do not themselves provoke antibody formation.

Autocoupling haptens

The injection of dinitrobenzene into an animal with the intention of producing antibodies would be a futile venture. However, the injection of dinitrochlorobenzene into the animal would not be futile, since this compound can combine with tissue proteins and create new antigens to which the animal responds. Haptens that spontaneously complex with existing tissue proteins or polysaccharides are sometimes referred to as autocoupling haptens (Fig. 3-4). Poison ivy, poison oak, poison sumac, contact dermatitis to leather products, dyes, and cosmetics, and allergy to penicillin and

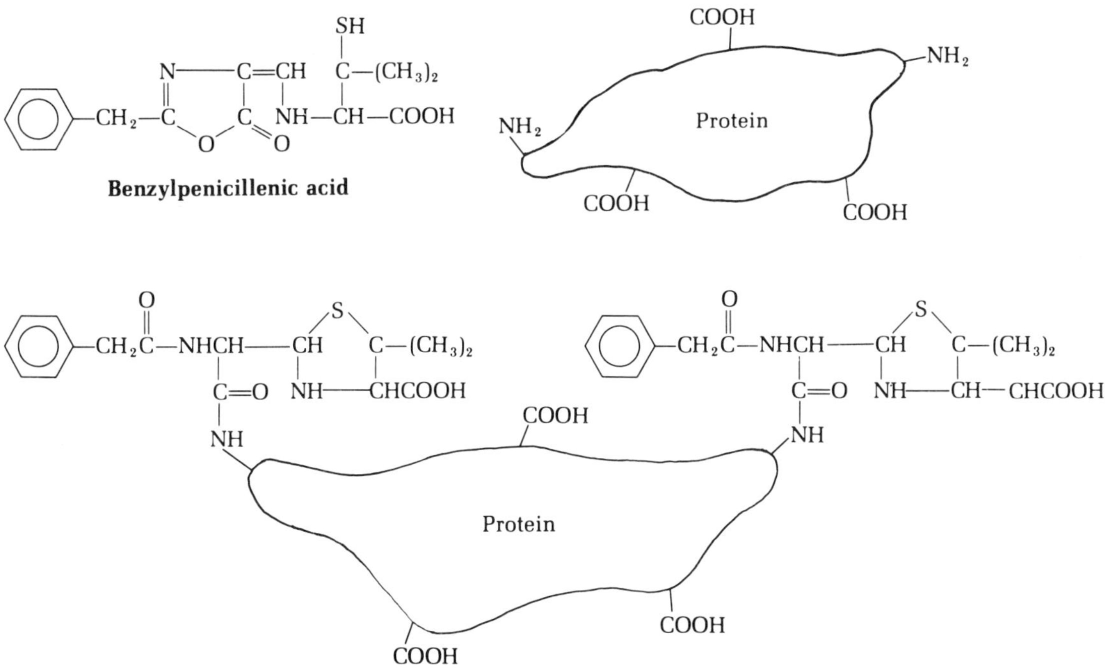

Benzylpenicillenic acid

Fig. 3-4. Benzylpenicillenic acid is one of many decomposition products of penicillin G. This acid can form peptide bonds with the amino groups of tissue proteins, creating neoantigens in which the penicillin derivative is most closely related to penicillenic acid. Conjugates of penicillin derivatives can also form easily by –S–S– exchange with the sulfur atom in the thiazolidine portion of the antibiotic structure, but these are less important as allergens.

other pharmaceuticals develop as the result of neoantigen formation with such autocoupling haptens. It is not absolutely essential for a hapten to establish a covalent bonding with its Schlepper (carrier antigen); firm ionic bonding may be enough to maintain the hapten so closely associated with the antigen that it appears as a new antigenic determinant to antigen-handling cells.

ADJUVANTS

Extensive modification of a simple, nonantigenic molecule may actually elevate it to a state of antigenicity by creating antigenic determinants where none existed previously. Adjuvants may produce the same apparent effect. Adjuvants (from the Latin *adjuvare,* meaning to help) are substances that improve the immune response, and if an adjuvant were used with an extremely feeble antigen, it might, by enhancing the response to it, appear to confer antigenicity on a nonantigen. This would only be an illusion; adjuvants are only stimulants of existing antigens. Immunopotentiation by adjuvants is more generally recognized by their capacity to improve immunoglobulin titers or to extend the immunoglobulin response over a greater period of time than when antigen is administered in the absence of adjuvant. Adjuvants also stimulate lymphokine production (T lymphocyte responses) as well as the immunoglobulin response (B lymphocyte).

Successful adjuvants maximize the following aspects of the immune response: (1) the duration of antigen exposure, (2) stimulation of antigen processing by macrophages and other cells of the reticuloendothelial system, and (3) stimulation of B and T lymphocytes or the cooperative activities between them and phagocytic cells. Adjuvants such as the aluminum and calcium salts precipitate the antigen so that it is presented to the animal in an insoluble form. This extends the half-life of the antigen in the immunized animal and encourages phagocytosis. Lanolin, mineral oil, and other oils or waxes form antigen-in-oil emulsions in which the aqueous, antigen-containing phase is held basically outside the animal's physiologic milieu. As the oil droplets gradually disintegrate, antigen is gradually released from its depot, thus extending the period of antigen exposure. Macrophages, which engulf these antigen particles, become primed by antigen ingestion and transmit a message as yet uncoded that traps lymphocytes in neighboring lymph nodes. This improves the exposure of lymphocytes to antigen, which is absorbed from tissues into the lymphatic canals. Vitamin A, mycobacteria, and corynebacteria are all good lymphocyte trappers. Other adjuvants, including nucleic acids and bacterial endotoxins, may stimulate B lymphocytes directly, possibly by altering their permeability to antigens. Other adjuvants such as beryllium and Freund's complete adjuvant function as T cell stimulants. Most adjuvants encourage germinal center development in lymphoid tissues where phagocytic cells and lymphocytes are positioned near each other, presumably permitting closer cooperation between the cells involved in the immune response. Beryllium salts and Freund's complete adjuvant, two of the most successful adjuvants for laboratory use, cannot be used on human subjects because they encourage disfiguring granuloma formation. Calcium phosphate or hydroxide gels and aluminum salts are the adjuvants most frequently used in human medicine.

IMMUNOGLOBULINS

Antigens were not recognized until recently to stimulate lymphokine production, but the induction of antigen-specific reactive substances in blood by antigens has long been recognized. These antigen-specific substances or antibodies, now more descriptively referred to as immunoglobulins, are formed in response to each determinant site possessed by the antigen. Consequently, an antiserum is truly a mixture of several antibodies, and each antibody is capable of reacting only with its corresponding determinant. This discriminating ability of immunoglobulins is well recognized—immunization with diphtheria toxoid induces immunity to diphtheria, not to other diseases—and has been of great benefit to analytical scientists in many disciplines. An antigen present in a complex mixture of substances can be identified simply by adding an antiserum directed against that antigen to the mixture and noting whether a serologic reaction develops.

Of course, there are limits to the specificity of antibodies, and antigens or haptens that are nearly identical may be cross-reactive. An antiserum prepared to an antigen conjugated to the hapten *p*-chloraniline will react with *p*-methylaniline, *p*-nitroaniline, and aniline to almost the same extent. Cross-reactive antigens such as the heterophil antigens mentioned earlier need not be absolutely identical to each other, but they must be very similar to each other. An interesting challenge to this concept of one antigenic determinant–one antibody specificity has recently been offered with evidence that some antibody molecules may react with more than one antigen or hapten and at the same time.

Immunoglobulin G

Immunoglobulin G (IgG) has been more extensively studied than any other immunoglobulin, and since many of its characteristics are shared by the other antibody molecules, it serves as the model for any discussion of immunoglobulin structure (Table 3-2). This immunoglobulin is the dominant antibody in most antisera, representing 75% to 85% of the total; consequently, references to gamma globulin, antibody, or 7S gamma globulin are taken as references to IgG even though other 7S gamma globulin antibodies are known. IgG in adult human serum is present at a level of 1275 ± 280 mg/100 ml. This concentration is achieved and maintained by the higher synthetic capacity (28 mg/kg of body weight/day) and longer half-life (25 to 35 days) of IgG compared to the other antibodies. The IgG molecule has a molecular weight of about 150,000, of which 2.5% is in the form of carbohydrate. The molecule is globular, has a low electrophoretic mobility at pH 8.6, and is situated in the gamma fraction of the serum proteins. On ultracentrifugation it sediments as a 7S molecule. These features have led to the many synonyms for IgG.

Bence Jones protein. Structurally, IgG consists of four peptide chains that exist as

Table 3-2. Characteristics of immunoglobulins

Characteristic	*IgG*	*IgA*	*IgM*	*IgD*	*IgE*
Percent of total	75-85	5-10	5-10	< 1	< 1
Concentration (mg/100 ml serum)	1275 ± 280	225 ± 55	125 ± 45	3	0.01-1
Molecular formula	$\gamma_2\kappa_2$ or $\gamma_2\lambda_2$	$\alpha_2\kappa_2$ or $\alpha_2\lambda_2$	$(\mu_2\kappa_2)_5J$ or $(\mu_2\lambda_2)_5J$	$\delta_2\kappa_2$ or $\delta_2\lambda_2$	$\epsilon_2\kappa_2$ or $\epsilon_2\lambda_2$
Half-life (days)	25-35	6-8	9-11	2-3	Unknown
Comment	Passes placenta	Secretory type known	Dissociates with —SH treatment	Biologic role uncertain	Identical to allergic reagin
	Subclasses IgG1 thru IgG4	α-Chain allotypes exist	Formed early after antigen exposure		Unstable at 56°-60° C for 30-120 min
	γ-Chain (Gm) allotypes		Secretory type known		

paired sets of two different peptides, one approximately twice as large as the other. The larger peptides, the heavy (H) chains, are joined to each other by one or more disulfide bonds. Each H chain is linked to one of the two light (L) chains by a single disulfide bond. The interchain —S—S— bond that unites the L and H chain originates at a terminal or penultimate cysteine in the carboxyl terminal end of the L chain. Both the H and L chains have intrachain disulfide linkages as well, customarily two in each L chain and six in each H chain (Fig. 3-5).

The amino acid sequences of both the L and H chains are known. Naturally this determination was simpler for the L chain because of its molecular weight of only 22,000; however, the sequencing of the L chains was simplified by the discovery that

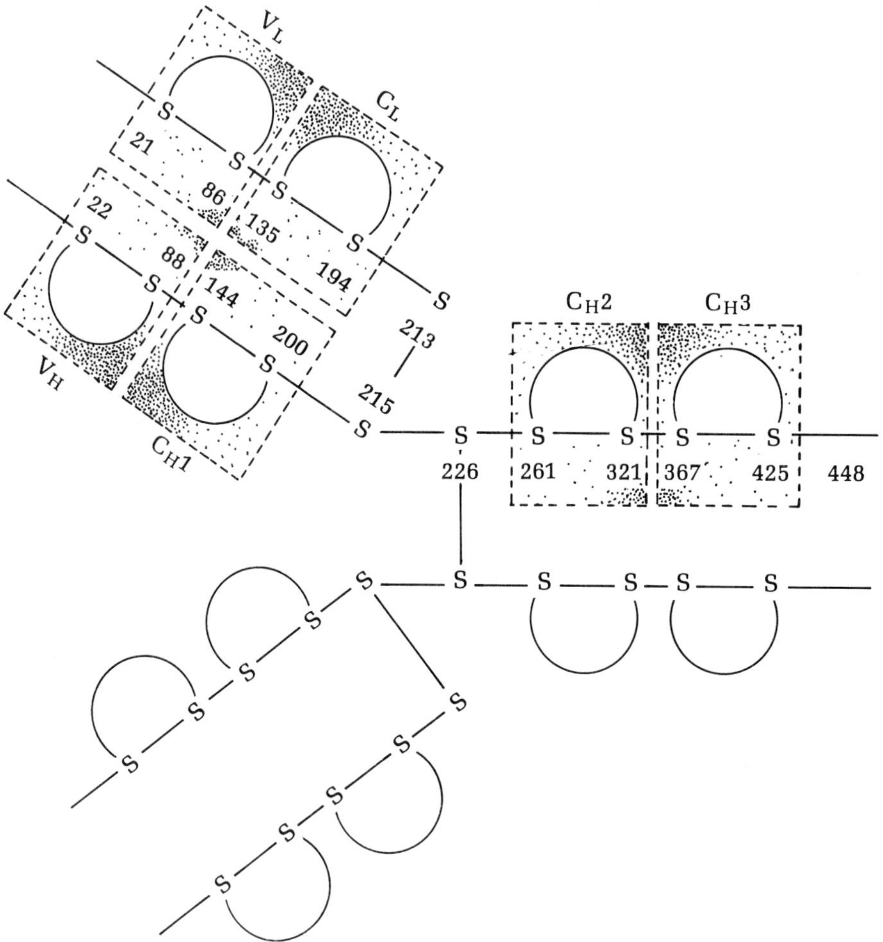

Fig. 3-5. Structure of IgG represented here consists of two L chains of 213 amino acid residues and two H chains of 448 residues. Variable amino acid sequencing, designated by V's, is characteristic of the amino portion of the four peptides. Constant sequence portion of L chains consists of its carboxyl terminal half and is designated C_L. H chain has three so-called constant domains, C_H1, C_H2, and C_H3, joined by regions of variable sequence. Position of disulfide loops is indicated in each chain. Numbering of bottom half of the molecule is exactly the same as upper half, although not indicated.

L chains and Bence Jones proteins are identical. Bence Jones protein is found in the blood and/or urine of most patients with multiple myeloma, a disease that can be considered a plasma cell neoplasm. The formation of abnormal plasma cells in the neoplastic state is frequently associated with a loss of their ability to produce H chains, resulting in a surplus of L chains in the blood, which are excreted in the urine. Bence Jones proteins (L chains) are characterized by solubility in dilute acid at room temperature and above 80° C but insolubility between 60° and 80° C. This facilitates their identification in urine and the diagnosis of plasma cell neoplasms (multiple myeloma). Urine that tests positive for Bence Jones proteins provides an excellent source of relatively pure L chains, and these have been used as the starting material for amino acid sequencing studies.

Allotypes: variable and constant regions. Immunologic studies revealed early in the analysis of Bence Jones proteins that two major subclasses existed—the κ and λ types. Chemically, each is a peptide of 214 amino acids and has two internal cystine loops (Figs. 3-6 and 3-7). In κ-chains this is located at amino acids 134 and 194 and amino acids 22 and 88, creating two loops of approximately 60 amino acids each. In λ-chains these loops are at residues 135 and 194 and 21 and 86. These two peptides have other interesting structural homologies. The carboxyl terminal half of all κ-chains, even those from different persons, have nearly identical amino acid sequences, whereas the amino terminal halves display considerable variation in their amino acid sequence. This same condition exists for λ-chains; for example, the sequence of amino acids 210 through 214 of practically all λ-chains is Pro-Thr-Glu-Cys-Ser, with Cys 213 serving as the bridge to the H chain. There is, of course, some variation in sequence of the constant portion of κ- and λ-chains from others of their subclass, but many of these can be accounted for by

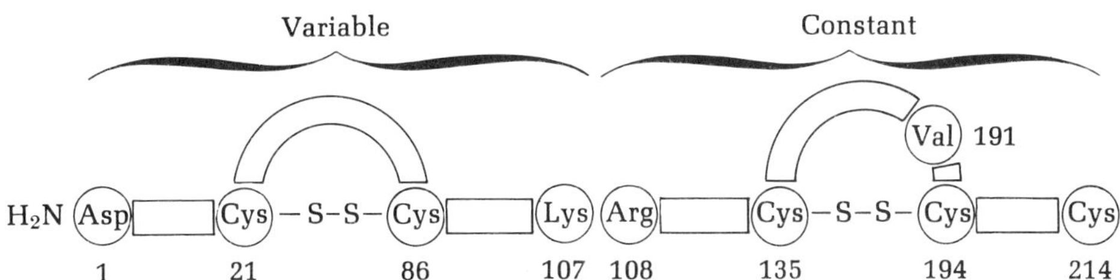

Fig. 3-6. This κ-chain consists of 214 amino acid residues, 107 of which are in the variable region and a like number in its constant sequence region. Residue 191 is the site of the Inv factor.

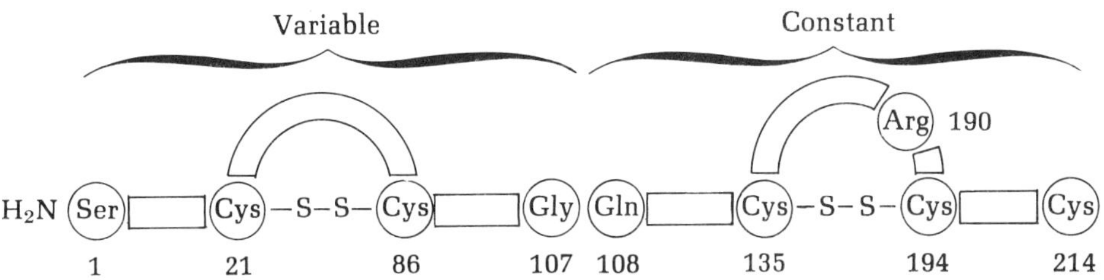

Fig. 3-7. The close relationship of the λ- and κ-type L chains can be observed by comparing to Fig. 3-6. The Oz determinant is located at position 190.

amino acid additions or deletions and, when these are ignored, serve to accent the homology of these peptides. Not only does a strong homology of the constant regions exist within κ- and λ-chains, but there is also a considerable similarity of the constant regions between these L chain subclasses. The variable regions within the κ and λ subclasses have some gross similarities, as indicated by the cysteine-cysteine loops, but they are basically dissimilar.

Within the λ subclass of L chains, further distinctions can be made on the basis of a specific amino acid substitution in position 190 (constant region). If this position is occupied by lysine, the chain is of the Oz+ type; if occupied by arginine, it is of the Oz− allotype. This substitution of a single amino acid creates λ-chain antigenic allotypes. κ-Chain allotypes are referred to as Inv 1, Inv 2, and Inv 3, with the possible existence of an Inv−. Inv 3 has the amino acid valine at position 191, and Inv 1 has a leucine located at that position. It is always possible that other allotypes of L chains will be recognized by antisera that react with only certain antigenic determinants in these chains.

The H chains of human IgG are known as γ-chains to distinguish them from the H chains of the other immunoglobulins. The entire amino acid sequence of several human γ-chains has been determined and provides an interesting parallel to the sequence studies of L chains. The first 100 to 110 amino acid residues at the amino terminal end exhibit considerable variation from one H chain to another, just as L chains are hypervariable in the same region. However, proceeding toward the carboxyl terminus of the γ-chain, three regions of similar amino acid sequence, connected by short units of variable sequence, are encountered (Fig. 3-5). These major divisions are referred to by the abbreviations V_H or V_γ for the variable sequence zone and C_H1, C_H2, and C_H3 or $C_\gamma1$, $C_\gamma2$, and $C_\gamma3$ for the constant sequence zones, each of which is composed of approximately 100 amino acid units.

Four major subclasses of human IgG have been recognized and are designated IgG1 through IgG4. These varieties of IgG vary from one another in the number of interheavy chain disulfide bonds. These are usually located between C_H1 and C_H2 in an area near the hinge region. The hinge region is the zone where H-L chain disulfide linkage occurs and where there is actually a bend in the linear structure of the H chain due to the inclusion of several proline residues in the chain. IgG1 has two interheavy chain disulfide linkages, IgG2 has three, IgG3 has four, and IgG4 has but one. Allotypes or antigenic varieties of the γ-chains exist, are presently 24 in number, and are designated Gm1, Gm2, Gm3, etc. These Gm allotypes are not uniformly distributed among the subclasses—Gm1 is present only in IgG1 and not other subclasses. IgG3 always has either Gm determinant 5 or 21 but not both. With few exceptions, these Gm factors are situated in the carboxyl terminal half of the γ-chain and result from the substitution of amino acids in specific positions; for example, Gm5 has phenylalanine at residue 296 and 436, and in Gm21 these are replaced by tyrosine. The amino acids responsible for Gm determinants are known in only a few instances.

Within a given individual, IgG κ- and λ-type L chains are usually present in a ratio of approximately 2:1. The IgG subclasses all exist simultaneously in an individual, and as a consequence there can be 2 (L chain subclasses) × 4 (H chain subclasses) or eight varieties of IgG in an individual, with no reference as yet made to allotypic variations in the γ-chain. If these are included in this consideration and we accept five Gm allotypes as reasonable, then 8 × 5 = 40 different IgG molecules. If each of these were formed against each of five determinants in an antigen, then there would be over 200 varieties of IgG in a single serum. Since each of these differs from the others in amino acid composition and/or sequence, each is an electrophoretically distinct molecule. When we add to this the great variations in amino acid sequences of the V_H and V_L regions, it becomes clear why IgG presents itself as such a broad spectrum of electrophoretically different proteins.

The variation of amino acid order in the V_H and V_L regions is responsible for the ability of an antibody to combine with the specific antigen that induced its formation. If there were no variable regions in the molecule, then all immunoglobulins would be nearly identical, and there would be no accounting for antibody specificity. Since the two L chains and two H chains all have a variable portion and since the hinge region of the γ-chains forces the molecule into a wishbone shape, there are then two major variable zones in the IgG molecule, or two antigen-combining sites. There is excellent support for this concept of two reactive centers (valence sites) in the IgG molecule. This was first determined on immunologic grounds and then supported by structural studies of IgG by Porter and Edelman, Nobel Prize winners in 1972. Edelman's major contribution was related to the tetrapeptide 2H-2L chain structural determination of IgG, and Porter fragmented IgG into its two antigen-binding fragments (Fab) and a third easily crystallized fragment (Fc) by papain proteolysis of the molecule. Each Fab unit consists of an entire L chain and approximately half of the H chain, the region referred to as the Fd fragment. Proteolysis of IgG with pepsin occurs at a slightly different point than when papain is used and produces the $F(ab')_2$ and Fc′ fragments.

Immunoglobulin M

Immunoglobulin M (IgM) is a macroglobulin with a molecular weight near 800,000 and a Svedberg number of 19. It is present in human serum at a level of 125 ± 45 mg/100 ml, where it represents roughly 9% of the total gamma globulin. This immunoglobulin has a half-life of 10 days and is synthesized at a rate of only 5 to 8 mg/kg/day. The carbohydrate content of IgM is about 10% of its total weight and is attached to the H chains. IgM can be referred to as a gamma globulin, but its location after serum electrophoresis bridges both the gamma and beta regions. For this reason IgM has been described as a β_2M or γ_1M molecule.

The chemistry of IgM is similar to that of IgG and the other immunoglobulins with important exceptions. Because IgM has a molecular weight five times that of IgG, the original notion was that it consisted of five IgG units held together by disulfide bonds. This concept was strengthened by the discovery that dilute solutions of reducing compounds such as 2-mercaptoethanol would disaggregate IgM into five 7S units, each with a molecular weight of 180,000 (Fig. 3-8). These 7S units each contained two L chains and two H chains, and the L chains were identical to the L chains in IgG; that is, they were κ- or λ-chains. However, the H chains of IgM differ from the H chains of IgG, first, in bearing more carbohydrate but more importantly in antigenicity. Antisera to γ-chains do not customarily react with H chains from IgM. Accordingly, IgM H chains are designated as μ-chains. The chemical formula of IgM was thought to be $(\mu_2\kappa_2)_5$ or $(\mu_2\lambda_2)_5$. Sulfhydryl reduction of IgM yields the 7S unit or γMs unit, which is structurally $\mu_2\kappa_2$ or $\mu_2\lambda_2$. The γMs fragment can combine with antigen but produces no physical change in the appearance of the antigen (Chapter 6). Trypsin digestion of γMs units and sulfhydryl reduction produce fragments corresponding closely with the fragments formed from IgG, and to identify them as originating from IgM the suffix μ is added. Thus we have Fcμ, Fabμ, Fdμ, $F(ab')_2\mu$, etc. Since there are five $F(ab')_2\mu$ units from each mole of IgM, IgM has 10 antigen-combining sites.

J chain. Another important feature of IgM is its content of J chain (Fig. 3-8). The J chain has a molecular weight of only 24,000 and joins the five tetrapeptide

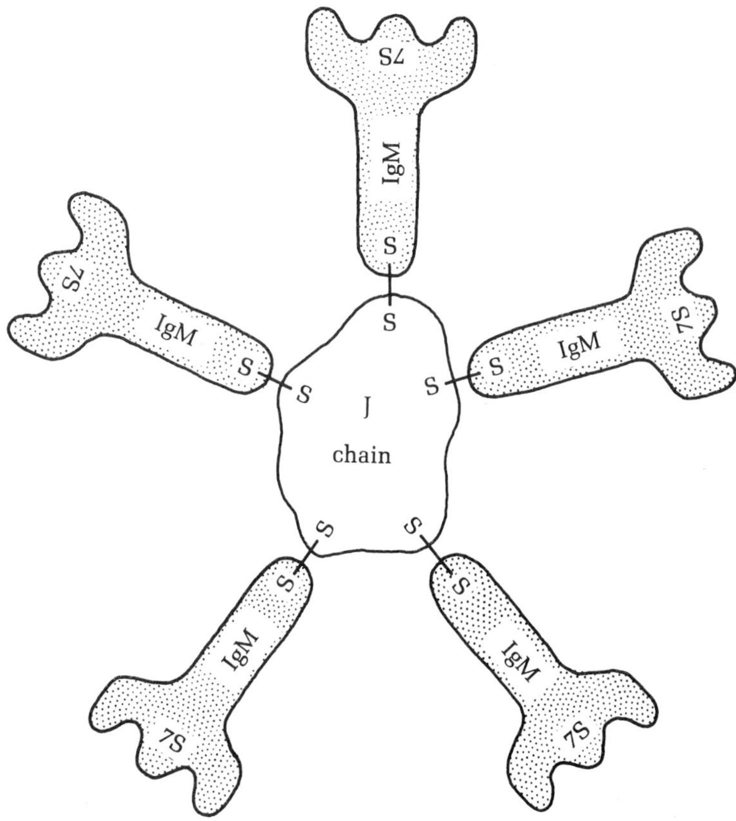

Fig. 3-8. IgM consists of five sets of 7S units held in assembly by the J chain. Each 7S unit consists of two L chains, either κ or λ, and two H chains, the μ-chains.

structures of the IgM molecules together. The J chain is attached to the Fc portions of the five μ-chains by disulfide bonds, and only one J chain is present per IgM molecule. Thus the molecular formula for IgM is best expressed as $(\mu_2\kappa_2)_5$J or $(\mu_2\lambda_2)_5$J. Allotypes of J chains or μ-chains are not yet known. A secretory form of IgM has been described recently. Its distribution in body fluids parallels that of secretory IgA, and its formula is represented by $(\mu_2\kappa_2)_5$ SC·J or $(\mu_2\lambda_2)_5$ SC·J.

Immunoglobulin A

Serum immunoglobulin A. Immunoglobulin A (IgA) in serum has a basic molecular weight of 160,000 and a sedimentation coefficient of 7S, but due to the ease with which IgA combines with itself through disulfide bond exchange, polymeric forms of serum IgA are well known. Serum IgA has a half-life of only 6 to 8 days and is synthesized at a rate of 8 to 10 mg/kg/day. These factors account for its rather low level in serum (225 ± 55 mg/100 ml). IgA distributes itself between the true γ- and β-regions of the serum electrophoretic profile and is sometimes referred to as the γA or β_2A immunoglobulin.

The L chains of IgA are of the κ or λ type, but the H chains are unique to IgA and are designated as α-chains. Each α-chain (mol wt 46,000 to 52,000) bears carbohydrate consisting of about 6000 dal-

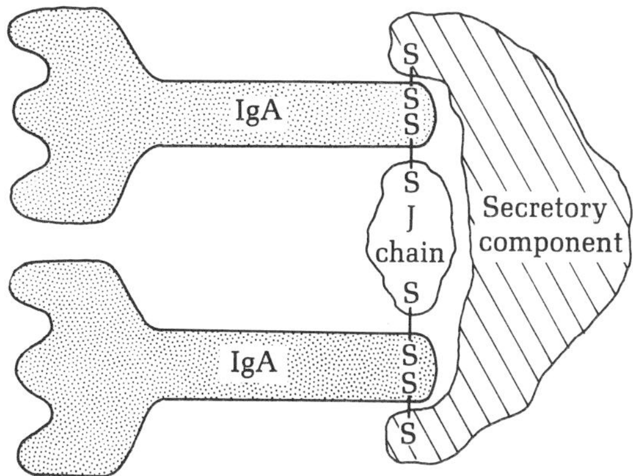

Fig. 3-9. Secretory IgA exists as an IgA dimer complexed with J chain and secretory component. The individual proteins are not represented to scale—IgA molecules are the largest.

tons, which accounts for about 9% of the total weight of the molecule. Allotypes of the α-chain, the Am1 and Am2 determinants, are known. Enzymatic digestion of serum IgA yields Fabα or $F(ab')_{2\alpha}$ units, but Fcα units are difficult to isolate due to their sensitivity to further digestion by papain or pepsin.

Secretory immunoglobulin A. The ratio of IgG and IgA in serum approaches 6:1, but in milk, nasal mucus, saliva, intestinal and respiratory mucus, and other external secretions, IgA is present in a higher concentration than either IgG or IgM. This is due to a peculiar secretory form of IgA (Fig. 3-9) in these fluids and not to an excretion of serum IgA into these external fluids. Secretory IgA can be expressed as $(\alpha_2\kappa_2)_2$SC·J or $(\alpha_2\lambda_2)_2$SC·J, in which α refers to the H chains, κ and λ to the L chains, SC to the secretory component, and J to the J chain. The H chains of IgA are antigenically different from the H chains of other immunoglobulins and deserve a special abbreviation. Since the L chains of IgA are identical to those in other antibodies, the same Greek symbols are used to identify them. Two of these tetrapeptide units of IgA are held together by a J chain. This dimer, synthesized and unified in plasma cells near the external mucous membranes, enters or attaches to the surface of adjacent epithelial cells and acquires the SC peptide. SC is a molecule with a molecular weight of 85,000 that, like the J chain, attaches to the Fcα portion of the protein. SC seems to protect secretory IgA from enzymatic digestion, a feature that may be very important in extending the duration of secretory IgA in the intestine and thus extending the protective benefits of IgA on the surface of the mucous membrane. Although serum IgA is devoid of SC, there is no critical evidence that SC aids excretion of secretory IgA onto mucosal surfaces.

Immunoglobulin D

A fourth immunoglobulin, immunoglobulin D (IgD), is so sparse in normal human serum that it was not discovered until it was detected in a patient with a myeloma that was producing IgD. Many myeloma patients produce and excrete excessive amounts of whole immunoglobulin molecules as well as Bence Jones protein. This myeloma protein had H chains that could not be identified as γ, μ, or α and were thus labeled δ. IgD has the usual κ- or λ-type L chains. IgD has a molecular weight of 180,000, a half-life of only 2 to 3 days, and a synthetic rate of 0.4 mg/kg/day. Since

IgD accounts for only 3.0 mg/100 ml of serum and has no known protective role, its contribution to a person's well-being is uncertain.

Immunoglobulin E

Like IgD, immunoglobulin E (IgE) is barely detectable in normal human serum, but unlike IgD it is known to have a vital role in disease, not as a protective force but as a causative agent. IgE is synonymous with reagin, an antibody in the serum of allergic persons. IgE is unique in several respects, including a sensitivity to heat denaturation when held at 60° C for 30 minutes to 3 hours and an inability to display visible serologic reactions.

Allergic reagin (IgE) is present in normal serum in concentrations of less than 1.0 mg/100 ml, but values 10 times this have been found in sera of highly allergic persons. This immunoglobulin has the characteristic tetrapeptide structure in which either κ- or λ-chains are incorporated with ϵ-chains to provide the formula $\epsilon_2\kappa_2$ or $\epsilon_2\lambda_2$. The ϵ-chain has a molecular weight of 75,000, which elevates the molecular weight of the tetrapeptide IgE by 40,000 over that of IgG. Ten percent of IgE is in the form of carbohydrate. Enzyme digestion of IgE liberates the expected Fab and Fc units plus some lower molecular weight molecules. The important role of IgE in hypersensitivity is the major topic of Chapter 8.

LYMPHOKINES

Antigenic or haptenic stimulation of T lymphocytes induces a new activity that is measured most easily when these sensitized lymphocytes are placed with other tissue cells and the antigen (hapten). For years it was felt that these new activities of T lymphocytes could be measured only when the T cell was in direct physical contact with the antigen and host cell, but this is now known to be erroneous. The T cells excrete peptides known collectively as lymphokines, and their effects can be measured in vitro. Individual lymphokines are responsible for the following activities: macrophage migration inhibition, macrophage aggregation, monocyte and macrophage chemotaxis, target cell destruction, T lymphocyte blastogenesis, viral resistance (interferon), cloning inhibition, and possibly others (Table 3-3). All of these can be considered as effector molecules of T

Table 3-3. Lymphokines

Lymphokine	*Function*	*Comment*
Migration inhibition factor (MIF)	Prevents macrophage migration	
Macrophage aggregation factor (MAF)	Agglutinates macrophages	Probably same as MIF
Macrophage activating factor	Summons "angry" macrophages	May be identical to MIF
Chemotactic factor	Attracts macrophages	Other T cell lymphokines attract neutrophils and eosinophils
Lymphotoxin	Destroys target cells	May consist of a family of proteins
Blastogenic factor	Initiates cell growth	Synonymous with mitogenic factor and lymphocyte transformation factor
Interferon	Confers protection on host cells against intracellular parasites	Possibly a family of proteins

cells in the same sense that immunoglobulins are effectors from B lymphocytes and plasma cells.

Transfer factor

Transfer factor (TF) is not properly considered a lymphokine, since the latter is formed in response to an antigenic stimulus and appears to be a low molecular weight protein, whereas TF is probably a polynucleotide and may be a normal component of T cells. However, the biologic role of TF is so intimately connected with lymphokines that its discussion here is appropriate.

TF was described by Lawrence as a substance present in cell-free extracts of leukocytes from the blood of a person with a tuberculin sensitivity that could be used to transfer that sensitivity to a previously tuberculin-negative individual (Fig. 3-10). Later it was found that leukocytes from persons with a delayed skin hypersensitivity to any antigen could transfer sensitivity to that antigen. The type of leukocyte responsible for this activity was later identified as the T lymphocyte. It was also found that incubation of these T lymphocytes with the antigen caused the release of TF into the suspending medium, where it was relatively free of other cellular materials, and it was assumed that this would facilitate the chemical identification of TF. This supposition has not yet been realized. It is known that TF will pass dialysis membranes that retain molecules greater than 10,000 in molecular weight. Efforts to destroy TF in these dialysates with trypsin, DNAse, RNAse, or combinations of these enzymes failed. Fractionation of concentrated preparations of TF resulted in the localization of TF in a nonantigenic low molecular weight fraction that is nearly free of protein. The ultraviolet absorption spectrum and faintly positive biuret test suggest a polynucleotide-polypeptide composition of TF. The heat sensitivity of TF is consistent with a double-stranded RNA

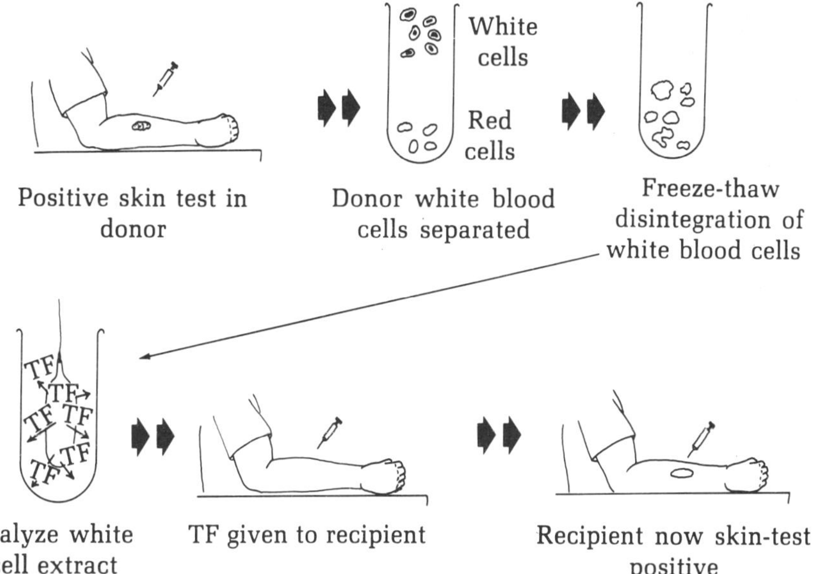

Fig. 3-10. Lymphocytes separated from peripheral blood of a person with a T cell–dependent (delayed-type) skin reaction to a specific antigen can be used as the source of transfer factor. This molecule will diffuse through the pores of a dialysis bag and can be used to convert a normal individual to the same reactive status as the TF donor.

structure as opposed to a single-stranded RNA structure that is more heat resistant. The ribonucleotide bases adenine, guanine, and cytosine have been identified in TF, but uracil has not. Conceivably this could confer RNAse resistance on the lymphokine.

TF is a moelcule of considerable medical importance because it appears to confer certain T lymphocyte functions on recipient lymphocytes. There is considerable evidence that immunity to several viral and fungal diseases as well as to tumor cells is dependent on lymphokine production; consequently, injections of TF may transfer immunity to persons with specific T cell deficiencies. Initial trials of such immunologic cures have been promising, and

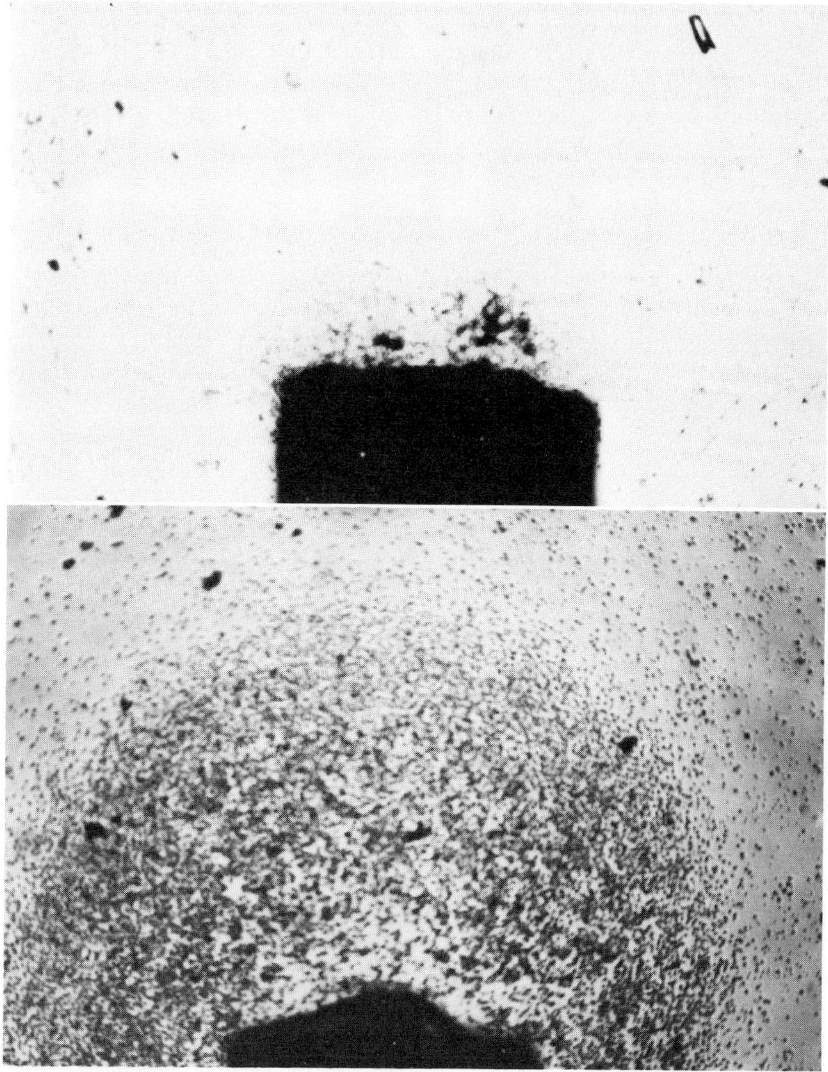

Fig. 3-11. Top: Migration of macrophages from a tube in which the macrophages were incubated with the histoplasmin-sensitized lymphocytes and histoplasmin has been inhibited by MIF produced by the lymphocytes. Bottom: This migration was not inhibited when histoplasmin was replaced by tuberculin.

there is even an expectation that at least certain forms of cancer may be amenable to TF therapy.

Migration inhibition factor

When the T lymphocytes of an animal previously exposed to an antigen are incubated in culture with the antigen and tissue macrophages, the macrophages are incapable of displaying their normal pseudopodial mobility. This inhibition of macrophage migration is due to the elaboration of a soluble migration inhibition factor (MIF) by the previously sensitized lymphocytes. Mixing normal lymphocytes with normal or sensitized macrophages in the presence or absence of antigen results in normal mobility (Fig. 3-11). Sensitized lymphocytes incubated with normal or sensitized macrophages in the absence of antigen have no effect on macrophage migration. From these experiments it can be concluded that it is only the sensitized lymphocyte in the presence of antigen that excretes MIF. This MIF functions on macrophages from either normal or antigen-exposed animals.

MIF production is suppressed by antibiotics such as puromycin that inhibit protein synthesis, and MIF activity is destroyed by chymotrypsin; MIF is thus believed to be a protein. It has a molecular weight near 25,000, migrates as a prealbumin, and is resistant to nucleases but sensitive to neuraminidase, thus classifying the molecule as a glycoprotein whose activity is dependent on intact sialic acid residues and peptide bonds. It is resistant to exposure to 60° C for 30 minutes.

MIF and MAF (macrophage aggregation factor) are probably identical. MAF activity is sometimes displayed in vitro in the MIF test, where the immobile macrophages are held in clumps, or in tube tests, where large numbers of macrophages (10^6/ml) are incubated with antigen and sensitized lymphocytes at 37° C for several hours. This test is observed as positive when large clumps of the macrophages are seen. The lymphokine responsible for macrophage aggregation has the exact characteristics of MIF.

Macrophage activating factor

The ability of T lymphocyte products to call forth a macrophage with an improved phagocytic activity is due to a substance described as a macrophage activating factor. This substance cannot be distinguished from MIF. More recent studies indicate that macrophage activation can also be induced by a macrophage RNA-antigen fragment.

Chemotactic factor

Lymphokines that are chemotactic for macrophages, neutrophils, and eosinophils are elaborated by T lymphocytes incubated with their sensitizing antigen. The factors that attract neutrophils and eosinophils are as yet largely uncharacterized, but preliminary studies indicate they differ from the better known macrophage chemotaxin. For example, the eosinophil leukotaxin depends on the presence of antigen-antibody complexes, a feature not required for macrophage chemotaxis. The macrophage and neutrophilic attractants also differ in electrophoretic mobility.

The chemotaxin for macrophages has a molecular weight near 25,000, is resistant to neuraminidase, is stable at 56° C for 30 minutes, and is slightly less acidic than MIF on electrophoresis (albumin as compared to prealbumin). Otherwise little is known of the biochemical nature of this molecule.

Lymphotoxin

When a T lymphocyte is exposed to a foreign cell, it acquires the ability to liberate a cytotoxic protein, lymphotoxin, that is responsible for the destruction of that cell. This requires several hours, and during this period the foreign cell, generally referred to as the target cell, can be seen to lose its normal morphology, swell, become spherical, cease motility, develop intracellular vacuoles, and eventually rupture. Lymphotoxin collected from antigen or phytohemagglutinin-stimulated T lymphocyte cultures initiates this same sequence of events. Lymphotoxin has never been isolated in highly purified form, but crude preparations are resistant to DNAse, RNAse, neuraminidase, and trypsin. Although it is resistant to trypsin, lymphotoxin is believed to be proteinaceous in nature. Its molecular weight has been estimated from 35,000 to 85,000, and there is a possibility that lymphotoxin is a family of proteins. Lymphotoxin is stable at 56° C. Electrophoretically, it is a beta globulin. There is considerable species variation in the chemical nature of lymphotoxins, and the preceding description is of the human and guinea pig proteins.

Blastogenic factor

Antigen-stimulated T lymphocytes release a substance into culture fluids capable of initiating cell growth in unrelated lymphocytes. This can be measured by an increase in amino acid incorporation by the normal lymphocytes or by their accelerated incorporation of radiolabeled purines or pyrimidines. The agent responsible for this activity has been referred to variously as blastogenic factor, mitogenic factor, or lymphocyte transformation factor. As yet, it is poorly characterized, it is heat labile at 56° C, it is resistant to destruction by RNAse and DNAse, and it is nondialyzable.

Interferon

A spectrum of proteins synthesized by T lymphocytes that can confer viral resistance on neighboring host cells is known as interferon. It is described in detail on p. 165.

Miscellaneous lymphokines

Molecules potentially able to meet the criteria of lymphokines include skin reactive factor and lymph node permeability factor, which are considered in Chapter 9. A factor that reduces the cloning capacity of tissue culture cells and one that inhibits the proliferation of human tissue culture cells are two additional lymphokines of which little is known.

BIBLIOGRAPHY

Benacerraf, B., and McDevitt, H. O.: Histocompatibility–linked immune response genes, Science **175**:273, 1973.

Benjamini, E., Michaeli, D., and Young, J. D.: Antigenic determinants of proteins of defined sequences, Curr. Top. Microbiol. Immunol. **58**:85, 1972.

Bernier, G. M.: Structure of human immunoglobulins: myeloma proteins as analogues of antibody, Prog. Allergy **14**:1, 1970.

Bradley, J.: Immunoglobulins, J. Med. Genet. **11**:80, 1974.

Butler, V. P., Jr., and Beiser, S. M.: Antibodies to small molecules: biological and clinical applications, Adv. Immunol. **17**:255, 1973.

Buxbaum, J. N.: The biosynthesis, assembly and secretion of immunoglobulins, Semin. Hematol. **10**:33, 1973.

Capra, J. D., and Kehoe, J. M.: Hypervariable regions, idiotypy, and antibody-combining site, Adv. Immunol. **20**:1, 1975.

Crumpton, M. J.: Protein antigens: the molecular bases of antigenicity and immunogenicity. In Sela, M., ed.: The antigens, New York, 1974, Academic Press, Inc., vol. 2.

Dayton, D. H., Jr., and others, eds.: The secretory immunologic system, Washington, D.C., 1970, U.S. Government Printing Office.

de Weck, A. L.: Low molecular weight antigens. In Sela, M., ed.: The antigens, New York, 1974, Academic Press, Inc., vol. 2.

Fudenberg, H. H., Pink, J. R. L., Stites, D. P., and Wang, A. C.: Basic immunogenetics, New York, 1972, Oxford University Press, Inc.

Gally, J. A.: Structure of immunoglobulins. In Sela, M., ed.: The antigens, New York, 1973, Academic Press, Inc., vol. 1.

Granger, G. A.: Lymphokines—the mediators

of cellular immunity, Ser. Haematol. **5**:8, 1972.

Greaves, M. F., Owen, J. J. T., and Raff, M. C.: T and B lymphocytes: origins, properties and roles in immune responses, Amsterdam, 1973, Excerpta Medica.

Heremans, J. F.: Immunoglobulin A. In Sela, M., ed.: The antigens, New York, 1974, Academic Press, Inc., vol. 2.

Hong, R.: The immunoglobulins, Clin. Immunobiol. **1**:29, 1972.

Ishizaka, K.: Chemistry and biology of immunoglobulin E. In Sela, M., ed.: The antigens, New York, 1973, Academic Press, Inc., vol. 1.

Jolles, P., and Paraf, A.: Chemical and biological basis of adjuvants, New York, 1973, Springer-Verlag New York, Inc.

Kochwa, S., and Kunkel, H. G., eds.: Immunoglobulins, Ann. N.Y. Acad. Sci. **190**:5, 1971.

Koshland, M. E.: Structure and function of the J chain, Adv. Immunol. **20**:41, 1975.

Landsteiner, K.: The specificity of the serologic reactions, rev. ed., New York, 1962, Dover Publications, Inc.

Levin, A. S., Spitler, L. E., and Fudenberg, H. H.: Transfer factor therapy in immune deficiency states, Ann. Rev. Med. **24**:175, 1973.

McCluskey, R. T., and Cohen, S.: Mechanisms of cell-mediated immunity, New York, 1974, John Wiley & Sons, Inc.

McDevitt, H. O., and Landy, M., eds.: Genetic control of immune responsiveness, New York, 1972, Academic Press, Inc.

Metzger, H.: Structure and function of gamma M macroglobulins, Adv. Immunol. **12**:57, 1970.

Milstein, C., and Pink, J. R. L.: Structure and evolution of immunoglobulins, Prog. Biophys. Mol. Biol. **21**:209, 1970.

Natvig, J. B., and Kunkel, H. G.: Human immunoglobulins: classes, subclasses, genetic variants and idiotypes, Adv. Immunol. **16**: 1, 1973.

Nossal, G. J. V., and Ada, G. L.: Antigens, lymphoid cells and the immune response, New York, 1971, Academic Press, Inc.

Pink, R., Wang, A. C., and Fudenberg, H. H.: Antibody variability, Ann. Rev. Med. **22**: 145, 1971.

Reichlin, M.: Amino acid substitution and the antigenicity of globular proteins, Adv. Immunol. **20**:71, 1975.

Scharff, M. D., and Laskov, R.: Synthesis and assembly of immunoglobulin polypeptide chains, Prog. Allergy **14**:37, 1970.

Smith, G. P., Hood, L., and Fitch, W. M.: Antibody diversity, Ann. Rev. Biochem. **40**: 969, 1971.

Tomasi, T. B., Jr.: Secretory immunoglobulins, N. Engl. J. Med. **287**:500, 1972.

Tomasi, T. B., Jr., and Grey, H. M.: Structure and function of immunoglobulin A, Prog. Allergy **16**:81, 1972.

Case histories

CASE 1. HETEROPHIL ANTIGENS: INFECTIOUS MONONUCLEOSIS

S. B., a 20-year-old female college student, consulted her physician because of a sore throat that had persisted for 4 days. She felt feverish and had a headache for a day or two prior to developing the sore throat. Physical examination revealed a modest bilateral enlargement of cervical lymph nodes, pharyngeal inflammation and edema, and a temperature of 101.2° F. Infectious mononucleosis was considered a strong possibility in the differential diagnosis when throat cultures showed normal flora and white blood cell counts revealed a prominent lymphocytosis (68% lymphocytes). A serologic test for heterophil antibody was requested. The results were Paul-Bunnell titer 1:3584 and differential absorption by guinea pig kidney 1:1792. The serologic findings were confirmatory, and a diagnosis of infectious mononucleosis was established.

Questions

1. Discuss heterophil antigen associated with serum sickness and infectious mononucleosis as well as Forssman antigen.

2. What is the Paul-Bunnell test and its interpretation?
3. Describe differential antibody absorption in infectious mononucleosis.
4. What is the prospect for specific serologic tests to detect infectious mononucleosis?

Discussion

Heterophil antibodies are those that react with apparently unrelated antigens of diverse sources. People receiving injections of horse serum, for example, develop antibodies that clump (agglutinate) sheep and beef red blood cells, and a small percentage of apparently normal individuals have antibodies that will agglutinate sheep red blood cells. The Forssman antigen was originally described as an antigen on guinea pig cells, except erythrocytes, that would induce the formation of antibodies that would agglutinate sheep red blood cells. Persons with infectious mononucleosis have similar antibodies. In human medicine the term "heterophil antibody" usually refers to one that will agglutinate sheep red blood cells. Since there are several of these, they must be distinguished before they can be used to diagnose disease.

The Forssman antigen has been partially characterized. It is truly heterogenetic, being present in corn, *Diplococcus pneumoniae,* sheep red blood cells, chicken, carp, toad, tiger, whale, and horse tissues. Resistance of the antigen to heat indicates it is a polysaccharide. Since extensive purification results in a loss of antigenicity, the possibility exists that the Forssman antigen is actually a hapten. Chemically, it is similar to human blood group A antigen. The heterophil antigen in horse serum and that associated with infectious mononucleosis are largely uncharacterized.

Most of the attention given to heterophil antigens has been in terms of their antibodies. In 1932 Paul and Bunnell discovered that the serum of patients with infectious mononucleosis would clump sheep red blood cells and suggested this as a diagnostic aid for the disease. The sheep cell agglutinin in normal human sera can rarely be diluted more than 1:28 and still retain activity; so that elevated titers were of some aid, but they did not distinguish true Forssman or serum sickness agglutinins from those of mononucleosis. This has come about by the use of differential absorption of these antibodies by guinea pig kidney and beef cells, known as the differential or Davidsohn differential absorption and is applied to sera that have a presumptive titer (unabsorbed serum plus sheep erythrocytes) greater than 1:28. Guinea pig kidney removes the "serum sickness" antibody but not that (or only very little of that) associated with mononucleosis. Bovine erythrocytes remove the serum sickness antibody and most of the mononucleosis and Forssman antibody.

Heterophil titers in infectious mononucleosis have reached 1:14,336, but figures between 1:28 and 1:3584 are more typical. After the third week of the disease, 100% of all patients have a titer of at least 1:14 after guinea pig kidney absorption, rising from 76% in the first week. Forssman antibody titers range up to 1:112 and are deleted by kidney absorption. Serum sickness titers range between 1:56 and 1:224 and are largely eliminated by absorption.

The prospect for a specific serologic test for infectious mononucleosis is dim. The current thoughts about the etiology of the disease include the Epstein-Barr virus as a possible agent. Antibodies against the Epstein-Barr virus persist for years, but the heterophil antibodies do not, which suggests that the Epstein-Barr virus is not the etiologic agent of mononucleosis. All patients do not develop heterophil antibodies, even though their diagnosis is almost certain based on other criteria. Until the etiology of the disease is known, the development of specific serologic tests is remote.

REFERENCES

Chervenick, P. A.: Infectious mononucleosis, Disease-A-Month, p. 1, December, 1974.

Davidsohn, I.: Test for infectious mononucleosis, Am. J. Clin. Pathol., Tech. Suppl. **2:** 56, 1938.

Paul, J. R., and Bunnell, W. W.: The presence of heterophile antibodies in infectious mononucleosis, Am. J. Med. Sci. **183:**90, 1932.

CASE 2. CROSS-REACTIVE HAPTENS

H. R., a 43-year-old alcoholic, entered the hospital with a temperature of 103.2° F, pulse rate of 140, respiratory rate of 30, and white blood cell count of 23,000 with 99% polymorphonuclear neutrophilic leukocytes. Bilateral respiratory rales and an x-ray film indicated severe lung congestion consistent with pneumonia. H. R. was well known to the emergency room personnel for his frequent admissions over the past several years for anaerobic abscess, pneumonia, and a stab wound. Penicillin treatment of these conditions had created a penicillin hypersensitivity in H. R. With this knowledge, the attending physician administered sodium cephalothin, a penicillin substitute. The patient had a severe anaphylactic reaction (Chapter 8) in which the blood pressure could not be measured and respirations were rapid and weak. Epinephrine was administered and the patient regained consciousness, became well oriented, and seemed almost fully recovered within 30 minutes.

Questions

1. Is cephalothin antigenic or haptenic?
2. How can an allergic reaction follow the first exposure to cephalothin?
3. What, if any, is the relationship between the previous allergy to penicillin and the cephalothin reaction?
4. How do species differences in immunologic responsiveness affect the marketing of potentially antigenic therapeutic agents intended for human use?

Discussion

Allergic reactions to penicillin are usually dependent on the development of antibodies to penicillin. Penicillin is not an antigen; it is a hapten of the autocoupling type. The reactive hapten is not penicillin per se, but penicillenic acid, a degradation product that can covalently link to the ϵ-amino groups of proteins to form penicilloyl-protein derivatives. Antibodies to such derivatives are responsible for the allergic reactions to penicillin.

Allergic reactions to cephalothin are, like those to penicillin, dependent on its haptenic qualities rather than its antigenicity because cephalothin and other simple chemical derivatives of 7-aminocephalosporanic acid are not antigens. The basis for the development of allergic shock to cephalothin on its first use in a patient who is allergic to penicillin has definitely been determined to result from the structural similarity of the two antibiotics (Fig. 3-12). The thiazolidine ring of penicillin and the dihydrothiazine ring of cephalothin are not unlike chemically and are both fused to a beta lactam ring that emphasizes their similarity. The result of this is that antibodies formed against the penicillin derivative cross-react with cephalothin or cephalothin derivatives and vice versa. Penicillin-directed antibodies that are already present would thus trigger an allergic reaction to cephalothin or any structurally related compounds on the first exposure to them.

The episode described emphasizes the need for physician awareness of the chemical nature of therapeutic agents. Structural similarities between low molecular weight haptenic compounds is only one consideration. Materials proved to be nonantigenic in laboratory animals may prove antigenic in man. It is generally agreed that dextrans with a molecular weight below 50,000 are very rarely antigenic for rabbits or man. Larger dextrans, which were initially thought to be nonantigenic in rabbits and thus presumed not to be in man, were used during World War II as blood volume expanders with unfortunate results. The dextrans proved to be allergenic in man, possibly because they were cross-reactive with

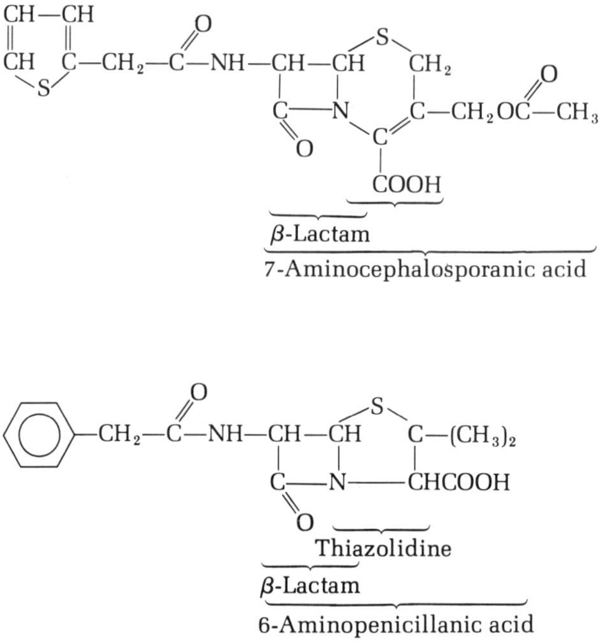

```
CH—CH        O
||   ||     //         S
CH   C—CH2—C—NH—CH—CH     CH2         O
  \S/              |    |     |         //
                   C——N      C—CH2OC—CH3
                    \\    \  //
                     O     C
                           |
                          COOH
                  β-Lactam
                  7-Aminocephalosporanic acid
```

```
             O
            //            S
(C6H5)—CH2—C—NH—CH—CH      C—(CH3)2
                 |    |     |
                 C——N——CHCOOH
                  \\
                   O
                     Thiazolidine
                 β-Lactam
                 6-Aminopenicillanic acid
```

Fig. 3-12. Structural relationship of penicillin and cephalosporin.

antibodies formed against polysaccharides of the normal human flora. (Dextrans are produced commercially from bacteria in the genus *Leuconostoc.*) It is also probable that certain antigenic impurities in the preparation of these dextrans, plus their own antigenicity for the human species, contributed to these allergic reactions. Because of species differences in responsiveness to antigens and haptens, it is often impossible to prove that the human animal will tolerate a therapeutic agent that is nonallergenic in several species of laboratory animals.

REFERENCES

Batchelor, F. R., Dewdney, J. M., Weston, R. D., and Wheeler, A. W.: The immunogenicity of cephalosporin derivatives and their cross-reaction with penicillin, Immunology **10**:21, 1966.

Grieco, M. H.: Cross-allergenicity of the penicillins and the cephalosporins, Arch. Intern. Med. **119**:141, 1967.

Thoburn, R., Johnson, J. E., III, and Cluff, L. E.: Studies on the epidemiology of adverse drug reactions. IV. The relationship of cephalothin and penicillin allergy, J.A.M.A. **198**:345, 1966.

chapter 4

Immunity

Resistance to infectious diseases can be examined from the viewpoint of the host and the forces the host can muster to repel invaders, or it can be examined from the viewpoint of the pathogen, including the type of disease it produces and the specific forms of opposition it must overcome to do so. Both of these will be considered in this chapter together with additional attention directed to the practical aspects of prophylactic and therapeutic immunization.

NATURAL RESISTANCE

The term "natural resistance," often equated with inherited or innate immunity, refers to the ability of an individual to resist infections through the normally present body functions of all members of his species. Natural resistance does not include resistance resulting from a previous exposure to a pathogenic organism or its toxic products; this is acquired immunity. Natural resistance relies on the nonadaptive or normal activities of our phagocytic cells, blood and tissue proteins, certain smaller molecules of blood and tissue, and the basic permanency and integrity of our cells and tissues. The meaning of natural resistance may become clearer as we consider the external and internal forces of which it is composed and compare it to acquired immunity.

External defense system

The first resistance forces encountered by an invading microbe are those actually outside the physiologic milieu of the body, and hence they are categorized as the external defense system. These activities do not represent a system in the sense of a consorted interplay of activities, and indeed the activities function independently of one another. Nevertheless, these forces are, by and large, highly effective against a heterogeneous battery of pathogens or potential pathogens. This is witnessed by the general good health of most infants prior to the development of their acquired immunity.

The first body surfaces contacted by most pathogens are the skin and mucosae. The keratinized outer layers of the skin constitute a highly effective structural barrier against invasion. It is generally believed that intact, healthy skin can be breached by relatively few pathogens—the treponeme of syphilis and the bacillus causing tularemia are two possible examples. However, the skin is more than a mere anatomic barrier against bacteria and fungi, for it is known that lactic acid in sweat and the unsaturated fatty acids in secretions from the sebaceous glands are antibacterial. The saturated fatty acids in these same secretions are fungistatic. Drying of delicate organisms such as the gonococcus or meningococcus contributes to their poor recovery from skin deliberately painted with these bacteria, but the primary disinfectant action of skin is a chemical phenomenon.

The mucous membranes are structurally more susceptible to penetration than is skin and, being moist, would theoretically permit a long-term survival of microbes on their surface. However, mucosal tissues are protected by several antimicrobial activities. The first of these is the mucous slime itself, a gelatinous-like bioadhesive excreted by and coating the mucosal epithelium. Microorganisms impinging on this film in the lung, for example, as the result of inhalation, are held a few micra away from the underlying vital tissue. The cell layer beneath this mucous film is ciliated and the cilia constantly sweep the mucus upward at a rate of 10 to 20 mm/minute. Within a short period of time the organisms and mucus are carried into the throat and, except for instances of extensive mucus formation, are swallowed. Another important protective activity also occurs in the mucous film—phagocytosis. A special kind of phagocytic cell known as the alveolar macrophage roams over the surface of the mucus. The major function of this cell appears to be the phagocytic destruction of inhaled objects.

Other mucosal surfaces have slightly different protective devices. In the male genitourinary system the periodic flushing with urine, which is normally somewhat acidic, provides both a mechanical and chemical protection to the mucous surfaces. The same may be stated for the female urinary tract. The reproductive tract of the mature woman appears to have a thicker underlying cell bed than in the prepubescent female. These cells synthesize and store glycogen; as the cells die, the glycogen is degraded to lactic acid, creating a bacteriostatic environment in the vagina. The mucosal surfaces of the eye are partially protected by the tendency to weep when objects of any size enter the eye, and this is an effective cleansing action.

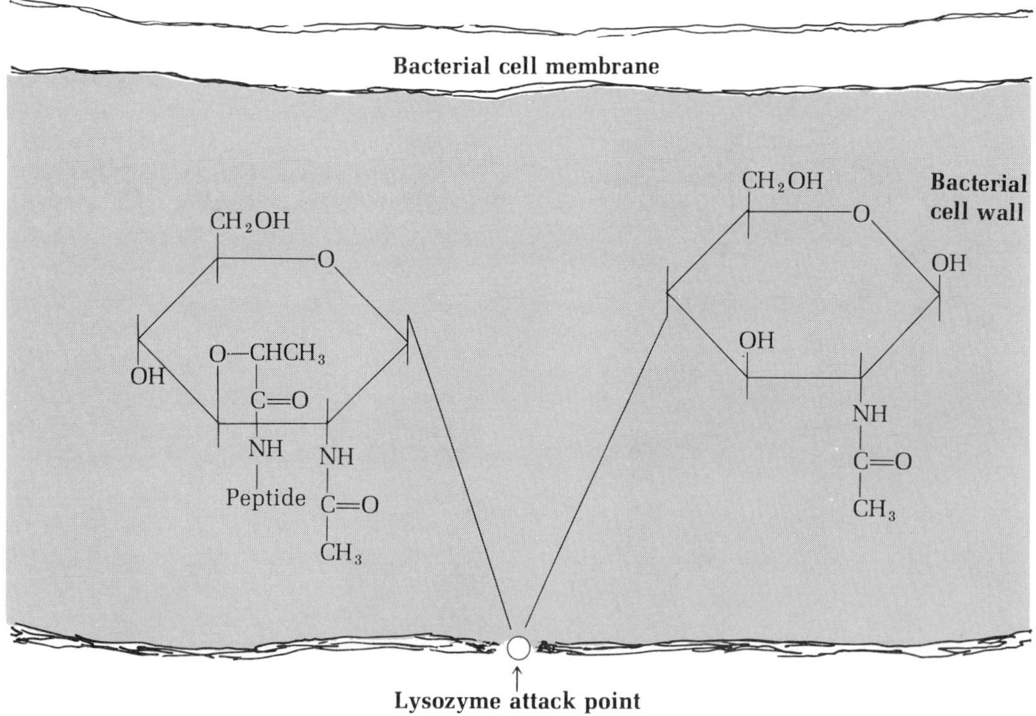

Fig. 4-1. Lysozyme-vulnerable point in cell membrane of gram-positive bacteria is the β-1, 4-glycosidic bond that unites muramic acid and *N*-acetylglucosamine. When this bond is hydrolyzed, the cell lyses. This lysozyme substrate is also present in gram-negative bacteria but is protected from the enzyme by lipids.

Far more important, especially when microorganisms enter the eye without being borne on particulate matter and when weeping is not induced, is the action of an enzyme known as lysozyme. Lysozyme is present in high concentration in tears but is also found in nasal mucus (where Fleming, the discoverer of penicillin, first identified lysozyme in 1922), urine, plasma, and within phagocytic cells. Lysozyme has an isoelectric point near pH 11.0, and most bacteria have acidic isoelectric points; this ionic dissimilarity may promote the union of the enzyme with the bacteria. On the surface of gram-positive bacteria the substrate for lysozyme is available in the cell wall (Fig. 4-1). In gram-negative bacteria the enzyme substrate is also present, but it is largely shielded from the enzyme by lipid. As a consequence, gram-negative microorganisms are highly resistant to lysozyme, but gram-positive bacteria are not. Lysozyme cleaves a β-1,4-glycosidic bond that unites *N*-acetylglucosamine and muramic acid (lysozyme is a muramidase). This exposes the underlying cell membrane to osmotic forces that rupture the cell. It is interesting that contagious pinkeye and many urinary tract infections are caused by the lysozyme resistant, gram-negative bacteria.

The digestive system, like the respiratory and genitourinary systems, is considered external to the body. No antimicrobial activities of any consequence are localized in the upper portion of the digestive system until the stomach is reached, where the pH may be as low as pH 1.0. This is not only an unfavorable environment for the growth of microorganisms but is actively lethal. Organisms that are markedly aciduric or protected inside poorly masticated pieces of food escape this acidity and are passed to the small and large intestine, both of which represent ideal growth environments for many organisms. Fortunately these regions of the alimentary canal are heavily colonized with the normal flora, a hetero-

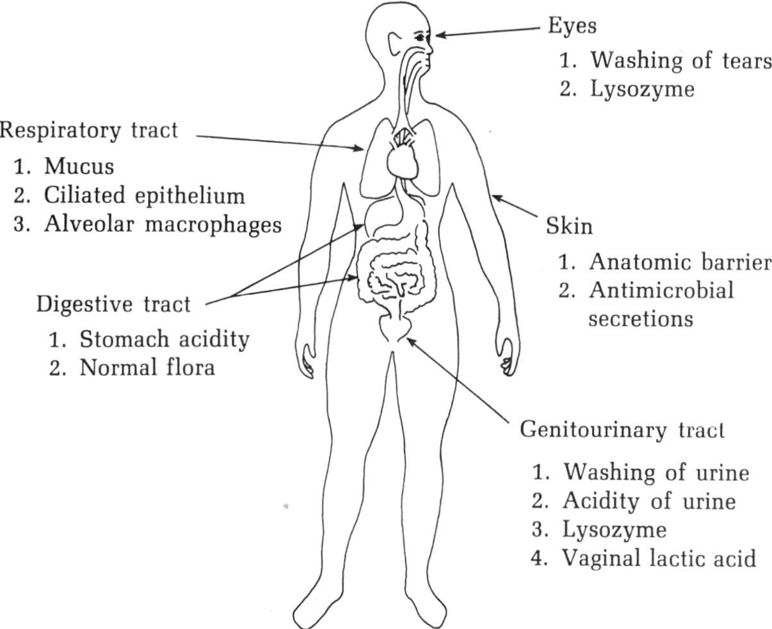

Fig. 4-2. Innate resistance factors that function on external surfaces of the body are indicated.

geneous collection of basically noninvasive bacteria. This population is quite stable and minimizes the opportunity for other, including the pathogenic, organisms to establish themselves in the intestine. Properties of the normal flora responsible for this include certain acid end products and antibiotic-like substances. The protective influence of the normal flora can also be demonstrated in other regions of the body such as the nasopharynx and the vagina.

A summary of external defense forces is presented in Fig. 4-2.

Internal defense system

Successful pathogens that escape the external defense system and penetrate into the true physiologic interior of the host may do so by virtue of their own invasive properties, by entrance through wounds or scratches, or by being ingested in food, milk, water, etc. Even when inside the host, the pathogen must still avoid a series of defense forces before it can establish an infection.

Foremost among the elements of the internal armory is phagocytosis (Table 4-1). Polymorphonuclear neutrophilic leukocytes, the circulating and tissue macrophages, and other phagocytic cells were discussed fully in Chapter 2, as was the engulfment process itself. It is probably sufficient for the present to emphasize that the phagocytic destruction of bacteria is a primary event in controlling and preventing infections by this type of parasite. Phagocytosis is promoted by several factors, among which the naturally present opsonins can be mentioned. Although originally defined as heat-labile substances that encouraged phagocytosis, the term has now been broadened in scope to include virtually any substance that improves phagocytosis. Many serum proteins serve as opsonins, apparently by coating the particle or cell to be phagocytosed, altering its surface charge, and making it more approachable by phagocytic cells. Another important stimulant of phagocytosis is leukotaxis (chemotaxis). Local tissue damage by the invading pathogen may liberate trypsinlike tissue enzymes that activate the complement pathway at C3. Alternatively, the activation of plasminogen to plasmin, such as by streptokinase from *Streptococcus pyogenes*, may begin complement activation at C1. Or as a third possibility, the polysaccharide capsule or endotoxins from the invading organism may activate complement at C3 via the properdin pathway. The exact mechanism of complement activation is of little serious consequence because the end result is the same—the neutrophilic chemotaxins C3a, C5a, and C5,6,7 are all formed, as is a C3-derived opsonin. Chemoattractants released by the neutrophils or by soluble factors excreted by the invading bacteria draw monocytes to the scene of the infection. In the tissues the monocytes transform into the highly phagocytic macrophages.

Macromolecules in blood may have antiviral or antibacterial properties. Glycoproteins, transferrin, and fetuin are all antiviral. Beta lysin, leukin, plakin, and other poorly described proteins are antibacterial. In tissues, polyamines and basic polypeptides are known to play a protective role against bacteria. Among these are the his-

Table 4-1. Internal defense system

Phagocytosis	Neutrophils Monocytes Macrophages
Leukotaxis	C3a C5a C5,6,7
Opsonins	C3 factor Miscellaneous proteins
Complement activation	Properdin pathway (polysaccharides) C1, enzymatic activation C3, enzymatic activation
Macromolecules	Glycoproteins Transferrin Lysozyme Various polyamines

tones, protamines, spermine, and spermidine (Table 4-1).

It is obvious that the external and internal defense forces do not function at the same level of efficiency in all individuals. It is generally recognized that such features as race, sex, nutritional status, hormonal influences, age, climate, fatigue, and alcoholism markedly influence the level of our natural resistance. Even in the human animal, where it is virtually impossible to prove that any two chosen individuals have had the exact same exposure to pathogens, statistical studies of persons in restricted environments such as prisons or mental hospitals have revealed that the black and white races have a different susceptibility to several infectious diseases. For example, Negroes are more susceptible to tuberculosis but more resistant to diphtheria and influenza than Caucasians.

The influence of nutrition on infection is easily demonstrated. Phagocytic cells of the malnourished person function at only 10% to 30% of the efficiency of these same cells in the well-nourished individual. Reduction of the trace element level (Cu, Zn, Fe, Mn, etc.) in the diet of rats reduced their lysozyme levels by 33% to 74%. Children with rickets (vitamin D deficiency) have twice the complications from whooping cough as children on normal diets. In general, undernourished individuals suffer more frequent episodes of infectious disease, the disease is more severe, and their recovery is unduly prolonged. A possible exception is presented by the intracellular parasites. Because of their extensive or, in the case of viruses, total reliance on healthy host cells for their replication, they apparently cause somewhat less severe disease in the malnourished individual whose cells are unable to metabolize at the optimal rate for viral replication.

Hormonal modifications of natural resistance are also readily recognized. Diabetics are unquestionably more susceptible to staphylococcal, streptococcal, and several fungal diseases. Insulin deficiency has an effect on the integrity of cell membranes, and this may render them more susceptible to disease. The corticosteroid hormones are known to reduce the inflammatory response and to depress phagocytosis. The thickening of the vaginal epithelium of the adult woman has already been mentioned as an age-hormone adjustment in the body's defense system. Pregnant women, as determined in the era before vaccines were available, have a higher incidence of poliomyelitis than nonpregnant women of the same age group. Many of these features just listed modulate both natural resistance and acquired immunity.

ACQUIRED IMMUNITY

The immunity an individual develops during his lifetime is traditionally discussed under the heading of acquired immunity. Unlike natural resistance, which is a broad-spectrum type of resistance not directed against any particular pathogen, acquired immunity is expressed most typically against a specific pathogen and develops as a result of exposure to that specific pathogen. When the acquired immunity is based on the acquisition of new defensive devices by the exposed host, actively acquired immunity is the result. When the immunity results from the activities of some other individual and the immune system is transferred to the host, the host then displays a passively acquired immunity.

Acquired immunity can be classified as follows:

- Acquired immunity
  - Actively acquired
    - Natural
    - Artificial
  - Passively acquired
    - Natural
    - Artificial

Macrophages

Acquired immunity, regardless of its subclass, is based on the activities of three major cell types: the macrophages, the B lymphocytes, and the T lymphocytes (Fig. 4-3). Exposure of a host to antigens of a pathogenic or potentially pathogenic organism initiates a series of adaptive responses in these three cell types. Phagocytic cells, by virtue of their inherent cytophagic ability, ingest and degrade the antigen. Portions of the antigen are passed to B and T lymphocytes. This stimulates growth and division in these cells so that the immunoglobulin-forming plasma cells are formed from the B lymphocytes. T cells also undergo lymphocyte transformation and elaborate their protective lymphokines. Among these is a product that summons forth a more aggressive macrophage known as an activated macrophage. The activated macrophage is not only more actively phagocytic but is more fully endowed with hydrolases and other enzymatic functions, making it more lethal for its phagocytic victims. It is also recognized that this vigorous new phagocytic activity is not unidirectional against only the organism initiating the response but is nonspecific and encompasses whatever foreign threat may be present. In fact, this is a characteristic of most T cell responses.

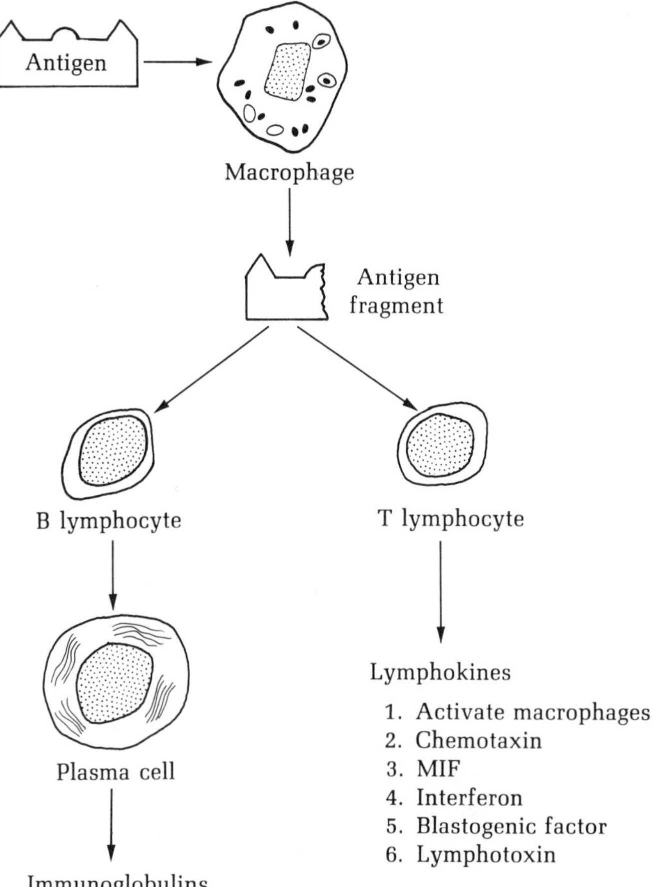

Fig. 4-3. Simplified presentation of sequence from antigen exposure to synthesis of protective lymphokines and immunoglobulins.

After a T cell has been exposed to a certain antigen, only that special antigen will catalyze lymphokine formation and secretion. However, the lymphokines express their protective functions against unrelated antigens as well as the specific antigen.

Other lymphokines associated with immunity are chemotactic factor, macrophage inhibition factor, lymphotoxin, interferon, and possibly blastogenic factor. Chemotactic factor draws monocytes into the arena where the T cell has contacted the antigen, macrophage inhibition factor holds the macrophage at the scene of infection, and lymphotoxin causes a cytolytic destruction of at least certain types of foreign cells. Blastogenic factor activates surrounding T cells to join in the secretion of these and other lymphokines. These substances were discussed more fully in Chapter 3; only interferon will be discussed in detail here.

Interferon

In the original descriptions of interferon it was suggested that interferon was a virus-induced substance that was helpful in limiting or preventing a viral infection. Now it is known that many intracellular parasites serve as interferon inducers—viruses, rickettsiae, mycoplasma, and certain protozoa for instance. The most active fraction of these parasites is their double-stranded ribonucleic acid (ds RNA). Recognition of this fact explained the ability of certain toxic chemicals of biologic or synthetic origin to induce interferon synthesis. Some of these materials, such as bacterial endotoxins or toxic doses of antibiotics, destroy host cells and release ds RNA. Others, such as complex polysaccharides, anionic polymers of maleic anhydride, or acrylic acid, mimic the repetitive structure and ionic behavior of ds

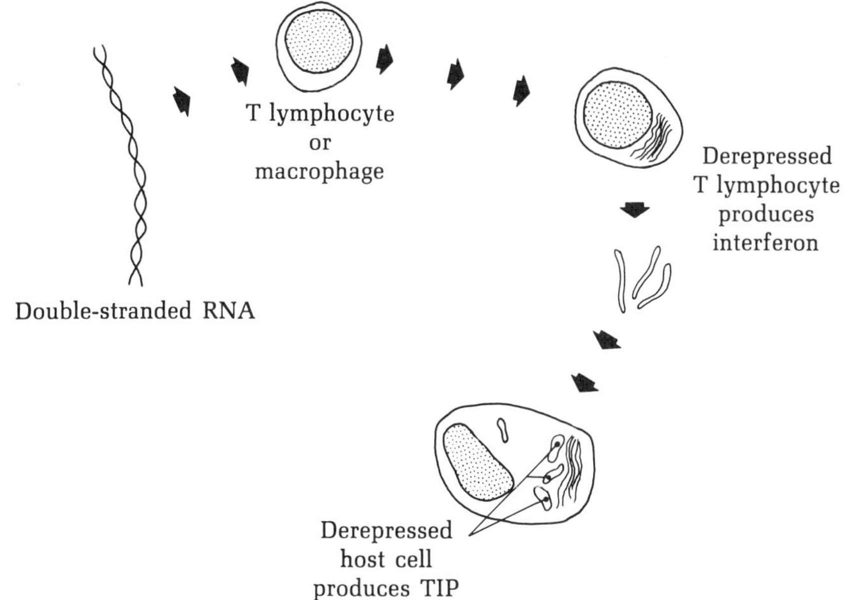

Fig. 4-4. Several uncertainties surround the exact pathway by which interferons are produced and the manner in which they function. One hypothesis indicates that double-stranded RNA stimulates T lymphocytes and/or macrophages to produce interferon, which derepresses other host cells that are then enabled to synthesize a translation inhibitory protein (*TIP*), which is the final effector molecule preventing replication of intracellular parasites.

RNA. Among the most active synthetic RNA pairs is a dimer of polyinosinic acid and polycytidylic acid (poly I·C). Thus there are a variety of interferon inducers, many of which are not antigenic. Unfortunately many of them, including poly I·C, are too toxic for human use.

In addition to the discoveries that many nonviral agents are satisfactory interferon inducers is the recognition that interferon can suppress the replication of several intracellular parasites, including viruses, rickettsiae, protozoa, and mycoplasma. The exact biochemical mechanism by which this is accomplished remains obscure, but it is believed that interferon, excreted by stimulated lymphocytes or other cells, enters adjacent cells and derepresses them to permit their synthesis of a translation inhibitory protein (Fig. 4-4). This novel protein restricts translation of foreign messenger RNA but has only a slight effect on host RNA, so the host cell retains its vitality while parasite replication is aborted. Although there is not complete satisfaction with this hypothesis among virologists and biochemists, it does account for the nonspecific nature of interferon. That is, one species of virus administered as an interferon inducer would permit the host to resist disease caused by many different intracellular parasites. The action of interferon is host cell directed, not parasite directed.

Another feature of interferons that is unlike that of immunoglobulins is the lower molecular weight of interferons, perhaps as low as 18,000, but some forms as large as 100,000 have been reported. Since several cell types, including T cells, macrophages, and several tissue culture cell lines, can produce interferon, it is possible that interferon activity is present in several similar molecules, rather than a single molecule. Interferons are stable at pH 2.0 at 4° C for 18 hours, which distinguishes them from the acid-labile immunoglobulins (Table 4-2). The time course for the development of macrophage-, lymphokine-, and immunoglobulin-based immunity is presented in Fig. 4-5.

Immunoglobulins

The protective antibodies, opsonins, antitoxins, and neutralizing antibodies that comprise but one element of actively acquired immunity may be formed as the result of overt clinical disease or an un-

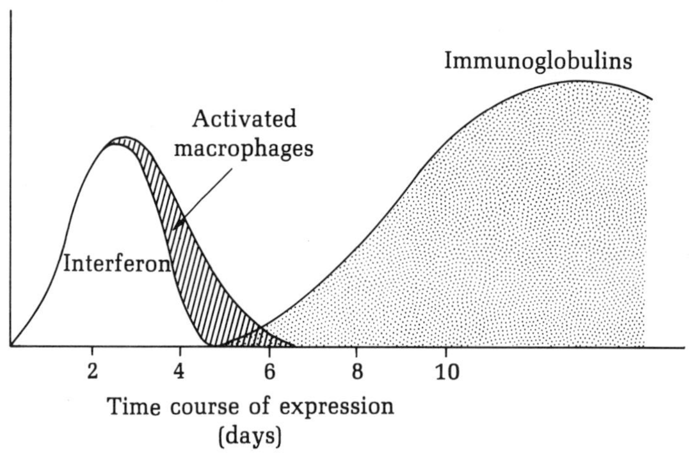

Fig. 4-5. Prior to the time immunoglobulins appear in the blood, protective interferons and activated macrophages have been engaged in host defense.

recognized, subclinical illness (Table 4-3). A subsequent encounter with the same pathogen finds the host well prepared against reinfection. This is classified as naturally acquired active immunity. Immunization with vaccines or toxoids (artificially acquired active immunity) is a safer and more economical means of acquiring protection against the ubiquitous pathogens. Thus we have killed or inactive vaccines for poliomyelitis, whooping cough, and the typhoid fevers. Attenuated vaccines, which are vaccines composed of living organisms of reduced virulence, are in use against poliomyelitis, rubella, yellow fever, smallpox, tuberculosis, and rabies. In those instances in which the disease is more accurately classified as an intoxication, that is, due to specific toxins of the pathogen, toxoids are used as the immunizing principle. Because of the time needed to reach protective levels of these immunoglobulins, immunity is not achieved until 5 to 14 days after the immunization. These immunizations are considered artificial means of acquiring immunity, as opposed to the natural means of developing and recovering from an actual infection. Since one's own cells participate in both forms of active immunity, the immune state may persist for months or years without reactivation by booster exposures to the antigen.

Passive immunity via immunoglobulins can also be acquired naturally or artificially. The former condition exists when maternal IgG transgresses the placental barrier from the mother to the unborn child and confers the mother's immunity related to that immunoglobulin class on the child. Some postnatal protection may be delivered to the nursing infant through the mother's milk and its secretory IgA.

Table 4-2. Comparison of interferons and immunoglobulins

	Interferons	*Immunoglobulins*
Inducers	ds RNA, polyanionic macromolecules	Antigens of all types
Cellular origin	T cells, macrophages, and others	Plasma cells
Molecular weight	18,000-100,000	150,000-900,000
Isoelectric point	Near 7.0	Near 8.0
Production	A few minutes after induction	IgM early, others slightly later
Duration of production	A few days	Months or even years
Specificity	Host cell directed	Parasite directed
Stability	Stable at pH 2.0	Labile at pH 2.0
Potential use	Prophylactic	Prophylactic and therapeutic

Table 4-3. Comparison of active and passive immunity

	Active immunity	*Passive immunity*
Source	Host cells	Another's cells
Method of induction	Disease, clinical or subclinical (natural) Immunization (artificial) by vaccines (killed or attenuated)	Transplacental antibody or colostrum (natural) Injection of antisera (artificial) Transfer factor injection (artificial) Adoptive transfer of lymphoid cells
Appearance	5-14 days	Immediate
Duration	Months or years	Variable, usually brief
Reactivation	Easy by boosters	Possible, but risk of anaphylaxis
Use	Prophylactic	Prophylactic and therapeutic

Unfortunately the heaviest flow of antibodies from the mammary glands is in the colostrum, which is seldom given to the newborn infant. A few days after birth the maternal milk decreases in antibody content, and the developing digestive functions of the child further restrict the role of these antibodies. Nevertheless, maternal milk-borne antibodies may give low-level surface protection to the intestinal mucosa.

Artificial means of receiving passive immunity rely on the injection of the gamma globulin fraction or whole hyperimmune serum into the person needing this protection. The benefits are instantaneous and persist according to the half-life of the immunoglobulin. For the intraspecies transfer of IgG this is about 30 days, so the immunity might extend over several weeks or a few months depending on the dose and the potency of the antiserum administered. The half-life of interspecies globulin transfers is only a few days and has the risk of causing serum sickness or, on reinjection, anaphylaxis (Table 4-3).

IMMUNITY AND INFECTIOUS DISEASE

Immunity and bacterial disease

Unfortunately there are only a few instances where it can be stated positively that a certain property of a bacterium is responsible for its pathogenicity. These are the diseases in which potent exotoxins are known to cause virtually all of the symptoms of the disease and in which the corresponding antitoxins confer total immunity on the host. Diphtheria, tetanus, and gas gangrene are such diseases, and although the latter has a multiple bacterial etiology, protection can be achieved through circulating antitoxins.

In a few other instances it is known that a certain surface antigen is nearly synonymous with virulence. Sometimes this is a capsular antigen, as with the pneumococcus, whose polysaccharide slime layer repels phagocytes. Anticapsular antibodies negate this antiphagocytic activity and provide immunity to the host. Other "virulence antigens" may be structural portions of the bacterial cell wall, and immunity to these agents is dependent on neutralizing antibodies directed against these antigens.

Two conditions amply illustrate the role of phagocytosis and immunoglobulins in antibacterial immunity. In chronic granulomatous disease where there is a failure of phagocytic cells to kill the bacteria that they ingest, repeated infections with common bacteria is the rule. In the hypo- or agammaglobulinemias an increased susceptibility to bacterial infections is also observed.

Immunity and viral disease

Several features of viruses as human pathogens affect the capacity of the host to develop a satisfactory immunity. One of these is antigenic drift, which means the gradual loss of certain antigens of the parasite through natural mutation and selection. If the existing population has protective activities designed to attack and repulse the pathogen on the basis of antigens no longer extant, then it is obvious the new antigenic mutants have a decisive invasive advantage. It is largely on this basis that pandemics of viral influenza arise periodically. Another feature of influenza virus that eases its infectivity is its ability to parasitize primarily the outer respiratory mucosa. Here the virus is located outside the major immune functions of the host. A third protective device of viruses is the ability, as exemplified by herpes simplex virus (cold sore or fever blister virus), to establish themselves intracellularly and be transmitted from host cell to daughter cell without ever leaving their intracellular residence. After periods of dormancy or latency the viruses emerge in a sporadic eruption and return to their latent condition in which they are refractory to attack by immunoglobulins, macrophages, or

T cells. A fourth characteristic, not of viruses per se but of viral diseases, is that what we think of as a single disease may have a multiple etiology. Symptoms typical of the common cold can be produced by roughly 100 different rhinoviruses plus numerous strains of coxsackievirus and adenovirus. The possibility of producing a satisfactory vaccine against the common cold becomes an exercise in mathematical futility.

Recovery from a viral disease is probably dependent on interferon production as much or more than on activation of macrophages or immunoglobulin synthesis. Hypogammaglobulinemic children develop and recover from the usual viral diseases of childhood in the normal way. Children with immunodeficiencies in their phagocytic system suffer no increase in incidence or severity of viral illnesses, but children with T cell deficits do. For example, smallpox vaccination can prove fatal to the child with Nezelof's syndrome, a congenital, athymic disease. These facts substantiate the generalization that T cell functions are the key to host resistance against viral disease. Of course, this is a generalization and these are exceptions. One important type of exception is provided by those viruses that must pass through the vascular system before they reach their primary target organ. One can consider the neurotropic viruses as a group—some enter the body through bites of animals (rabies virus), mosquitoes (the several encephalitis viruses), or the intestine (poliomyelitis). In each instance the virus must pass through blood or tissues before entering neural tissues. If specific immunoglobulins in the blood coat the virus particle and prevent its cell receptors from attaching to intended victim cells, the viral disease, or at least its devastating neural phase, cannot develop. Thus circulating immunoglobulins may be critical to immunity and yet play a small role in recovery from viral disease.

Immunity and mycotic disease

Our knowledge of the basis for resistance to fungal disease is poorly developed. Many molds and yeasts are resistant to intraphagocytic destruction. Immunoglobulins seem hardly more protective against systemic fungal agents than against dermatophytes. Failures in the natural development of the thymus and its attendant T cell functions are probably more conducive to fungal diseases than failures in any other portion of our immune armory. Unfortunately this is the best generalization in the present state of our knowledge.

Immunity and parasitic disease

Animal parasites span such a broad range of anatomic and physiologic forms that it is not realistic to consider them as a group. For protection against the protozoan tissue forms such as the malarial parasites, toxoplasma, and others, a defensive role for humoral antibodies and interferon has been suggested. It is unknown if any of the usual immune systems can provide protection against the tissue-invading helminths—the parasites are too large to be phagocytosed and seem to be little affected by T or B lymphocyte activities. Intestinal protozoa and helminths reside outside the range of the major host's defensive forces.

Two of the world's most prevalent diseases are caused by animal parasites—malaria and schistosomiasis. Some resistance is naturally present and some can be acquired against these diseases; immunologists working in the realm of animal parasite diseases are very hopeful of significant accomplishments in the near future.

IMMUNIZATIONS

Since most active immunizations are begun and completed in childhood, the American Academy of Pediatrics has established a schedule of such immunizations for normal infants and children dwelling in the United States. The following discussion is based on the academy's report in 1973 (Table 4-4).

Active immunization

Protection against the following diseases through a prophylactic immunization program is advised: diphtheria, whooping cough (pertussis), and tetanus, poliomyelitis, measles, rubella, and mumps. Routine smallpox vaccination is no longer recommended (Table 4-4).

Diphtheria, pertussis, and tetanus (DPT). The first vaccination given the young child is the DPT vaccine administered at 2, 4, and 6 months of age with later booster injections. DPT preparations contain the toxoids of *Clostridium tetani* and *Corynebacterium diphtheriae* and killed cells of *Bordetella pertussis.* It has been known since the studies of von Behring over 75 years ago that specific circulating antitoxins would neutralize the exotoxins of the diphtheria and tetanus bacillus and confer protection against their lethal effects. The amount of diphtheria antitoxin required for protection is between 0.01 and 0.1 unit/ml, and such quantities in the blood can be determined very simply by the Schick test. Normal human skin reacts slowly to injections of diphtheria toxin to produce a tender erythematous reaction known as the positive Schick test. If a person has greater than 0.03 unit of antitoxin/ml of blood, this test is negative. Since tetanus toxin has no effect on human skin, no simple appraisal of immunity such as the Schick test can be used, but it is well known that the present toxoid will confer protection (after the series of injections) for 7 to 12 years.

The killed *B. pertussis* organisms in the DPT preparation consist of the capsule variant most clearly associated with human virulence, the phase I type. This phase I capsular antigen has never been characterized. These bacteria play two important roles in this triple vaccine: (1) the induction of specific antipertussis immunity and (2) a pronounced adjuvant effect on the other two antigens. This adjuvant effect is reflected by a circulating lymphocytosis and heightened antibody titers plus other immunologic phenomena. Most DPT preparations containing additional adjuvants—aluminum hydroxide or aluminum phosphate gels—are clearly superior to fluid preparations.

It is interesting that no other vaccines used against bacterial diseases are recommended by the American Academy of Pediatrics. In the case of the vaccines for several enteric diseases this is understandable—the vaccine for typhoid and paratyphoid fevers is of dubious value, and modern sanitation has probably done as much to reduce the incidence of typhoid fever in the United States as immunization. The risk for cholera is low, and its vaccine confers only a tenuous immunity and even that has an expected duration of only 3 to 6 months. However, these features do not apply to bacille Calmette-Guérin (BCG) vaccination. BCG, under the auspices of WHO and UNICEF, has been administered to over 250 million individuals since 1950. The organism, an attenuated culture of *M. tuberculosis* variety *bovis,* was attenuated by Calmette and Guérin through 13 years of cultivation on bile-containing media. It is administered intradermally to tuberculin-negative individuals and produces a small lesion that heals slowly over a period of approximately 1 month as host resistance

Table 4-4. Recommended pediatric immunizations

DPT	At 2, 4, and 6 mo with boosters at 1½ yr and at entrance to school; tetanus booster at 16 yr
Poliomyelitis (oral vaccine)	Same as DPT
Measles	At 1 yr (may be given with rubella and mumps)
Rubella	After 1 yr, before puberty in females
Mumps	After 1 yr

NOTE: Smallpox, BCG, and other vaccinations are recommended for international travel, medical personnel, and other conditions.

develops. Considerable proof of the success of this vaccine is available in the immunologic literature, not only for protection against tuberculosis but also suggesting an important role in the control of leprosy, dermal infections by *M. ulcerans*, and most recently in the control of certain forms of cancer.

Poliomyelitis. The first successful vaccine for active immunization against poliomyelitis relied on the use of the formaldehyde-inactivated virus developed by Salk. This vaccine was comprised of a mixture of the three antigenic types of poliovirus and was administered intramuscularly. Because of a failure to completely inactivate all of the virus in certain of the early vaccines, a few tragic examples of vaccine-induced disease developed. Presently used inactivated polio vaccine does not have this hazard. Even so, the active attenuated or oral polio vaccine is preferred. There are several reasons for this, one of which is the simpler, painless method of administering the virus on a sugar cube. Much more important is the type of immunity offered by the oral vaccine. Since it is composed of an active virus and is ingested, it mimics very closely the normal sequence of polio infection: first an infection of the intestinal mucosa and then entrance into the vascular system. The attenuated virus does not invade the neural system, but by virtue of the intestinal and vascular phase of its infection, a local intestinal and systemic immunity results. In contrast the Salk vaccine offers only systemic immunity, and Salk vaccinees could have an intestinal infection and serve as carriers of fully virulent poliovirus. Another possible advantage of the oral vaccine is that during the intestinal phase of its infection, virus excretion might serve as an "accidental" vaccine for close personal contacts.

Measles. Attenuated strains of active measles virus produce protective antibodies in approximately 95% of all 1-year-old children receiving the vaccine. The Edmonston B strain vaccine has now been replaced by more attenuated strains. This has reduced the incidence and extent of the febrile episodes typically following measles vaccination and eliminated the need for the accompanying injection (0.02 ml/kg body weight) of measles immune globulin. Measles vaccination of all children is recommended. The disease is far more serious than generally recognized; it can produce encephalitis with permanent brain damage or death.

Rubella. Rubella, also known as German measles, causes a milder infection of children than the regular or hard measles just described. In addition it is a less contagious disease than hard measles. Despite these facts, immunization of adolescent females with rubella virus has a high medical priority. This is based on the finding that rubella virus infection of an expectant mother in the first trimester of her pregnancy is accompanied by a rubella virus infection of the fetus with dire consequences. The virus interferes with normal embryogenesis, and if the fetus is not aborted or stillborn, the child is apt to be seriously deformed. Cataracts, deafness, anemia, developmental abnormalities of the heart, microcephaly with permanent brain damage, and other major defects have been associated with in utero rubella virus infections.

Live rubella vaccination is recommended for both male and female children after 1 year of age and before puberty. Pregnant women should never be given the vaccine, and other adult women should be carefully evaluated individually as regards unknown or expectant pregnancy before being given the vaccine.

Mumps. Attenuated mumps virus vaccine has been available in the United States since 1967. An important aspect of mumps prophylaxis is that it obviates orchitis, which occurs in 20% of postpuberal males who develop natural mumps. A single dose of the vaccine will confer protection on 95% of the vaccinees and has few complications. The mumps vaccine can be administered successfully in combination with measles and rubella vaccines in a single injection.

Other vaccines. Several other vaccines of proven worth are available and recommended under special circumstances. These include vaccines for influenza, rabies, smallpox, Rocky Mountain spotted fever, typhus, and yellow fever. Vaccines of lesser value might include those for cholera, plague, and typhoid fever. Currently under trial is a vaccine for hepatitis B.

Passive immunization

Passive immunization continues to play a significant role in infectious disease control, but there have been obvious adjustments in its application in the last two decades (Table 4-5). Until recent times passive immunization was limited almost exclusively to tetanus and diphtheria, with occasional uses in cases of botulism or gas gangrene. Antiserum therapy was also used in pneumococcal pneumonia and a few other diseases. The antisera used were of equine or bovine origin or possibly from rabbits. Incidents of serum sickness and even anaphylaxis coupled with a low therapeutic efficacy and the emergence of the antibiotic era lessened the need for immunoglobulin therapy of the old type.

Newer developments in immunoglobulin therapy include the preparation of human hyperimmune sera and the consequent decrease in allergic reactions from their use. Second, the use of hyperimmune sera against measles, mumps, vaccinia, and rubella viruses to modify the severity of the responses to attenuated vaccines or to modify the severity of disease in very young infants exposed to or developing these infections can be mentioned. The recognition of hypogammaglobulinemic persons has created a continued need for antiserum therapy. Perhaps most dramatic of all, since it is outside the realm of infectious disease, is the use of human anti-Rh sera to prevent the development of Rh antibodies in women delivering Rh-positive babies. This is an expected part of perinatal medical care and should reduce hemolytic disease in newborn infants due to maternal-fetal Rh incompatibility (Chapter 7).

Passive immunization can also include adoptive immunization, the reconstitution of immunologically deficient persons with thymus or bone marrow, and the injection of transfer factor to activate dormant T cells. These procedures are discussed in Chapters 9 and 12. A future prospect is passive immunization with interferon or other specific lymphokines.

BIBLIOGRAPHY

Acton, J. D.: The lymphoreticular system and interferon production, J. Reticuloendothel. Soc. **14**:449, 1973.

Alexander, J. W.: Host defense mechanisms against infections, Surg. Clin. North Am. **52**:1367, 1972.

Allison, A. C.: Immunity against viruses, Sci. Basis Med. Ann. Rev. p. 49, 1972.

Carr, I.: Biological defence mechanisms, Oxford, 1972, Blackwell Scientific Publications, Ltd.

Carter, W. A., and De Clercq, E. D.: Viral

Table 4-5. Passive immunizations

Measles	Hyperimmune globulin immediately after exposure or with weakly attenuated vaccines
Rubella	Pregnant women exposed to rubella
Infectious hepatitis	Immediately after exposure
Tetanus	Immediately after injury if not immunized or outdated immunization
Rh disease	Within 72 hr after delivery
Hypogammaglobulinemia	Pooled human gamma globulin

infection and host defense, Science **186:** 1172, 1974.
Edsall, G.: Principles of active immunization, Annu. Rev. Med. **17:**39, 1966.
Faulk, W. P., Demaeyer, E. M., and Davies, A. J. S.: Some effects of malnutrition on the immune response in man, Am. J. Clin. Nutr. **27:**638, 1974.
Gontzea, I.: Nutrition and anti-infectious defence, Basel, 1974, S. Karger, AG.
Grossberg, S. E.: The interferons and their inducers: molecular and therapeutic considerations, N. Engl. J. Med. **287:**13, 79, 122, 1972.
Hayward, A. R.: Development of the immune response, Clin. Allergy **3**(suppl.):559, 1973.
Jackson, G. S., Herman, R., and Singer, I., ed.: Immunity to parasitic animals, New York, 1969, Appleton-Century-Crofts, vols. 1 & 2.
Nelson, D. S.: Macrophages and immunity, Amsterdam, 1969, North-Holland Publishing Co.
Rodgers, R., and Merigan, T. C.: Interferon and its inducers: antiviral and other effects, CRC Crit. Rev. Clin. Lab. Sci. **3:**131, 1972.
van Furth, R., ed.: Mononuclear phagocytes, Philadelphia, 1970, F. A. Davis Co.
WHO Scientific Group: A survey of nutritional-immunological interactions, Bull. WHO **46:**537, 1972.
WHO Scientific Group: Oral enteric bacterial vaccines, WHO Tech. Rep. Ser. No. 500, 1972.
WHO Scientific Group: Cell-mediated immunity and resistance to infection, WHO Tech. Rep. Ser. No. 519, 1973.

Case histories

CASE 1. INTERNATIONAL IMMUNIZATIONS

J. B., a 45-year-old archeologist, was invited on a "dig" in central Nigeria. His previous travel abroad had beeen limited to excavations in 1964, 1965, and 1966 near Roskilde, Denmark. He was excited about the possibility of opening an African chapter in his career; however, he was greatly concerned about the need for immunizations and consulted his family physician. His International Certificate of Immunization revealed only smallpox immunization in 1964. His physician's inquiries revealed that he had been in the U.S. Army in 1945 and 1946. He was uncertain about the immunizations he had received either in the service or in civilian life. Accordingly, his physician scheduled the following immunizations: smallpox, typhoid fever, tetanus, poliomyelitis, yellow fever, and cholera.

Questions

1. What is the current status of smallpox immunization in the United States, and what is the recommendation for international travel?
2. Why are typhoid and cholera immunizations recommended when it is known that they are of dubious, short-term value?
3. Will a full immunization course or only a tetanus booster be required for protection against that disease?
4. What geographic areas of the world are at risk for yellow fever?
5. What is the need for poliomyelitis vaccination in middle-aged adults with an unknown history of polio immunization?

Discussion

Smallpox. The American Academy of Pediatrics no longer recommends routine smallpox vaccinations for children. The rationale for this is the estimated cost of $150,000,000 per annum for smallpox surveillance and control of the disease in the United States, where the last confirmed case was diagnosed in 1949. The U.S. Public Health Service no longer requires a validated smallpox certificate for those entering the United States from smallpox-free areas. At the present time smallpox is considered endemic in only two regions of Asia and Africa. Sporadic importation of smallpox into Europe has occurred only some dozen times in the past 5 years, and quarantines and mass smallpox immunization have limited the spread of the disease. However, these measures have not prevented smallpox death in the Yugoslavian outbreak, for example.

American physicians, like those of most European nations, recommend vaccination on exposure, the prophylactic and therapeutic use of vaccinia immune globulin, and chemoprophylaxis and chemotherapeutics with *N*-methylisatin-β-thiosemicarbazone. Critics of these substitutes for generalized vaccination point to the fact that chemoprophylaxis with substituted thiosemicarbazones may be a satisfactory procedure for preventing overt smallpox in exposed persons, but that the therapeutic efficacy of these compounds has yet to be determined. The same criticism is offered against the use of vaccinia immune globulin. A massive immunization program can be mounted and be successful after smallpox disease is recognized. In New York City 6.3 million persons were immunized within a few days after a "smallpox scare." The suitability of smallpox immunization after exposure is based on the inordinately long incubation period of the disease, often as long as 30 days. Within this time vaccination can confer immunity on the person. However, as in the Yugoslavian epidemic, there can be no guarantee that all persons needing the vaccine can or will receive it in time to prevent their death. In terms of cold numbers this risk must be compared to the knowledge that of our present U.S. population, about five deaths per year could be attributed to complications following smallpox immunization. In the long run, medical statisticians believe this to be a greater risk than to vaccinate after exposure.

For international travelers entering regions where smallpox is endemic, vaccination is still recommended. In terms of this specific case it is believed that Nigeria has been free of smallpox since 1972. International traffic between central African nations is increasing, and the possibility of a nonimmune person being exposed is sufficiently great to advise vaccination. Although J. B. was vaccinated in 1964, the policy of a revaccination every 10 years (if needed, as described previously) would require his immunization at this time.

Tetanus. Fluid tetanus toxoid boosters are recommended every 10 years. Persons engaged in dangerous occupations where wound contamination with soil is very probable are obviously at a greater risk than the average individual and are doubly advised to maintain their tetanus immunization program. Military tetanus immunization allowed only the fluid booster to be given to J. B.

Poliomyelitis. J. B. was not certain as to his status concerning polio vaccinations but hesitantly recalled receiving at least a portion of the Salk injection series. In the United States adults such as J. B. are unlikely to be exposed to polio. Although the incidence is rising slightly, there were only 19 cases in 1971. Medical personnel and travelers to nations with limited control of polio should receive the oral polio vaccine. This is given as three separate immunizations—one for each antigenic type of virus —over a period of about 3 months, that is, 6 to 8 weeks between immunizations.

Yellow fever. The yellow fever attenuated vaccine was developed by Max Theiler, and he received the Nobel Prize for this in 1951. In the United States the 17D, chick embryo–grown vaccine is used. It must be administered by a WHO-approved Yellow Fever Vaccination Center, and it is a rare physician who has actually given the vaccination. It consists of a dose 0.5 ml administered subcutaneously. Immunity following vaccination persists for 10 years.

The Dakar or French strain vaccine is more neurotropic than the 17D strain, and its use is complicated by a 5% incidence of meningoencephalitis. Complications following the administration of the 17D strain are unusual, but since the vaccine is egg-derived, persons who are highly allergic to eggs may develop an immediate hypersensitive reaction.

Cholera. Cholera vaccines are of very limited efficacy. No more than 50% of the vacinees are protected and then only for a period of 3 to 6 months. Consequently, vaccination within a month of departure for foreign travel is advised. The International Certificate of Vaccination (international health card) confirming cholera vaccination is invalid after 6 months. The vaccine is given twice within a period of about 1 month and may provoke considerable local discomfort, generalized fever, and headache due to the high endotoxin content of the vaccine.

REFERENCES

Cvjetanovic, B., and Uemura, K.: The present status of field and laboratory studies of typhoid and paratyphoid vaccine, Bull. WHO **32**:29, 1965.

Gangarosa, E. J., and Faich, G. A.: Cholera, the risk to American travelers, Ann. Intern. Med. **74**:412, 1971.

Regamey, R. H., and Cohen, H., eds.: International symposium on smallpox vaccination, Basel, 1973, S. Karger AG.

Scheibel, I., Bentzon, M. W., Christensen, P. E., and Biering, A.: Duration of immunity to diphtheria and tetanus after active immunization, Acta. Pathol. Microbiol. Scand. **67**:380, 1966.

CASE 2. RABIES

As M. D., a 55-year-old housewife with a history of allergies, was placing her 5-iron in her golf bag, an animal lunged from under her motorized golf cart and bit her on the ankle. The animal had brown fur, a hairless or nearly smooth tail, and moved rapidly. After biting her, the animal ran into some rocks that were used to fill an abandoned well. A conservation agent was called for assistance in retrieving and/or identifying the animal, but he was not successful in this effort. M. D. contacted her physician who initiated the rabies immunization series.

Questions

1. What is the relative role of domestic and wild animals in the transmission of rabies?
2. How is the diagnosis of rabies determined in lower animals?
3. What is the currently preferred method of rabies prophylaxis?
4. In what way does an allergic predisposition influence the rabies immunization program for an individual?
5. Under what conditions is antirabies serum administered?

Discussion

Human rabies has decreased in the United States to only one case per year. In domestic animals the incidence of rabies has also fallen sharply, but this has been accompanied by the prominence of rabies in wild animals, especially skunks, foxes, and bats. Urban dwellers thus run little risk of exposure to rabies, but residents of rural areas or any persons exposed to wild animals have a slightly higher risk. The animal involved in the case under discussion could have been a muskrat, weasel, opossum, or other animal.

Under ideal circumstances, lower animals suspected to have rabies should be impounded and observed for the development of rabies, which is believed to terminate invariably in death. Central nervous tissue can then be stained for Negri bodies or subjected to immunofluorescent examination. The latter method is also applied to the animal's brain when the animal has been killed and will identify rabies virus in putrefied or other damaged tissues that are unsuitable for the histologic identification of rabies virus inclusion bodies. The tissue preparation is flooded with antirabies virus serum and then with a fluorescent antiserum to the gamma globulin of the rabies virus serum (Chapter 6). This indirect fluorescent antibody procedure is sensitive, rapid, and inexpensive. Its outcome can determine if rabies prophylaxis need be initiated.

In those instances in which the suspected animal is not captured and in which tissue examination is not possible, postexposure prophylaxis is recommended. This is especially the case with wild animal bites, bites of unvaccinated domestic animals, or severe bites from an unusual behaving animal. Postexposure rabies prophylaxis was pioneered by Pasteur on the assumption that the long incubation time of rabies would permit a suitable immunity to be developed in the interlude between the bite and symptoms of disease. This has been repeatedly confirmed and is the basis for the numerous Pasteur Institutes throughout the world.

The original Pasteur rabies vaccine consisted of an emulsion of dried spinal cord taken from rabid rabbits. Although this is almost universally described as an attenuated vaccine, there is no evidence that the virulence of the virus was itself weakened while maintaining infectivity. Preparations dried for several days consisted of inactive virus, and this initiated an immune response that allowed the vaccinee to resist later injections containing active virus. The original Pasteur vaccine and the Semple phenol-inactivated vaccine are given in 14 daily injections. The lengthy immunization schedule and the high content of rabbit brain and spinal cord antigens in the Semple and Pasteur vaccines have been closely associated with neuroparalytic reactions occurring at an incidence of about 1 in every 8500 vaccinees. This prompted the development of the Flury chick embryo or HEP (high egg passage) vaccine that avoided the problem of allergic encephalitis. Since 1971, 90% of those receiving rabies prophylaxis in the United States have been given the DEV (duck egg) vaccine. Erythema, pain, tenderness, and pruritus at the inoculation sites are common with DEV. These may become more severe after 8 to 10 doses have been administered. Atopic individuals (those with allergies) should be observed carefully for systemic reactions and may require antihistamine and adrenergic drug support.

Rabies immune serum may also be advised concomitant with vaccination if the bite wounds are severe or near central nervous tissue as on the head, face, and neck. In fact, there is good evidence that hyperimmune rabies antiserum in combination with vaccination is the best prophylactic course. With dual prophylaxis of this type, active vaccination is continued for 21 days. Unfortunately equine antirabies serum, which is the only preparation available in the United States, induces serum sickness in 20% of its recipients. Appropriate skin testing is necessary to reduce the risk of anaphylactic shock (Chapter 8).

REFERENCES

Center for Disease Control, Advisory Committee: Collected recommendations of the Public Health Service advisory committee on immunization practices, Morbidity and Mortality **21**:1, 1972.

Greenberg, M., and Childress, J.: Vaccination against rabies with duck-embryo and Semple vaccines, J.A.M.A. **173**:333, 1960.

WHO Expert Committee: Fifth report of the expert committee on rabies, WHO Tech. Rep. Ser. No. 321, 1966.

chapter 5

Complement

Complement was initially described as a substance in peritoneal fluid and sera that cooperated with antibodies in the lytic destruction of bacteria (bacteriolysis—Pfeiffer's phenomenon). Shortly after this Bordet observed that complement was essential for immune hemolysis and, as in the initial discovery, confirmed that complement was thermolabile. Recently the discovery that complement displays a battery of protective and potentially harmful biologic functions has confirmed the importance and increased the interest in complement. Several features of complement are now fully agreed on.

1. Complement is present in all normal mammalian sera, and its concentration in sera is not changed by immunization procedures.
2. Complement consists of a complex of nine major blood proteins that act in sequence, all nine of which are required in serologic reactions that terminate in cell (antigen) lysis.
3. Thermal destruction of complement is accomplished by keeping sera at 56° C for 30 minutes, at which temperature the activity of immunoglobulins is not influenced. Aging sera for longer times at lower temperatures will also destroy complement.
4. Complement activation by antibody-antigen combination is possible only with immunoglobulins of the IgM class and the IgG1 and IgG3 subclasses. Other classes of antibodies do not normally activate or are very poor activators of complement.
5. Species barriers in the activation of complement are only rarely encountered. For example, normal guinea pig or normal rabbit sera are able to react with human IgM and vice versa.
6. Complement is activated by all serologic reactions involving IgM and the proper subclasses of IgG, even if not required to display that type of serologic reaction. A fluid antigen and IgG1 would precipitate and simultaneously activate complement. This phenomenon is the basis for complement fixation tests.
7. During the activation of complement, several important biologic functions are expressed other than immune lysis. These include kinin formation, chemotaxis, opsonization, anaphylatoxin formation, immune adherence, and others.
8. Activation of complement by an alternate pathway not requiring antibody and elimination of the first three of the nine complement molecules is possible. This requires the participation of other serum proteins in what is known as the properdin pathway of complement activation.

PROTEINS OF THE COMPLEMENT SYSTEM

Classic activation pathway

Since the classic pathway of complement activation requires immunoglobulin-antigen combination, it is important to point out that neither serum, secretory IgA, nor IgE is able to catalyze the complement se-

Table 5-1. Characteristics of components of complement

	C1	*C2*	*C3*	*C4*	*C5*	*C6*	*C7*	*C8*	*C9*
Molecular weight	650,000	117,000	185,000	240,000	185,000	95,000	120,000	150,000	79,000
Sedimentation coefficient	18	6	6	10	9	6	5	8	4.5
Electrophoretic mobility	γ_2	β_1	β	β	β	β	β	γ	α
Serum concentration (μg/ml)	1000	30	1300	400	75	50	60	50	2
Comments	Composed of Clq (400,000 mol wt), Clr (170,000 mol wt), and Cls (100,000 mol wt); origin of esterase activity	Labile SH groups	Heat labile		Exists as complex with C6 and 7				

quence. IgM and IgG allotypes 1 and 3 are the best complement activators. There seems to be no restriction as to the chemical nature of the antigen, and this is due to the fact that it is the Fc portion of the immunoglobulin chain to which complement attaches. Antigens and the Fc portions of certain immunoglobulins do not have the needed receptors for the first component of complement.

The first of the nine components of complement, C1, is a large molecule (mol wt 650,000) and quite abundant in serum (1000 μg/ml), where it exists as a trimer (Table 5-1). Its three parts, Clq, Clr, and Cls, are held in association by Ca++, and the removal of calcium by chelating agents such as EDTA (ethylenediaminetetraacetic acid) dissociates the triad into its subunits. Clq is the largest of the subunits and has a molecular weight of 400,000. It is one of the most basic proteins in human serum and is responsible for the electrophoretic location of C1 in the γ_2-fraction of the serum proteins. Four Clq units attach to the Fc portion of antibody, and this binds Clr and Cls to the complex as well. It is thought that C1 may unite with two tetrapeptide units of antibody, and the nearness of such units to each other in IgM would account for its complement-fixing efficiency (Fig. 5-1).

Little is known about Clr, but Cls has been extensively studied. Cls behaves as a proenzyme until the time that it is fixed into the serologic reaction, and then it is activated to become an enzyme. Activated C1, written $C\overline{1}$, or activated $C\overline{1s}$ acquires an esterase activity similar to that displayed by the pancreatic proteoesterases trypsin and chymotrypsin. $C\overline{1}$ esterase, like trypsin and chymotrypsin, is capable of hydrolyzing *p*-toluene-sulfonyl-L-arginine methyl ester (TAME) and *N*-acetyl-L-tyrosine ethyl ester (ATEE). C1 esterase is also inhibited by diisopropylfluorophosphate and other compounds that attach to serine in the enzyme, another property common to trypsin and chymotrypsin. Although esters are abundant in the cell walls and membranes of many cellular antigens that are lysed by antibody acting in consort with complement, it is certain that $C\overline{1}$ esterase is not directly responsible for this

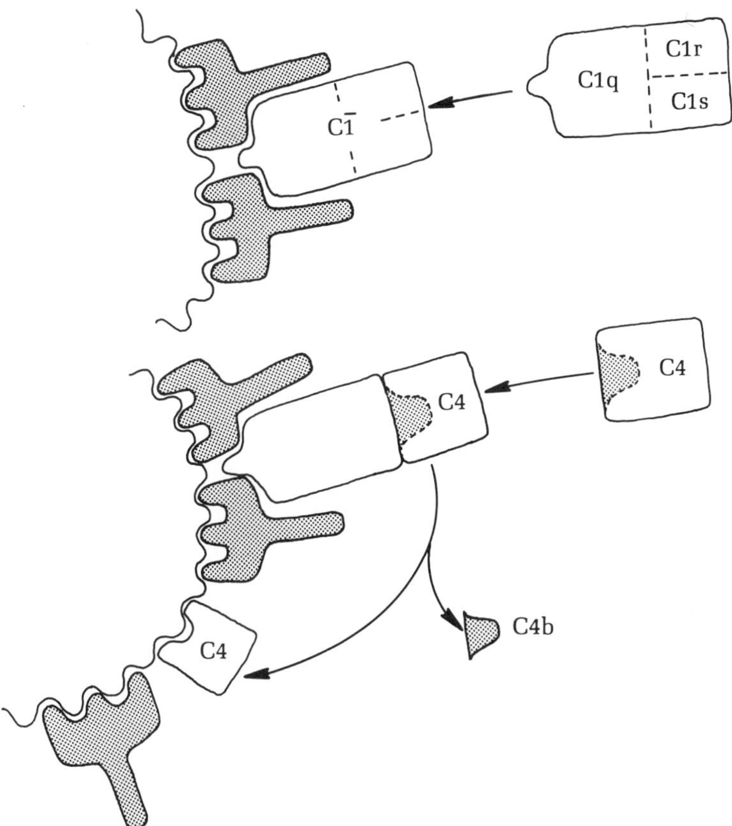

Fig. 5-1. In the activation of C1̄, the C1q, C1r, C1s complex is presumed to bridge two antibody molecules. Contact of activated C1 with C4 results in alteration of the latter so that C4 attaches to the antigen. The remaining complement components combine with C4 and do not attach to the antibody molecules.

lysis, since lysis requires the participation of eight additional components.

The next molecule in the complement series to become activated is C4. The numerical order of the first four components of complement to function is 1, 4, 2, and 3, and this evolved from the early fractionation methods of complement. Treatment of whole fresh serum (complement) with distilled water produces a precipitate (C1) and a soluble fraction (C2). This soluble portion, originally thought to contain but one substance, actually contained two subfractions, as does the precipitate. When all four of these proteins were precipitated in a partially purified form, it was found that part of the soluble fraction acted first (C1), followed by the two subfractions of the precipitate already designated as C4 and C2 and then the other component of the soluble portion (C3). In this way the functional and numerical sequence of complement came to disagree. Ultimately C3 was found to consist of five additional components, C5, 6, 7, 8, and 9, which are known as the late-acting components.

C4, like C1, is also quite abundant in serum, existing at a concentration of 400 μg/ml. It is a β-globulin with a molecular weight near 240,000. C4 is activated by C1̄ esterase and becomes C4̄ simultaneous with the release of some low molecular weight peptides from the original molecule. The activation of C4 refers not to the development or expression of a new enzymatic activity but to the acquisition of a new adhesiveness that allows $\overline{C4}$ to adhere to antigens. $\overline{C4}$ does not attach to the antibody or to $\overline{C1}$. In fact, $\overline{C1}$ can be eluted from the serologic complex, and $\overline{C4}$ will still combine with the antigen. The function of $\overline{C4}$ is to serve as a receptor for C2.

C2 is a β-globulin with a molecular weight of 117,000, about half that of C4. It is rather scant in serum, being present in quantities of only 30 μg/ml. C2 is easily inactivated by organic mercurials or other sulfhydryl reagents, indicating a requirement for intact –SH bonds for its activity. C2 is modified by $\overline{C1}$ and as $\overline{C2}$ exhibits an enzyme activity in the $\overline{C4,2}$ complex. $\overline{C2}$ attached to $\overline{C4}$ is referred to as C3 convertase because it converts C3 to an active form.

C3 is also labile, accounting in part for the thermal instability of complement. It is a β-globulin with a molecular weight of 185,000. It is found in serum at a level of 1300 μg/ml. The change in C3 produced by $\overline{C4,2}$ is a hydrolysis of the molecule into two major parts, C3a and C3b. C3a has a molecular weight of only 7500 and is liberated into the fluid phase. C3b is further altered to C3c and C3d. Until recently it was thought that C3b attached to the complement complex, but this may actually be C3d.

The remaining components, the late-acting complement components, function in the order C5, 6, 7, 8, and 9. There is a tendency for some of these proteins to aggregate with each other. This has handicapped critical biochemical studies, as has their scarcity in serum. For instance, C5 is present at a level of only 75 μg/ml; C6 at 50 μg/ml; and C7, 8, and 9 in only trace amounts. C5, 6, and 7 tend to exist as a triad, which has complicated a study of the individual molecules. C5 is heat labile, which has also interfered with its characterization. The molecular weights of these compounds are known, however, and range between 185,000 for C5 to 79,000 for C9. C5, 6, and 7 are β-globulins, C8 is a γ-globulin, and C9 is an α-globulin.

C5 is cleaved by $\overline{C4,2,3}$ to produce C5a and 5b, the latter of which is bound into the complex. C5a has a molecular weight of only 8500. Then C6 and 7 attach, followed by C8 and finally C9. As mentioned earlier, the cytolytic activity of complement is not demonstrated until all nine components have been involved. The critical change produced by C9 or the cumulative changes by each component have not yet been deciphered. Erythrocyte and bacterial cells subjected to complement-induced cytolysis develop eroded depressions about 80 to 100 μ in diameter in their outer membranes. These do not actually penetrate the membranes but are presumed to contribute to lysis.

Alternate (properdin) activation pathway

The classic pathway of complement activation is generally described as that pathway initiated by the reaction of antigens with certain immunoglobulins, eventually involving all nine of the proteins of the complement system. Actually, plasmin and certain other proteases can catalyze C1 activation, and since this prompts activation of the later proteins in the complement series, it represents a variation of the classic activation pathway. A key feature of the alternate pathway of complement activation is that the first three proteins, C1, 4, and 2, do not participate in the molecular cascade. This is possible because activators of the alternate pathway catalyze the conversion of a normal serum protein, properdin, into a biologically active form leading to the activation of C3.

Properdin was first described in the 1950s as a normal protein constituent of sera involved in complement activation. Because of the inaccurate claims as to the role of properdin in viral immunity and resistance to radiation disease, etc. and the unsuitability of purification procedures for labile molecules, it was not possible to accurately describe at that time how properdin functioned. At the present time this mystery is being unraveled, and firm evidence is available as to the chemical nature of properdin and its place in the alternate pathway of complement activation.

Properdin is a γ_2-globulin with a molecular weight of 180,000 due to the association of four subunits, each of which has a molecular weight of 45,000 (Table 5-2). The blood level of properdin, a glycoprotein containing about 10% polysaccharide, is 20 μg/ml. Properdin has the unique capacity to be activated by polysaccharides such as inulin, the polysaccharide capsules of bacteria and yeasts, bacterial endotoxins (which are lipopolysaccharides), zymosan, a cell wall fraction from yeast high in polysaccharide, and aggregated IgA. Activated properdin ($\overline{P}$) then interacts with C3 to form C3 PAse or C3 PA convertase (Fig. 5-2).

Table 5-2. Characteristics of proteins involved in alternate pathway of complement activation

	Properdin	*C3 proactivator*	*C3 proactivatorase*	*Cobra venom factor*
Abbreviation	—	C3 PA	C3 PAse	CoF
Synonyms	—	GBG, factor B	GBGase, factor D	—
Molecular weight	180,000	80,000	60,000	144,000
Sedimentation coefficient	5	6	3	5
Serum concentration (mg/100 ml)	2.5	35	?	Not found in serum
Electrophoretic mobility	γ_2	γ_2	α	—
Comments	Activated by polysaccharides; glycoprotein	Heat labile	Converts C3 PA to C3 activator	Complexes with C3 PA

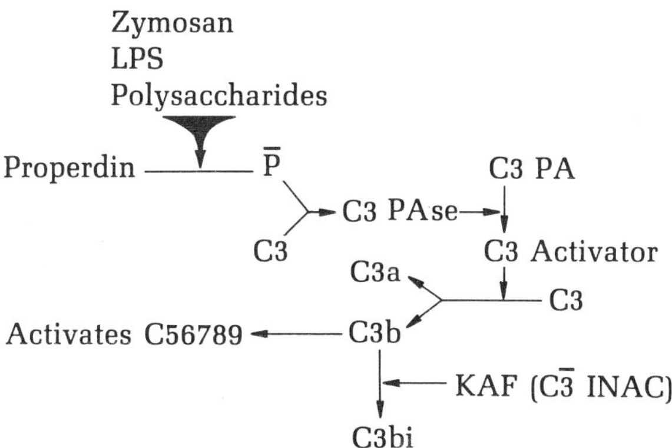

Fig. 5-2. Properdin or alternate pathway of complement activation begins with activation of properdin by polysaccharides or polysaccharide-containing materials such as zymosan or endotoxins (LPS) at C3 in complement cascade after intermediary formation of C3 PAse and C3 activator. Thereafter, alternate and classic activation pathways are identical.

C3 PA is a heat-labile β-globulin with many synonyms. It has been called factor B and glycine-rich β-glycoprotein (GBG). It has a molecular weight of 80,000 and exists in serum as a proenzyme, C3 proactivator, from which it derives its most commonly used label, C3 PA. When serving as the substrate for C3 PAse, C3 PA becomes the C3 activator. This transition is effected by the $\overline{P}$-C3 PA product C3 PAse, an α-globulin found in normal serum. A substance in cobra venom called cobra venom factor (CoF) also behaves as a C3 PAse. CoF is a large protein (mol wt 144,000) that complexes with C3 PA to act like C3 convertase or C3 activator. Patients with certain types of nephritis have a high molecular weight protein in their blood known as C3 nephritis factor (C3 NeF) that functions much like CoF. The activation of C3 by CoF and C3 NeF can be considered variants to the alternate pathway since properdin is not involved.

After the activation of C3 by C3 activator, CoF, or C3 NeF, the alternate pathway of complement activation is identical to the classic pathway and proceeds through C5, 6, 7, 8, and 9. Biologic activities arising from these late-acting complement components, or from C3, are thus released by both complement activating pathways.

BIOLOGIC FUNCTIONS OF COMPLEMENT

The foregoing discussion has emphasized in a molecular way the complexities of the complement system. Molecules of different size, different electrophoretic nature, and different cellular origin, totaling 10% of the serum globulins, have become united into an interlacing network of stepwise activation or change to produce with antibody a dramatic change in the structure of certain cell membranes terminating in cell lysis. At practically every stage in this molecular cascade, there is a release of key biologic activities that have nothing to do with cell lysis (Fig. 5-3).

Enzymes

At the C1 level a very important change occurs in relationship to subsequent changes of the molecules of the complement system, and that is the liberation of C1s esterase, an enzyme that can probably also express proteolytic activities. A second proteoesterase arises during the activation of C2 and the formation of the $\overline{C1,4,2}$ complex that catalyzes the change of C3 to $\overline{C3}$. This C3 convertase is not to be confused with the C3 activator, also called C3 convertase, that is formed in the properdin pathway. The properdin pathway also has the enzyme C3 PAse as an integral part of its sequence.

Chemotaxins

At least three chemotaxins are natural byproducts of the complement system. C3a and 5a are the two best characterized. Both are low molecular weight split products of C3 and 5, respectively, with leukoattractant functions for polymorphonuclear neutrophils. A chemotaxin is also liberated somewhere in the $\overline{C5,6,7}$ maze that is not C5a, but its exact origin and identity has not yet been determined. Trypsinlike tissue and blood proteases, including plasmin and streptokinase from *Streptococcus pyogenes*, can release C3a-like or C5a-like substances with chemotactic activity from their parent molecules. It is apparent that any or all of these molecules could contribute to the bodily defense system.

Anaphylatoxins

The leukotaxins C3a and 5a also possess anaphylatoxic activity. An anaphylatoxin may be defined as any low molecular weight compound, usually of natural origin, that will release histamine from mast cells. Histamine is a potent vasodilator and contracts smooth muscle, changes that are associated with erythema and edema. Such inflammatory behavior, regardless of its origin, is still debated as to whether it is a protective or destructive activity. Those favoring the latter view point to the local

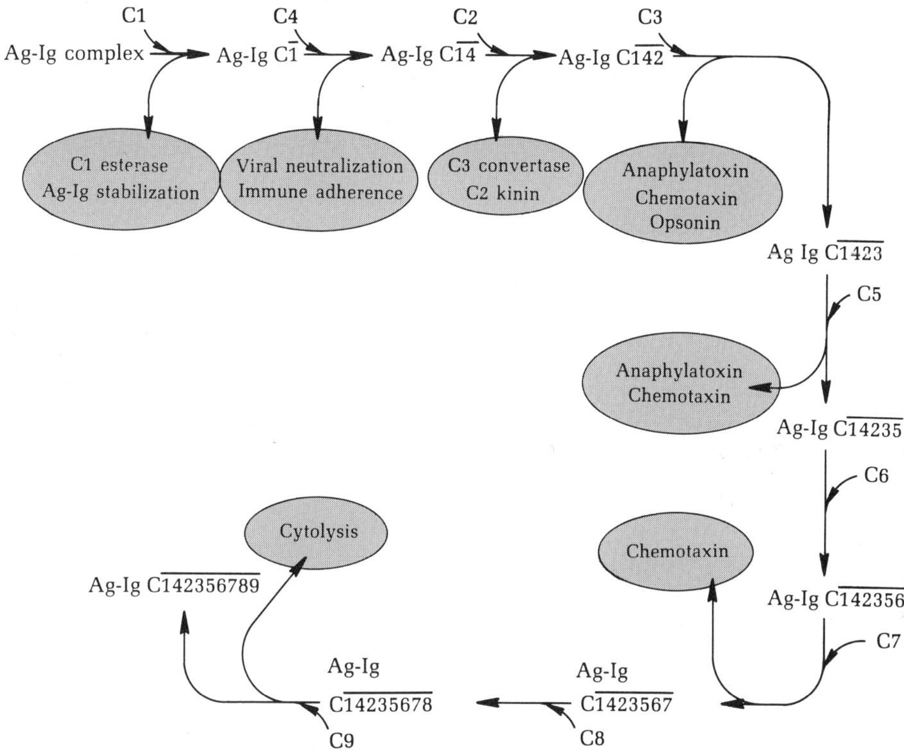

Fig. 5-3. Classic pathway of complement activation involves nine major components of the complement system. New biologic activities that arise during these activation steps are indicated in the inner portion of the diagram.

tissue damage, physical discomfort, alteration in blood flow, and other changes as evidence of tissue injury. Their opponents cite the cleansing action of tissue edema and the infiltration of granulocytes as obvious benefits of the inflammatory response. It is quite probable that each individual situation deserves its own evaluation as to the effect of inflammation, to which C3a and 5a may contribute.

Opsonization

The promotion of phagocytosis through chemotactic functions has already been mentioned as an activity of complement split products. Phagocytosis is also subject to stimulation by opsonins that modify the surface of the object to be phagocytosed so that it becomes more approachable by the phagocytic cell. Such an opsonic activity has been associated in the past with C3b. This probably deserves reevaluation in view of the more recent knowledge that C3b is enzymatically cleaved to form C3c and 3d.

Immune adherence

Another important protective function of complement can be noted at the C4 level with the appearance of a property known as immune adherence. Immune adherence is most easily detected when a homologous cellular antigen-antibody pair and complement are allowed to react in the presence of some indicator particle. The indicator particle can be an unrelated cell such as a yeast, bacterium, erythrocyte, or an inanimate particle such as carbon, latex, or polystyrene. During the serologic reaction it will be noted that the indicator particles attach and cling to the antigen. This is immune adherence, and it is attributed to changes in the structure of C4 that unmask polysaccharides, thus creating a gummy antigen-antibody-complement complex. This "stickiness," though usually measured by the use of indicator particles, can also be measured by an increased phagocytosis of the serologic complex. The efficiency of phagocytosis is improved when the subject particle is held firmly against a surface, allowing the phagocytic cytoplasm to force against, flow around, and engulf it. Immune adherence in vivo is believed to promote the adhesion of the complex to blood vessel walls, thereby enhancing phagocytosis.

Conglutinin and immunoconglutinin

Conglutinin and immunoconglutinin are associated with C3. Immunoconglutinins are antibodies that display a specificity for new antigenic determinants created or exposed in complement when it is fixed with antigen and antibody. These new sites appear to be largely in C3, but some experiments have suggested C2 and 4. Because of the several known proteolytic alterations in C3, it is not unlikely that neoantigens arise that are the stimulus for immunoconglutinin formation. These antibodies can be detected in animals injected with antigen-antibody-complement complexes and also appear spontaneously in individuals with chronic infections—that is, in persons who have antigens present after the time they have responded with specific antibodies. The resulting serologic reaction in vivo binds complement, exposes the new antigenic determinant sites, and stimulates immunoconglutinin formation. Since immunoconglutinins would contribute to the removal of the primary antigen, they can be considered as protective.

Conglutinin is a β-globulin normally found in bovine serum that can clump antigen and antibody complexes when complement through C3 has been bound into the complex. Conglutinin can demonstrate this activity only if C3 or some derivative of C3 has been modified by a normal serum enzyme called conglutinogen-activating factor (KAF). The word conglutinogen is used here in the sense of a substance that gives rise to a conglutinating activity. The suffix *ogen* does not refer to a proenzyme. KAF is actually an enzyme that has C3b (or possibly C3d) as its substrate. KAF is identical with $\overline{C3}$ INAC (inactivator); it has a molecular weight of 100,000 and is a β-globulin present in sera at a level of 25 μg/ml. The precise change that KAF causes in the C3-derived peptides is uncertain, but it permits the peptide, C3b or 3d, to combine with conglutinin. If C3 is attached to an antigen-antibody complex, the activity of conglutinin can be observed as an increased clumping or agglutination of the antigen.

Other activities

The addition of C1 to antibody molecules that have combined with antigen stabilizes the antigen-antibody combination so that it is not easily dissociated. This apparent change in the affinity of the immunoglobulin for antigen is presumably due to a readjustment in the ionic forces that hold the reactants together. In addition to the new expression of an immune adherence property, the addition of C4 to antiviral immunoglobulins does more to neutralize infectivity by the virus than does the simple virus-antivirus globulin combination. At the level of C2 incorporation into the complex a new kinin activity can be measured. Kinins are defined as substances that cause vasodilation and muscle contraction. Kinins, such as bradykinin, are most commonly polyamines or polypeptides. The C2 kinin may be a polypeptide released from C2 during the activation, but its true identity is uncertain. It is not bradykinin or closely related compounds because the C2 kinin is not neutralized by antagonists of bradykinin. Kinin activities contribute to the inflammatory response by causing erythema and edema.

Another feature of the complement, whose importance is as yet undetermined, is the attachment of C4 and 3b to receptors on neutrophils. Lymphocytes and macrophages also have receptors for complement fractions. These receptors could potentially relate to phagocytosis, antigen recognition, and/or immunoglobulin synthesis.

The complement system is also closely associated with the blood clotting system and its ability to release kinins. Plasmin, derived from the blood clotting pathway, can activate C1.

MODULATION OF COMPLEMENT FUNCTIONS

The first described complement inhibitor is that of the C$\bar{1}$ esterase. This protein is present in normal human serum at a level of 180 μg/ml. It has a molecular weight of 90,000 and is described as an acid-labile, heat-labile α_2-neuraminoglycoprotein, since it is unstable below pH 6.0, above 60° C, and contains 17% of its molecular weight as neuraminic acid. Several other glycoproteins such as those from egg white, soybean, pancreas, and blood are inhibitors of proteases; so this property of C$\bar{1}$ esterase inhibitor is not unexpected. C$\bar{1}$ INH, the presently accepted abbreviation for the C$\bar{1}$ esterase inhibitor, does not react with C1 in its proenzyme form but only after its activation.

The importance of C$\bar{1}$ INH as a modulator of complement functions is most sharply illustrated by those persons with the disease known as hereditary angioneurotic edema. People with this condition suffer sporadic attacks of subcutaneous edema, most frequently involving the eyelids, lips, neck, wrists, ankles, and other joints. This edema resolves itself spontaneously in 72 hours, is not especially uncomfortable, and would be primarily a cosmetic problem were it not that edema in the intestinal tract and other visceral tissues is painful and that edema in the throat can be so formidable as to impair normal respiration. The etiology of the disease is attributed to a genetic deficiency in C$\bar{1}$ INH that reduces the blood level of the inhibitor to about one sixth of the normal amount. A second type of individual who has the normal quantity of the inhibitor in his blood has also been found. In this case hereditary angioneurotic edema can be related to the fact that this molecule is dysfunctional. Spontaneous activation of the complement cascade, by serologic reactions or from plasmin (itself activated via the blood clotting system) in the absence of substantial quantities of functional C$\bar{1}$ INH presumably allows C2 kinin release and the edematous episode.

C$\bar{3}$ INAC(KAF), through its ability to enzymatically convert C3b (or 3d) to an inactive molecule, is a complement-regulating agent. A C$\bar{6}$ INAC has been described recently, but its nature and exact mode of action have not yet been unraveled.

C3a is subject to inhibition by a heat-stable γ-globulin in the blood. This large molecule (mol wt 300,000) also inhibits C5a, and because of the chemotactic and anaphylatoxic functions of these complement components, this inhibitor may have a very important role in regulating complement-associated activities.

ROLE OF COMPLEMENT IN DISEASE

Protection versus destruction

Like so many substances involved in human disease that have both detrimental and beneficial aspects, complement too is in an ambiguous position. It is obvious that bacteriolysis could function as an important part of the body's defense system, but it should be emphasized that many gram-positive bacteria are highly resistant to complement-induced lysis. Thus complement is probably noncontributory to the dissolution of streptococci and staphylococci, two of the most commonly encountered infectious bacteria. On the other hand, most of the gram-negative bacteria, mycoplasma, and even certain viruses are lysed by complement in coordination with specific antibody, and even destruction of other infectious organisms would be favored by the opsonic and chemotactic activity of complement.

Unfortunately complement-induced lysis of erythrocytes and leukocytes (most other mammalian cells are refractory to complement-mediated lysis) is characteristic of several forms of human anemia and leukopenia, including those associated with transfusion reactions, those of autoimmune origin, and hemolytic disease of the newborn (erythroblastosis fetalis). In the same way examples of undesired opsonic and chemotactic events related to complement activation have been observed in certain human allergies such as the Arthus reaction, immune complex pneumonitis, and glomerulonephritis where neutrophils appear to participate in host cell destruction. In these cytotoxic immune complex diseases, complement-derived kinins and anaphylatoxins may contribute to tissue edema and pathologic structural alterations.

The property of immune adherence and viral neutralization would seem to be solely protective; however, this need not be the case for the former where vascular obstruction, as seen in immune complex diseases, may contribute to host cell pathology.

Complement fixation

The activation of the complement pathway can be described in several ways—complement activation emphasizes its catalytic aspects; complement consumption indicates that complement is utilized or removed; and complement fixation suggests that complement is bound to the antigen-antibody system. This latter connotation is only partially true; indeed, some of the most significant characteristics of complement are related to the fractions that are liberated during activation of the various components. But the term "complement fixation" is still preferred to describe those serologic tests in which an exact amount of complement is added to what is believed to be an antigen-antibody system. If so, the complement is fixed into the serologic complex and is then unavailable to react with the sheep red blood cell–anti-red blood cell hemolysin system that requires complement for lysis of the cells. In this way one can determine if complement were fixed in the unknown system, a finding that reveals if the unknown antigen-antibody system was complete. In this way complement fixation tests have been used extensively to identify antigens or antibodies in human sera (Chapter 6).

BIBLIOGRAPHY

Alper, C. A., and Rosen, F. S.: Genetic aspects of the complement system, Adv. Immunol. **14**:252, 1971.

Alper, C. A., and Rosen, F. S.: Clinical applications of complement assays, Adv. Intern. Med. **20**:61, 1975.

Burkeholder, P. M., and Littleton, C. E.: Immunobiology of complement, Pathobiol. Annu. **1**:215, 1971.

Cooper, N. R.: Activation of the complement system, Contemp. Top. Mol. Immunol. **2**:155, 1973.

Frank, M. M., and Atkinson, J. P.: Complement in clinical medicine, Disease-A-Month, p. 1, January, 1975.

Gigli, I., and Austen, K. F.: Phylogeny and ontogeny of the complement system, Annu. Rev. Microbiol. **25**:309, 1971.

Hadjiyannaki, K., and Lachmann, P. J.: Hereditary angio-oedema: a review with particular reference to pathogenesis and treatment, Clin. Allergy **1**:221, 1971.

Humphrey, J. H., and Dourmashkin, R. R.: The lesions in cell membranes caused by complement, Adv. Immunol. **11**:75, 1969.

Inoue, K.: Immune bacteriolytic and bactericidal reactions, Res. Immunochem. Immunobiol. **1**:177, 1972.

Osler, A. G., and Sandberg, A. L.: Alternate complement pathways, Prog. Allergy **17**:51, 1973.

Ruddy, S., and Austen, K. F.: Inherited abnormalities of the complement system in man, Prog. Med. Genet. **7**:69, 1971.

Ruddy, S., Gigli, I., and Austen, K. F.: The complement system of man, N. Engl. J. Med. **287**:489,545,592,642, 1972.

Ward, A. P.: Biological activities of the complement system, Ann. Allergy **30**:307, 1972.

Case history

CASE 1. HEREDITARY ANGIONEUROTIC EDEMA

B. B., a 16-year-old white female, was admitted to the hospital because of repeated attacks of abdominal pain that she had experienced since early childhood. Although early childhood recurrences seldom exceeded two or three per year, since puberty the attacks had become more frequent and seemed to coincide with the menses. She also complained that severe facial edema, especially of the lips and eyelids, was interfering with her social life. The symptoms usually persisted for 2 or 3 days and then were repeated a month later. Intervening bouts seemed to be associated with mild physical exercise—she had given up guitar lessons because they caused her fingers to swell.

Questions

1. How is the immunologic and clinical diagnosis of hereditary angioneurotic edema established?
2. How does $C\bar{1}$ INH regulate this disease?
3. In what way is the complement cascade regulated by current therapeutic programs?

Discussion

A definitive diagnosis of $C\bar{1}$ INH deficiency on immunologic grounds cannot be made in the usual hospital or clinic. Assays for $C\bar{1}$ INH depend on the activity of the patient's serum in neutralizing the action of C1 esterase on synthetic substrates. Traditionally *N*-acetyl-L-tyrosine ethyl ester (ATEE) is used as the substrate for C1 esterase, which removes the ethyl ester group liberating the carboxyl group of tyrosine that is titrated with dilute alkali. The C1 esterase inhibitor, incubated with a sample of the esterase, would depress hydrolysis of the substrate. This test is not performed in the routine laboratory nor are immunodiffusion tests for the inhibitor. This means that the diagnosis is established on indirect laboratory evidence and clinical grounds. The former depends on low-complement activity in diluted sera of patients with hereditary angioneurotic edema compared to that of normal persons. Diagnostic features include familial distribution of the disease, anatomic distribution and frequency of the episodes, and response to therapy.

Transfusion of normal plasma to reconstitute the patient's level of $C\bar{1}$ INH is one of the most direct means of therapy. Angioneurotic edema is frequently treated just as any acute urticarial condition—with epinephrine and antihistamines. ϵ-Aminocaproic acid is a more specific drug because it is a specific esterase inhibitor.

REFERENCES

Donaldson, V. H., and Evans, R. R.: A biochemical abnormality in hereditary angioneurotic edema, Am. J. Med. **35**:37, 1963.

Fong, J. S.-C., Good, R. A., and Gewurz, H.: A simple diagnostic test for hereditary angioneurotic edema, J. Lab. Clin. Med. **76**:836, 1970.

chapter 6

Serologic reactions

The in vitro combination of an antigen with its specific antibody usually results in some physical change that is easily detected and serves as evidence of the serologic reaction. This physical change is not invariably observed; the two reagents may not be in the proper concentration or proportions to accumulate enough of the antigen-antibody product to make it visible. To guard against this possibility the antiserum containing the antibody is customarily diluted in a 2-fold or 10-fold dilution series, and each dilution is tested for its reactivity with a standard concentration of antigen. In some instances the concentration of the antigen is varied and tested against a constant, standard amount of antiserum. Regardless of which process is used, it may be possible to detect a difference in the amount of the serologic product formed in different tubes of the dilution series.

In the first few tubes, where the excess of immunoglobulin compared to antigen favors the formation of soluble or a sparse number of insoluble aggregates, only a slight reaction may be apparent. This zone, where the excess of antibody favors the formation of soluble complexes with antigen, is known as the prozone. This is followed by a series of several tubes in which steadily increasing amounts of the serologic product are formed and then an additional few tubes in which the product dwindles in amount. Usually the centermost tube or limited few tubes within this range will represent the equivalence point, the point where all of the available antigen has combined with its immunoglobulin. Consequently, the equivalence point is the point where the greatest amount of product is observable. This does not necessarily mean that all the molecules of antigen and antibody have been converted into a visible product. Indeed, throughout the dilution series, soluble antigen-antibody aggregates usually accompany the insoluble, visible aggregates. At the far right of the dilution series no serologic product will be visible; this is known as the postzone. It simply means the antibody has been diluted beyond its capacity to react with antigen.

The dilution series, in addition to providing us with a good opportunity to observe a serologic reaction if indeed it is bound to occur, also provides a means of estimating the amount of antibody in an antiserum. Certainly if an antiserum can be diluted 1:5120 and still retain serologic activity when dilution of a second antiserum beyond 1:80 no longer produces a positive test, then the first antiserum is approximately 64 times more potent than the second. The greatest dilution at which an antiserum (or antibody) will produce a positive test is known as its titer, and comparisons of antiserum titer are useful in evaluating the relative potency of antisera. Naturally this applies only when the two sera are tested under precisely identical conditions with the same antigen.

Several factors can prevent or restrict the amount of a serologic reaction that is observed in addition to the concentration of the reagents used. In some instances the dominant immunoglobulin class present in an antiserum may be relatively ineffective in producing a certain type of serologic reaction. Antibodies of the IgE class, for example, can combine with antigen but cause no observable change in its physical state. Combination of antigen and antibody is simply the first of what is accepted to be a two-stage serologic reaction. The second stage is designated as the aggregative phase and is the portion that develops the serologic test into a visible reaction, but for reasons unknown, IgE does not have this ability. Other antibodies, known as monovalent or incomplete antibodies, that may be of the same immunoglobulin class as complete antibodies may also impede or prevent the development of the usual serologic reaction. Such antibodies are often referred to as blocking antibodies because they can compete with ordinary immunoglobulins and block the full expression of the serologic reaction. It must be emphasized that blocking or monovalent antibodies are not yet known to differ in structure from the divalent (IgG, IgA, and IgD), tetravalent (secretory IgA), or decavalent (IgM) antibodies.

Just as monovalent antibody molecules fail to give evidence of themselves in the usual serologic reaction so also do simple haptens give the illusion that they do not participate in serologic reactions. Haptens possess but a single antigenic determinant and as such could not possibly cross-link antibody molecules. Cross bridging can occur when divalent (or multivalent) haptens are created by conjugating two hapten units to opposite ends of a serologically inert linear carrier. Then the full serologic reaction can develop. Binding of haptens in their original form with antibodies can be demonstrated by two other methods. The first of these requires that the hapten be labeled, perhaps with radioisotopes, so that it can be traced independently of its serologic activity. Incubation of the antihapten serum with its radioactive hapten to permit their combination is followed by some procedure that renders the antibody molecule insoluble. Ethanol or ammonium sulfate precipitation may be used as long as the free hapten is not coprecipitated. This is essential because counting of radioactivity in the precipitate will be used as proof of the hapten-antihapten combination, and contamination with free hapten would invalidate the results. A second procedure can be used when hapten-antigen conjugates are available. Complexes of this conjugate with antihapten will ordinarily be visible because the antigen in this case would be multivalent in regard to hapten. Formation of such a serologic complex with the conjugate would be inhibited if the antihapten were first saturated with hapten by a prior incubation before addition of the complex. Inhibition testing of this sort is useful with haptens or feeble antigens and is the basis of the serologic testing procedure for pregnancy.

Several physical factors will obviously influence the amount and rate of the serologic reaction. These include the pH and ionic strength of the medium in which the reaction is being performed, the presence of electrolytes, plus the time and temperature at which the reaction is conducted. Serologic reactions are reversible in solutions of high ionic strength, at either low or high pH or at elevated temperatures, so these conditions would minimize the extent of the observable reactions. Some antigens are heat labile and immunoglobulins are denatured near 65° C. Temperatures below this, 52° or 55° C, are employed to accelerate the reaction beyond that achieved at 37° C, the customary incubation temperature.

ANTIGEN (OR ANTIBODY) BINDING TESTS

As just described, serologic tests with haptens result in the binding of two hapten molecules to each molecule of IgG. Because of the serologic valence of the hapten, a continuation of the reaction to the formation of large, visible aggregates of the product does not occur, and no visible change in the hapten-antibody mixture is apparent. The fact that binding of the hapten to the antibody has occurred is determined by the hapten-inhibition reaction mentioned earlier or by radioimmunoassay. These two serologic procedures are also applied to the analysis of reactions between certain low molecular weight antigens and their antisera. It is often difficult to produce high-titered precipitating antisera to such antigens, and yet a need to quantitate these antigens is often met in clinical serology. A serologic method is often the most specific, sensitive, and rapid procedure available. To a lesser extent this applies to the detection of antibodies too. Radioimmunoassays are increasingly used for this purpose.

Radioimmunoassay

The arrangement of most radioimmunoassays (RIA) establishes a competition of a known amount of radiolabeled antigen (or hapten) and an unknown amount of the same antigen present in some biologic preparations with a limited, standard amount of antibody. The amount of antibody used is determined by an earlier titration with labeled antigen and is usually the amount of antibody or antiserum that will bind 70% of the antigen. A simple mathematical explanation of the reaction based on 100% binding will be used (Fig. 6-1). If it is assumed that only the IgG class of antibody is involved in the reaction, then 100 molecules of immunoglobulin will bind 200 molecules of antigen (hapten), since each IgG molecule has two binding sites. If a mixture of 200 molecules of radiolabeled antigen and 200 molecules of unlabeled antigen are incubated with the 100 molecules of IgG, it is obvious that half of the radiolabeled antigen will be displaced from the antibody, creating a bound/free ratio of 1:1. Thus in any experimental determination that results in a 50% diminution in binding of the radiolabeled antigen, the concentration of the unknown sample is exactly the same as the known. It follows logically that other bound/free ratios of antigen could be used to determine other concentrations of the unknown antigen.

A critical part of any RIA is clearly the problem of distinguishing between the bound and free portions of the labeled antigen (hapten). If the antigen forms a precipitate with the antibody, the unbound molecules can be removed simply by washing the precipitate. The difference in the amount of radiolabel added and that recovered in the precipitate is then the amount of free antigen. As a matter of practical application, RIA tests of this type are usually not performed. RIA tests are conducted more frequently with nonprecipitating haptens or, for reasons of economy, with antibody solutions diluted beyond their capacity to form a visible reaction. Under these conditions some physiochemical method must be used to separate the bound and free haptens.

There are at least a dozen different methods for separating antibody-bound antigens and free antigens, some of which are applicable only to certain antigens and others are wasteful, offer poor recovery of the antigen, or have other disadvantages. Only the most widely applied methods will be discussed.

When the antigen is of low molecular weight or when a hapten is used, advantage can be taken of the insolubility of immunoglobulins in 50% saturated ammonium sulfate to separate the free from the immunoglobulin-bound hapten. After the competition between labeled and unlabeled antigen has reached equilibrium, the mixture is adjusted to 50% saturation with ammonium sulfate. This precipitates the antibody and its bound antigen but leaves the unbound antigen in solution. Counting the radioisotope content of the precipitate and subtracting this from the amount of isotope added follows the same mathematical procedures discussed previously. Other precipitants than ammonium sulfate may be used—other sulfate salts and ethanol are examples. The only restriction is that they must not precipitate the free antigen or effect any dissociation of the bound antigen from the antibody. The original application of the Farr technique, the ammonium sulfate precipitation of soluble antigen-antibody complexes, was to de-

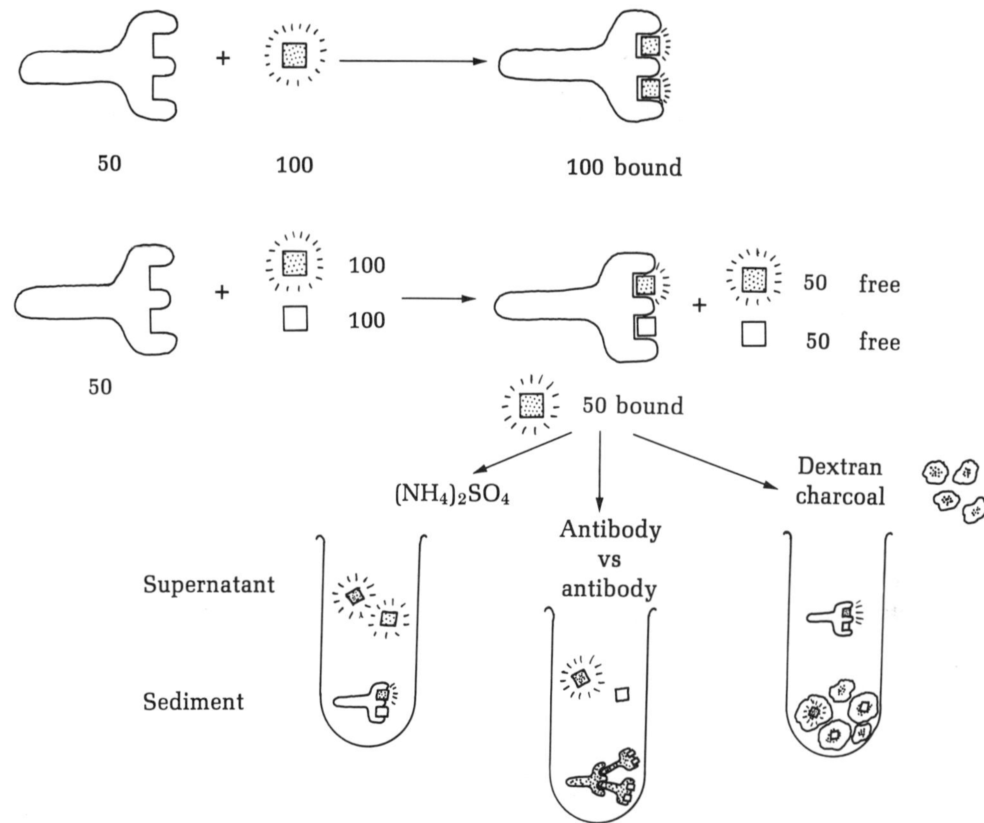

Fig. 6-1. A radioactive hapten is totally bound to its antibody when reaction mixture consists of 100 parts of hapten and 50 parts of immunoglobulin. Doubling the quantity of hapten by adding 100 parts of unlabeled hapten results in the binding of only 50 parts of radiolabeled hapten. Bound and free hapten are separable from each other by precipitation of the antibody by $(NH_4)_2SO_4$, as in the Farr technique, or by the antiglobulin method illustrated. Dextran-coated charcoal can be used to absorb the free hapten. Solid-phase radioimmunoassay, in which the antibody is attached to an insoluble carrier, is not illustrated.

termine nonprecipitating antibody, but its use in RIA is a valuable extension of the method.

A second method of precipitating soluble antibody-antigen complexes is by the double antibody procedure or antiglobulin method, sometimes referred to as an "immunologic sandwich." In this form of RIA testing it is necessary to know the species origin of the antibody being used in the assay and to have an antibody that will precipitate that species of gamma globulin. If the competitive binding portion of the assay utilizes a rabbit antibody, the experimentor needs an antibody against rabbit gamma globulin to complete the test. If the original antiserum is of goat origin, then an antibody against goat gamma globulin is needed. The primary antibody and its bound antigen are precipitated by the antiglobulin. The primary immunoglobulin serves both as an antibody and antigen and is the "meat" of the sandwich.

There is nothing mysterious about the ability of a gamma globulin to serve as an antigen. It meets all of the criteria of an antigen when injected into a foreign species. Gamma globulins contain antigenic determinants in their Fab and Fc portions, and the combination of the Fab portions with an antigen does not sterically block the attachment of antibodies to the Fc determinants. Advantage of this is taken in other double antibody procedures in the Coombs test and in histochemical precipitation.

A third RIA method is the one used most frequently in the clinical environment and is generally referred to as a solid-phase RIA. In this variation the antibody is already provided or converted to an insoluble form. In one form of the test the antibody is allowed to attach to the inner surface of polystyrene assay tubes by physical adsorption. Covalent linkage of the antibody to an insoluble carrier is ordinarily preferred, since this precludes dissociation of the antibody from the inert carrier. This is accomplished by coupling the antibody to cellulose, Sepharose, or Sephadex or by embedding it in porous glass beads or polyacrylamide particles as the solid-phase support. The cross-linked dextrans (Sephadex or Sepharose) and porous glass entrap the large antibody molecules within their matrix and yet still permit the entry and exit of smaller molecules by simple diffusion. After equilibrium is reached, centrifugation separates the bound from the free antigen. One possible advantage of solid-phase RIA is that treatment of the product with mild acid solutions will regenerate the antibody by dissociating the antibody-antigen complex, allowing the antibody preparation to be reused.

A fourth modification of RIA uses all reagents in their soluble form, and after the serologic reaction has been completed, the large molecular weight reactants (antibody-antigen complexes) are separated from the low molecular weight molecules (antigen) by the addition of dextran-coated charcoal. Charcoal is a classic absorbent. It is used to clarify smoke and vapors, to clean or whiten chemicals, and to remove undesirable odors or tastes. It is easily removed by filtration or centrifugation. It can be converted to a specific absorbent for small molecules by applying a dextran overcoat that is impermeable to macromolecules. The use of dextran-treated charcoal in RIA is in one sense the mirror image of the solid-phase procedure. In the former the free antigen is removed by its entrapment in the charcoal solid phase. In the latter the bound antigen is recovered on the solid-phase support.

Regardless of the exact experimental technique used, the great advantage of all RIA procedures is their great sensitivity (Table 6-1). There is no other serologic reaction used in the routine laboratory that approaches RIA in its ability to detect trace amounts of antigen (hapten). Commercially

Table 6-1. Relative sensitivity of serologic tests

Serologic procedure	*Antibody**	*Antigen†*
Radioimmunoassay	0.001	Picograms
Hemolysis	0.001-0.003	Not applicable
Passive agglutination	0.001-0.03	Micrograms
Complement fixation	0.01-0.1	Micrograms
Bacterial agglutination	0.01-0.1	Not applicable
Hemagglutination	0.5-1.0	Not applicable
Fluid precipitation	0.5-3.0	Micrograms
Immunodiffusion	3-100	Micrograms
Immunoelectrophoresis	>50	Micrograms

*Micrograms of antibody nitrogen per milliliter of antiserum required for positive tests.
†Smallest amount of antigen per milliliter that can be detected.

available RIA kits may detect as little as 1 nanogram (a billionth of a gram) or 1 picogram (10^{-12} gram or a trillionth of a gram) of antigen. This is obviously of great significance in following or determining the blood level of certain hormones or therapeutic agents that seldom exceed a few micrograms per milliliter. RIA procedures have the disadvantage of relatively great expense in terms of both the reagents and radioisotope counting equipment and the unavoidable hazards associated with radioisotopes. These features obviously have not been a serious handicap to the clinical application of RIA. RIA procedures currently in use for monitoring cardiovascular function include assays for digoxin, digitoxin, renin (angiotensin), and aldosterone. Reproductive functions can be estimated by RIA methods for follicle-stimulating hormone (FSH), luteinizing hormone (LH), human placental lactogen (HPL), testosterone, estrogen, and progesterone; hematopoietic function by vitamin B_{12}, folic acid, and immunoglobulin methods; and various metabolic functions by RIA for insulin, thyroxine (T_4), triiodothyronine (T_3), ACTH, cortisol, parathormone, human growth hormone (HGH), and thyroid-stimulating hormone (TSH). RIA kits are being developed for opiates, barbituates, amphetamines, and other abused drugs. Detection of hepatitis-associated antigens is another important application of RIA.

In view of the expense and potential hazards of RIA, the question of whether a suitable substitute exists is logical. At the moment, the answer is no, but the possibility that an equally valuable and sensitive test could replace RIA always exists. A potential candidate is the enzyme-labeled antibody method. Enzyme-linked antibody tests are already in vogue as histochemical procedures, but when an antigen is insoluble or can be easily insolubilized, the possibility for quantitative serology by this method also exists. This procedure is discussed briefly in the following section.

Serologic histochemistry

The ability to attach tracers to immunoglobulins and to detect the immunoglobulin (and thus its corresponding antigen) by the location of the tracer has proved itself to be a worthy modification of the serologic reaction. Such procedures are based on the ability of radioisotopes, fluorescent dyes, enzymes, or other easily detected molecules to attach to and preserve the activity of the immunoglobulin. Naturally the activity of the tracer molecule must also be retained after this conjugation. It is not mandatory that these tagged antibodies be used as histochemical reagents, and the radioallergosorbent test (RAST, Chapter 8) is an important example of a different application.

Fluorescent antibody procedures are microscopic procedures in which a fluorescent dye is used to track the antibody. Fluorescein and rhodamine B are two examples of such fluorochromes, although there are many dyes available that share the ability to absorb light energy (short blue and ultraviolet rays) and to emit a longer wavelength, visible light. Fluorescein emits a greenish yellow color, and rhodamine emits an orange-red color. These compounds in their isothiocyanate or sulfonyl chloride forms readily conjugate with the amino groups in immunoglobulins. Such amino groups tend to have little influence on the serologic activity of an immunoglobulin and can be masked with a fluorescent dye in such a way as to permit complete retention of immunoglobulin activity.

The application of fluorescent antibodies is either by the direct or indirect method (Fig. 6-2). In the direct procedure the antigen to be identified is placed on a glass slide, which is then flooded with a fluorescent antibody against that antigen. After a suitable incubation period in which serologic combination of the antigen and antibody takes place, the excess labeled antibody is removed by washing. The slide is then examined through a microscope that is placed

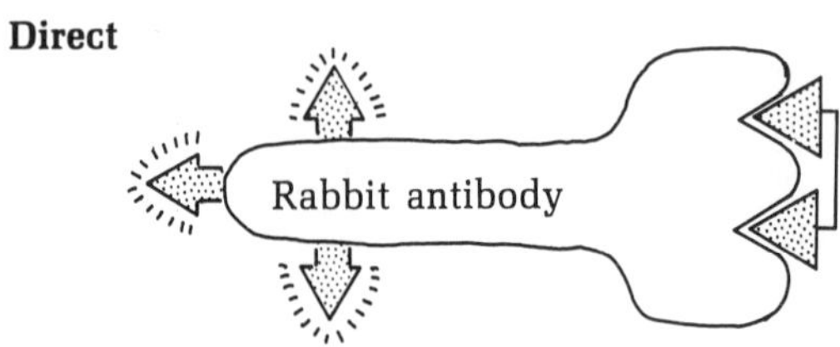

Labeled antibody is antigen directed

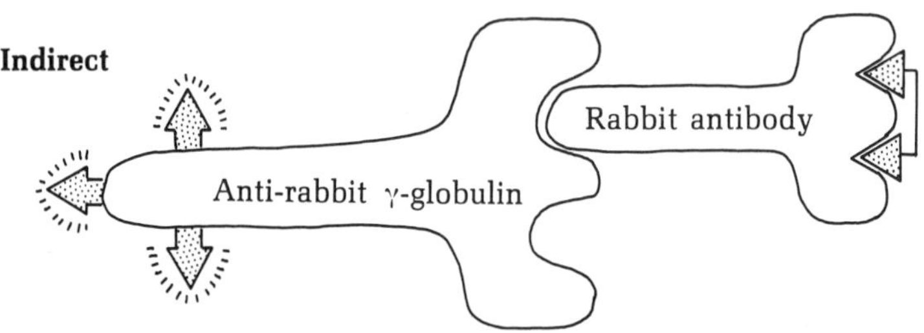

Labeled antibody is antibody directed

Fig. 6-2. In direct fluorescent antibody tests the labeled antibody is directed against the antigen. In indirect fluorescent antibody procedures the labeled antibody is an antiglobulin. Although this diagram does not so indicate, several molecules of fluorescent globulin can attach to the primary antibody, giving the indirect test a distinct advantage in sensitivity over the direct procedure.

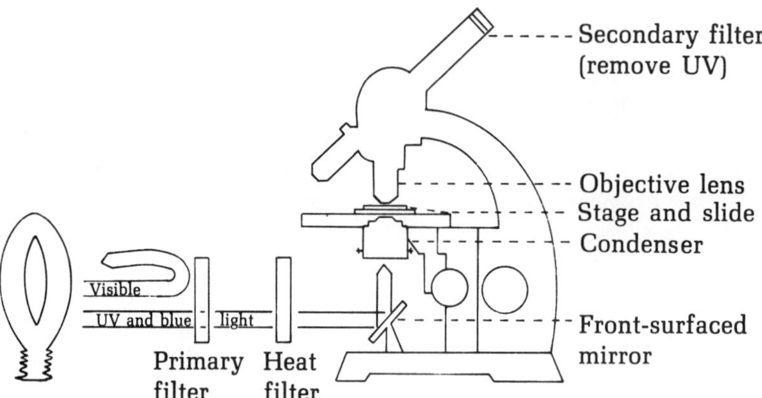

Fig. 6-3. To conduct fluorescent antibody test a microscopic assembly similar to that illustrated is required. A primary filter and a heat filter remove unwanted visible light and heat rays that are emitted from the light source, a hydrogen or mercury vapor lamp. Ultraviolet and short blue light that passes the filters is reflected from a front-surfaced mirror into a darkfield condenser. The condenser diverts light path away from objective lens, except that visible light, emitted by a fluorescent antibody molecule bombarded by ultraviolet rays, radiates in all directions and some of this enters the objective lens. Stray ultraviolet rays are removed by a secondary filter at the ocular lens.

in an ultraviolet microscopy alignment (Fig. 6-3). Here the ultraviolet and short blue light beam emitted from a mercury lamp is filtered to remove heat rays and most of the visible light. Thereafter, a front-surfaced mirror diverts the light into a darkfield condenser, which in turn diverts the light beam so that it does not enter the objective lens of the microscope. Objects on the microscope slide that absorb and radiate (visible) light can be seen because the light is radiated in all directions, and some of it enters the objective lens of the microscope. Any ultraviolet light that is accidentally refracted into the microscope is blocked by a filter in the ocular lens, so that these rays will not damage the eye of the viewer. In a positive fluorescent antibody (FAB) test the viewer sees points of green or reddish light against a black background. If an ordinary Abbe lightfield condenser were used, these colors would be seen against a bright white background. The human eye is very insensitive to color on an intense white field, so a darkfield condenser is preferred.

In immunofluorescent serology as in any serologic test, suitable controls are required. Here the control is known as the blocking test. The blocking test simply involves a preincubation of the antigen with a portion of unlabeled antibody prior to incubation with the fluorescent antibody. The attachment of the unlabeled antibody to the antigen blocks the attachment of the labeled antibody, thereby producing the negative control. Positive controls consisting of known amounts of antigen and a range of dilutions of the fluorescent antibody should also be incorporated into the experiment.

One handicap of the direct immunofluorescent antibody method is the necessity to have a supply of fluorescent antibody available to identify each antigen that might be encountered. This restriction is overcome by the indirect fluorescent antibody method.

The identification of antibodies in a person with syphilis will illustrate the indirect fluorescent antibody procedure. The test begins by flooding a slide containing *Treponema pallidum,* the spirochete that causes syphilis, with the patient's serum. These slides are available commercially or can be prepared from a commercially available suspension of the organisms. If the patient's serum contains antibodies, these antibodies will fix to the spirochete during this first incubation period. The slide is then washed to remove unreacted antibodies and flooded with a fluorescent antiserum directed against human gamma globulin. After this the slide is washed, dried, and examined by immunofluorescent (ultraviolet) microscopy. The inability to observe fluorescence is a negative test, and the presence of visible fluorescence is a positive test. Indirect fluorescent antibody testing is another application of the antiglobulin, double antibody, or immunologic sandwich technique. For clinical laboratory use, only one fluorescent antibody is needed, one directed against human gamma globulin. This will allow the identification of antibodies against virtually any medically important antigen. The blocking test should also be used as a control for the indirect fluorescent antibody procedure. It consists of incubation of the antigen-antibody complex with an unlabeled antihuman gamma globulin prior to the addition of labeled antiglobulin.

Direct fluorescent antibody procedures are customarily used to identify antigens—bacteria, viruses, etc.—in specimens collected from patients. Even if a bacterial pathogen is present with a mixture of other bacteria of the same morphology and gram staining characteristics, a specific fluorescent antibody will stain only that pathogen. Fluorescent antibodies have been used to identify group A hemolytic streptococci, *Neisseria meningitidis, N. gonorrhoeae, Brucella* species, *Hemophilus influenzae, Bordetella pertussis, Candida albicans, Histoplasma capsulatum, Blastomyces dermatitidis,* rabies virus, herpesvirus, influenza virus, etc. The application to the identification of viruses is especially important because fluorescent antibody tests are often positive when other staining procedures or cultural methods are negative. Fluorescent antibodies have also enabled the identification of plasma cells as the gamma globulin-producing cells and have helped to prove that a single plasma cell produces both the light and heavy chains for an immunoglobulin, that the cellular location of thyroid hormone is in the colloid, and that cell wall synthesis proceeds from the fission point in streptococci. Indirect immunofluorescence is more frequently applied clinically to the detection of antibodies in a patient's serum. Among others the following infectious diseases have been studied by the indirect method—syphilis, toxoplasmosis, herpesvirus, hepatitis virus, trachoma, and other virus infections, various types of infectious meningitis, and infectious mononucleosis. Indirect and direct fluorescent antibody methods have also been useful in studying the autoimmune diseases, those in which antibodies are formed against self-antigens.

A second variation of the labeled antibody as a histochemical reagent is the ferritin-labeled antibody. Ferritin is a protein with a molecular weight of 465,000 that bears about 23% of its weight as iron. This iron is localized in distinct micelles that are opaque to electrons, thus permitting the localization of a ferritin-labeled antibody under an electron microscope. Except for the type of microscopy involved, ferritin-labeled antibodies are used just like fluorescent antibodies.

Enzyme-labeled antibodies that produce a chromogenic end product can be applied to visible light histochemistry. One advantage of these enzyme-linked antibodies is that one molecule of the labeled antibody, because of the catalytic activity of the attached enzyme, will attack many molecules of substrate. Where a sensitive method of detecting this alteration in the substrate exists, there is the possibility of developing a sensitive enzyme-linked antibody method. This is the case with horseradish peroxidase, alkaline phosphatase, and glucose oxidase, and the use of these enzyme-labeled antibodies in quantitative immunochemistry is a genuine prospect in the future. Moreover, since some enzyme products are easily converted to electron-dense products, the adaptation of enzyme-labeled antibodies to electron microscopy has also been possible.

FLUID PRECIPITATION

The mixture of a true solution of antigen with its antibody (usually in the form of a whole antiserum) will result in the formation of a visible precipitate (Fig. 6-4). This is the result of the formation of an (approximately) alternating latticework of the two molecules until the point of insolubility is

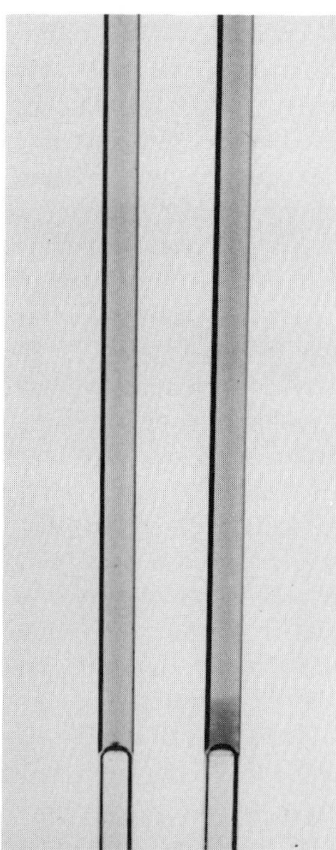

Fig. 6-4. In capillary precipitation the insoluble antigen-immunoglobulin complex settles to the bottom of the fluid mixture above the air space, as seen in the tube on the right. The tube on the left shows a negative reaction.

reached. If the interfacial or ring test is performed, a disc of precipitate develops at the plane where the antigen is layered over the antiserum (or vice versa). The ring test has the advantage that if the reagents are concentrated in excess of their equivalence concentration, diffusion during the test will eventually place them at a suitable concentration for precipitation. This usually takes only a few minutes. If the two reactants are mixed in a small tube or drawn into a capillary tube but are not in the optimal proportions, precipitation may be delayed for several hours. The necessity to test several dilutions of the antigen or antiserum is very real in this form of precipitation testing.

A medicolegal or forensic medical application of the precipitation test is seen in the identification of blood stains in the case of an unexplained death. This is done by mixing the unknown blood sample or an extract of cloth bearing the blood stain with a battery of antisera against blood from several different species of animals. Within the known limits of cross-reactivity of such antisera, a positive test will identify the species source of the blood. When precipitation occurs with the antihuman blood, the stain is of human origin. It is even possible to identify the blood type of human blood with specific anti-A or anti-B sera (Chapter 7).

C-reactive protein is an abnormal albumin found in the serum of individuals experiencing an inflammatory disease. This protein is not present in the blood of other persons. Fluid precipitation tests with anti-C–reactive protein provide a facile and inexpensive aid to the diagnosis of bacterial infections or certain forms of cancer.

QUELLUNG REACTION

The quellung reaction (from the German *Quellung*, meaning swelling) must be one of the least used varieties of the precipitation test. The test is based on the precipitation of anticapsular antibodies on the perimeter of bacterial capsules, resulting in a sharp definition of their outline under the microscope. Whether or not a sufficient number of antibody molecules combine with the capsule to produce a true swelling or increase in size is doubtful. This test can be performed and interpreted within a few minutes; consequently, it can provide a rapid means of identifying an encapsulated organism in a mixture of bacteria. Regardless of this, the replacement of antiserum by antibiotics and chemotherapy has caused the quellung test to dwindle in popularity. The test is admittedly difficult to interpret and could only be applied to *Streptococcus pneumoniae, Neisseria meningitidis,* and *Hemophilus influenzae* under routine circumstances.

IMMUNODIFFUSION (GEL PRECIPITATION METHODS)

Unless performed under sophisticated circumstances, fluid precipitation tests indicate only that a positive test has developed. Precipitation tests in gel can determine that several antigen-antibody systems have participated in the reaction, can identify unknown antigens in the mixture with known antigens, and can determine the concentration of known antigen. All of these features are not combined in a single type of immunodiffusion test; there are several modifications.

Ouchterlony-type immunodiffusion

One of the first gel precipitation techniques to gain popularity was the double diffusion test, so designated because both the antigen and antibody diffuse from separate reservoirs placed in an agar film. Purified agar or agarose replaces the usual bacteriologic grade of agar in these tests, since it forms clearer gels and is relatively free of sugar sulfates that combine ionically with cationic antigens. When a pure antigen and its corresponding antibody or antiserum are analyzed in the Ouchterlony test, a single line of precipitate will form in the gel between the two reservoirs. When two depots

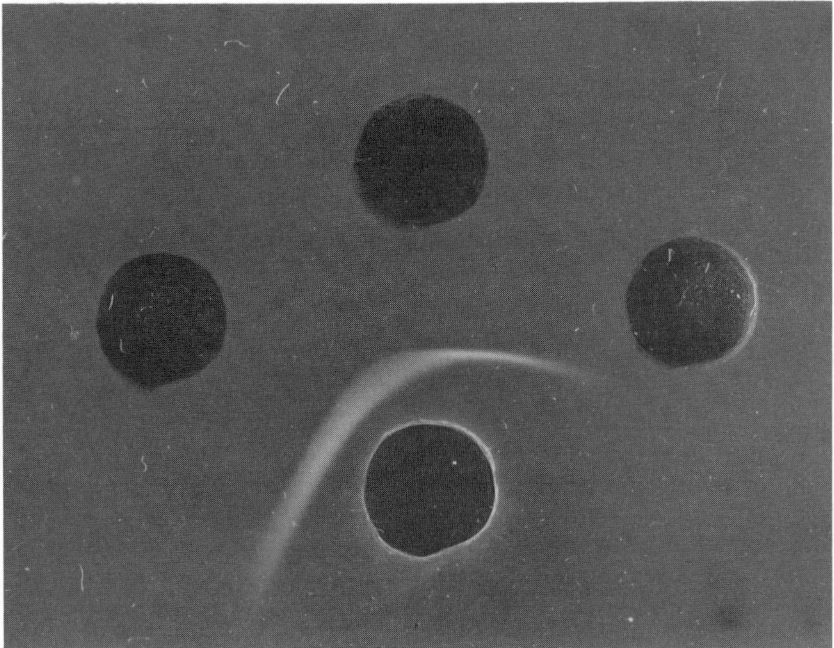

Fig. 6-5. Ouchterlony-type immunodiffusion reaction of identity. Antiserum was placed in the center well and the same antigen was placed in the two wells corresponding with the immune precipitate.

of the antigen are used in a triangular arrangement with a single well of antibody, a curved, single line of precipitate will develop (Fig. 6-5). This is in reality two separate precipitin lines that have fused at their point of contact into a smooth arc, known as a reaction of serologic identity. If two serologically unrelated antigens are placed in the two separate antigen wells and diffused against an antiserum that contains both of the corresponding antibodies, two intersecting lines of precipitate will develop. This is a reaction of nonidentity. A less frequent reaction of partial identity is seen when two partially related antigens combine with an antibody and produce a spurred reaction. The word "identity" in the description of these reactions is used in the sense of serologic identity, and it is understood that an antibody might not detect miniscule chemical differences in antigens, as between a toxin and its toxoid.

When a multiple antigen-antibody system is subjected to Ouchterlony-type immunodiffusion, it is highly unlikely that the diffusion rates of the several antigens, a property dependent primarily on molecular size and shape, would coincide. Even if the diffusion rates of two or more antigens should coincide, it is unlikely that their specific antibodies would exist at exactly the same concentration in the antiserum. For these reasons the probability that two antigens and their antibodies would precipitate on a single line is a statistically rare event, and separate precipitation lines are formed by each antigen-antibody system involved. Thus it is very simple to determine the number of antigens in a mixture by use of the Ouchterlony technique unless an unusually large number of precipitin arcs are formed within the space between the antigen and antiserum wells.

Double immunodiffusion tests can also be arranged in tubes so that the reactants diffuse into a plug of intervening agar (the

Oudin technique), but this is a physically cumbersome test to use and does not permit as easy an identification of antigens as the Ouchterlony method.

Counterimmunoelectrophoresis

Counterimmunoelectrophoresis is a double immunodiffusion test in which an electrical force is applied to accelerate the convergence and combination of antigen and antibody. The physical design of the test is basically the same as the Ouchterlony test; the antigen is placed in one well cut in an agar film and the antiserum in another. A major restriction is that the antigen and immunoglobulin must carry opposite ionic charges at the pH of the buffering system employed. Since a pH between 7.0 and 8.3 is customarily chosen, the gamma globulin molecules will bear a positive charge. Hence the test is limited to antigens with an acidic isoelectric point, that is, those antigens that will have a negative charge at a slightly alkaline pH. Under these circumstances the transmission of a direct electric current through the gel will force the antigen and antibody toward one another, causing them to precipitate more quickly than when only simple diffusion is in effect. Counterimmunoelectrophoresis is a time-saving procedure, but one that is limited largely to polysaccharide and virus antigens. Its primary application at the present time is in the diagnosis of viral hepatitis.

Immunoelectrophoresis

Immunoelectrophoresis must also be considered a double immunodiffusion process, but one in which electrical displacement of the antigens in a mixture precedes diffusion of the Ouchterlony type. Electrophoretic separation of antigens is accomplished on agarose or cellulose acetate films placed in an electrical field. Molecules of different net charge are displaced from the starting reservoir primarily according to their charge. Thereafter, a trough is cut in the agar film along the same axis as the electrophoresis, and the trough is filled with an antiserum containing antibody to one or more of the antigens. During a succeeding incubation period, precipitates develop as the result of ordinary immunodiffusion, each antigen and its antibody forming a separate arc.

Immunoelectrophoresis is most often applied clinically to the analysis of serum proteins. The serum sample is electrophoretically fractioned at pH 8.6, a pH in which there is extensive movement of the albumin (electronegative) to the positive pole and little movement of the gamma globulins. Immunodiffusion subsequently with an antiserum directed against whole human serum will identify all of the major serum proteins. The use of specific antisera against IgG, IgA, or IgM or against κ- or λ-type light chains identifies the molecules bearing these specific antigenic determinants. The intensity of the precipitation arc can be used as a crude quantitative estimate of the concentration of specific proteins and assist in the diagnosis of hypo- or hyperglobulinemias, although the more precise radial immunodiffusion procedure is a more secure basis for such diagnoses.

Radial immunodiffusion

Radial immunodiffusion, the Mancini technique, has developed rapidly into one of the most important serologic techniques used in the clinical laboratory. It is invariably used to measure the concentration of some antigen. This is done by measuring the area (or some parameter of the area) of the precipitation ring that the antigen produces as it diffuses from a well placed in an agar film that contains antibody specific for that antigen (Fig. 6-6). By the careful selection of monospecific antisera and the incorporation of a series of antigen standards in the test, the concentration of the unknown sample can be readily determined. Radial immunodiffusion is now used to measure the concentration of the human serum immunoglobulins and several important serum proteins—lipoproteins, transferrin, the C4 and 3 components of comple-

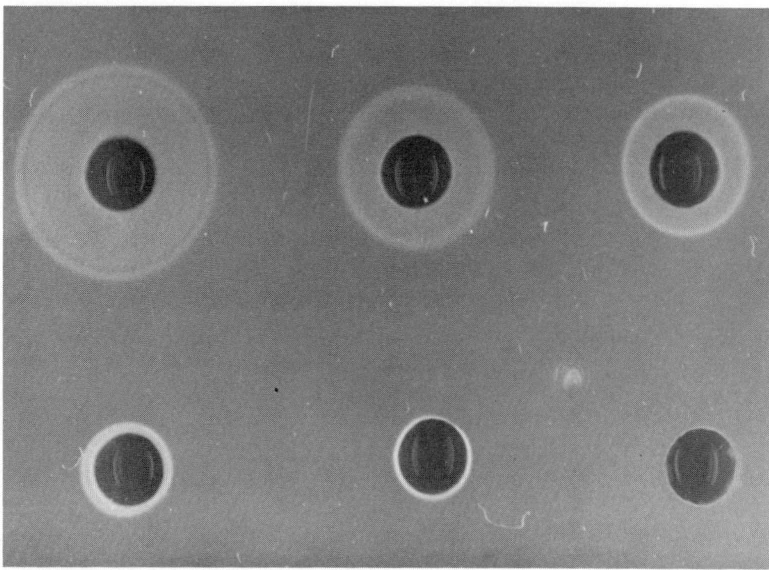

Fig. 6-6. Mancini (radial immunodiffusion) test. Antigen in upper wells was at a concentration of 10, 5, and 2.5, μg/ml reading left to right. In lower row only left well received antigen, 1.2 μg/ml.

ment, ceruloplasmin, α_1-trypsin inhibitor, lysozyme, etc.

Crossed immunoelectrophoresis

Crossed immunoelectrophoresis, the Laurell procedure, is a procedure in which a mixture of antigens is electrophoretically separated in one direction on an agar strip that is then transferred to a plate of agar containing antibody against the antigen mixture. A second electrophoretic separation is applied at 90 degrees to the direction of the original separation so that the antigens are drawn into the agar that contained the antibodies. Precipitation lines develop in long spear- or rocketlike probes as each antigen migrates into the antiserum gel. The area under the arc is a very accurate expression of the concentration of the antigen when appropriate standards of the antigen have been incorporated into the experiment. If one simply wants to determine the concentration of a single, known antigen, the original electrophoretic step may be omitted, and it is in this way that the Laurell method is used today.

Since crossed immunoelectrophoresis is basically a quantitative immunodiffusion method, its merits relative to radial immunodiffusion must be considered. The former requires additional equipment but is more rapid because the antigen and antibody are compelled to combine under electrophoretic force. Antigen choice is restricted to those with good electrophoretic mobility at pH 8.3 to 8.6, where the immunoglobulins are nearly immobile, a restriction not met in the Mancini procedure.

In all of the precipitation tests previously described, the dominant contributing immunoglobulin is IgG. Other immunoglobulins are feeble precipitators. The sensitivity of the various tests for detecting antigen will vary according to the particular dimensions and physical arrangement used. Microtechniques are almost invariably more sensitive and economical. Staining of the precipitation lines or the use of radioisotopes will significantly increase the sensitivity of these procedures. In the usual clinical situation, radial immunodiffusion can detect as little as 1.25 μg of antigen/ml.

Crossed immunoelectrophoresis is of similar sensitivity and the other tests are 3- to 30-fold less sensitive.

BACTERIAL AGGLUTINATION

Agglutination of bacteria by antisera is one of the oldest serologic tests available to the clinical laboratory; it was advanced as an aid to the diagnosis of bacterial infections by Widal in 1896. The older reference to bacterial agglutination as the Widal test to honor his discovery is gradually falling into disuse. The diagnostic capabilities of the agglutination test can be achieved from either of two directions: (1) unknown bacteria can be identified by known antisera maintained in the laboratory stock or (2) by using known bacteria, antibodies in a patient's serum can be identified.

An example of the first situation is often encountered in enteric bacteriology. More than 300 different species of *Salmonella* have been isolated from human patients with intestinal disease. The severity of these diseases range from outright typhoid fever to milder, subclinical diarrhea or abdominal distress. A complete bacteriologic identification of the enteric pathogen is dependent on the isolation of potentially pathogenic strains on plate cultures and the eventual determination of the genus and species by its fermentation of carbohydrates, formation of specific end products from amino acids, and other cultural and morphologic characteristics. Not only is this a time-consuming process requiring 3 or more days, but it is often frustrated by an inability to make an exact identification of the isolate due to a deviation of one or two of the biochemical tests from that produced by typical strains. If, at the first moment a potential pathogen is recognized, a serologic identification is attempted, considerable time and expense may be spared.

This is accomplished by emulsifying a small amount of the bacterial growth in a droplet of saline solution on a glass slide and adding a drop of antiserum known to agglutinate a certain bacterium. After mixing the reagents, the slide is observed for clumping of the bacterial cells, which would identify the bacterial species as corresponding with the antiserum (Fig. 6-7). Obviously this test is not going to be rapid and inexpensive if it is necessary to perform this reaction with each of the 300 *Salmonella* antisera. The number of tests is limited in two ways, first by removing those antisera to the unusual isolates that are very rarely encountered and second by using a series of polyvalent antisera. A polyvalent antiserum is a blend of antisera to several antigens. When a polyvalent antiserum yields a positive test, then the individual antisera contributing to the pool are tested until the bacterium is identified by its reaction with a single antiserum.

The ideologic goal in which the bacterium reacts with a single antiserum may never be achieved. This is true because of the extensive sharing of antigens between the *Salmonella* species. Preparation of monovalent antisera that will react with only a single antigenic determinant of these bacterial cells has been accomplished, and numbers and lettters have been used to denote these antigens. The cellular antigens are given numbers, and the flagellar antigens are given either letters or numbers. S. *typhosa* has the antigen formula 9, 12, Vi, and d, where 9 and 12 are the ordinary somatic antigens, Vi is a special somatic antigen associated with virulence, and d is the flagellar antigen. The several dozen other bacteria possessing antigens 9, 12, Vi, or d would be agglutinated by an antiserum to S. *typhosa*. However, only S. *typhosa* has the antigenic composition stated and would react with monospecific antisera to all four of these antigens.

Bacterial agglutination of cellular antigens with their antibodies produces a physically different aggregate of bacterial cells than the reaction between flagellar antigens and their antibodies. The former, referred to as the O type of reaction, is granular and compact, whereas the latter is loose and flocculent. In O type agglutination the cells

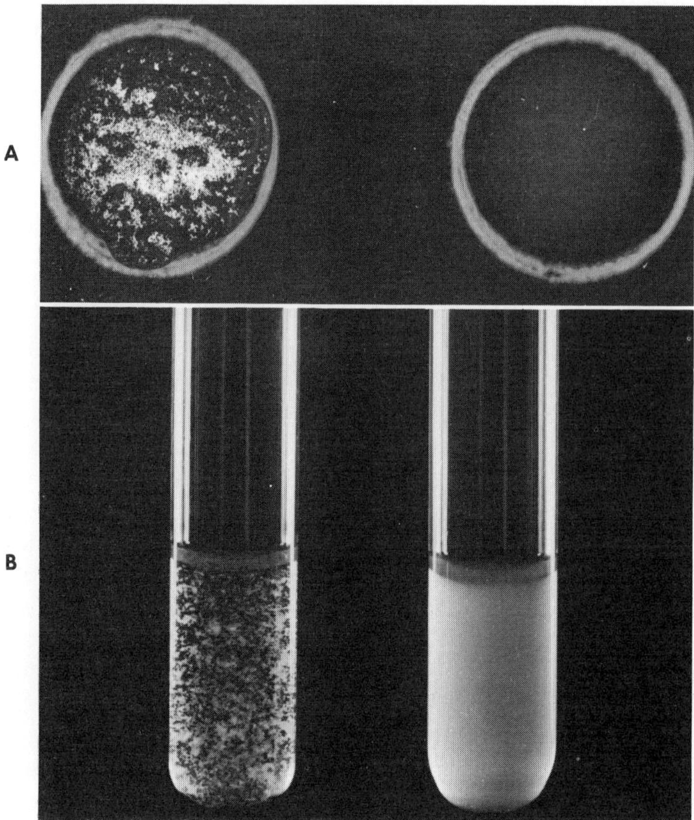

Fig. 6-7. **A,** Slide agglutination of bacteria is a rapid method of identifying unknown bacteria with known antisera or the reverse. **B,** Tube agglutination can be used for the same purpose and to quantitate the antibody content in an antiserum. In each case the positive test is seen on the left and the negative control on the right.

themselves are held in close physical contact by interlocking molecules of antibody. In the H type of reaction the flagella that extend from the cell surface combine with antibody, and this actually holds the cells some distance apart, causing the agglutinated mass to be less dense. The letters O and H are used to describe the somatic and flagellar types of agglutination; they stem from the German *Hauch,* meaning a film (of growth), and *ohne,* meaning without. Flagellated or *Hauch* bacteria will produce a thin film of growth on a moist culture plate, whereas *ohne Hauch* organisms cannot due to their lack of motility.

Although the slide agglutination test was used in the previous example as a qualitative test, it is possible to arrange a semiquantitative test by using measured volumes of antiserum and micropipets. There would be no advantage to this in the illustration presented, although some circumstances do require a more quantitative evaluation of bacterial agglutination. This is depicted in the second situation mentioned previously in which bacterial isolation procedures from a patient with a febrile, enteric complaint are regularly negative for pathogens. If in this situation the laboratory has an acute serum sample collected shortly after the person became ill and a convalescent serum sample taken 14 to 21 days later, a comparison of the agglutination titers of the two samples may be informative as to the patient's disease. If the acute serum titer is 1:80 with S. *typhosa* as the antigen and the convalescent serum titer is 1:1280, it can be assumed that during the interlude between the two serum collections, the person had an immunizing experience with S. *typhosa.* Of course, this statement applies only when potential cross-reactions with other antigenically related bacteria have been determined and proved to be harmonious with this result. In general, a 4-fold increase in titer between the acute and convalescent sample is considered supportive of the diagnosis. Notice that information from a single serum sample may be entirely misleading—a low titer may mean that the antibody response curve is still at the foot of its sharp rise, and a high titer could be due to prior immunization or disease. Many laboratories will perform the test only on paired serum samples for these very reasons.

IgM is the dominant immunoglobulin in most agglutination tests. This may be due to its greater valence than that possessed by other immunoglobulins and its tendency to dominate the response to polysaccharide antigens, which is the chemistry of most cell wall antigens. There is little that is unique about bacterial agglutination—erythrocytes, yeasts, fungal cells, sperm, protozoa, etc. are all agglutinable by their specific antibodies.

PASSIVE AGGLUTINATION

Agglutination of particulate objects such as bacteria, erythrocytes, latex, or polystyrene spherules can also be accomplished by antisera directed to extraneous antigens that are purposely attached to or adsorbed to the particle surface. In this way the coating of soluble antigens onto particulate carriers converts a precipitation test into an agglutination test. Agglutination tests have a greater sensitivity than precipitation systems, which accounts in large part for the popularity of these passive or indirect agglutination procedures. These tests can also be "inverted," so that the antibody is adsorbed to the particle and agglutination is created by incubation with the antigen. Both forms of the test as well as a modification based on inhibition are applied to medical problems.

Antibodies to thyroglobulin and to certain nucleic acid–containing antigens are developed by some patients with hypothyroiditis and lupus erythematosus, respectively, and can be detected by particles coated with the appropriate antigen. C-reactive protein (the antigen) is detected by the reversed procedure in which the antibody is attached to the particle. A reversed passive agglutination procedure is also used to estimate the amount of gamma globulin in human blood. Passive hemagglutination inhibition, in which chorionic gonadotropin in the urine of pregnant females is used to impede the reaction between this hormone attached to erythrocytes and its antibody, is the basis for serologic pregnancy testing, undoubtedly one of the most frequently performed serologic tests in the clinical immunology laboratory.

FLOCCULATION TESTS

The term "flocculation" as used in immunology has a double meaning. It refers to a form of precipitation test and equally to a type of agglutination test. In the first sense, flocculation test refers to a precipitation with certain equine or similar antisera in which precipitation occurs over a relatively limited zone of antibody concentration. This is in contrast to human and rabbit antisera that tend to precipitate over a broader dilution range. In medical immunology, flocculation is applied more often in terms of its second meaning as a special variety of agglutination testing practiced in syphilis serology. Serologic test for syphilis (STS) takes many forms, but the preparation of one type of "antigen" embodies the admixture of cholesterol and lecithin with an alcoholic extract of beef heart (cardiolipin). The alcoholic extract is a crystal clear solution, but when it is diluted in buffer, it acquires a milky opalescence as the lipid constitutents become insoluble. Under a microscope, minute rod-shaped particles can be seen that coalesce to form large aggregates when incubated with sera from persons with syphilis. These flocculation tests show good agreement with the diagnosis of syphilis, but since the antigen is a nonspecific antigen in the sense that it has no antigenic relationship with *Treponema pallidum,* positive STS results are usually confirmed by a second test using specific treponemal-derived antigens.

COMPLEMENT FIXATION

The complement fixation test is founded on two critical properties of the complement system—its participation with certain immunoglobulins to produce immunolysis and its ability to participate in a serologic reaction even though not required for that reaction. In the performance of the test an awareness of the heat lability of complement and its presence in all sera are also important.

The discussion of complement fixation tests is simplified if the test is fragmented into its two overlapping halves—the test system and the indicator system (Fig. 6-8). The test system is comprised of an antigen

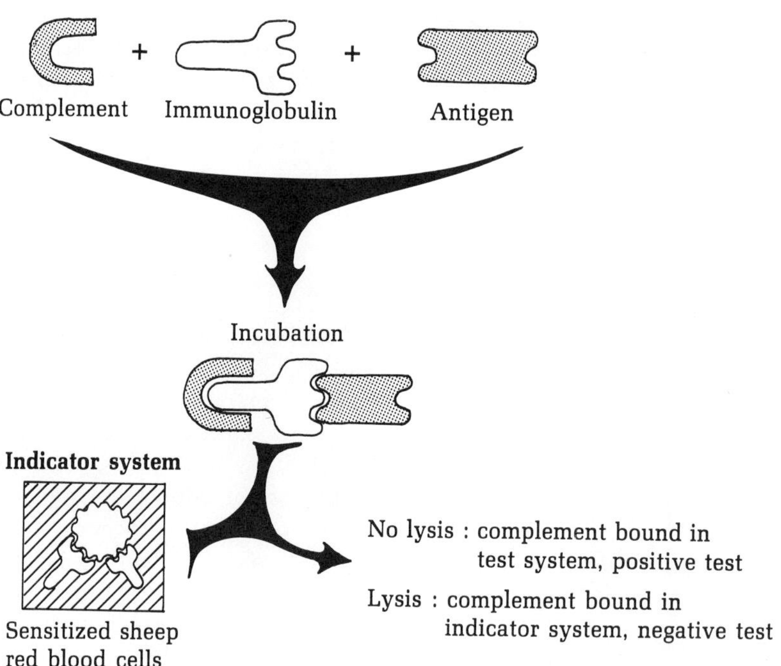

Fig. 6-8. Scheme of standard complement fixation test. When seeking to identify antibodies in a patient's serum, the serum is heat inactivated and incubated with the antigen and a standard quantity of complement. Thereafter, hemolysin and sheep erythrocytes are added. When complement is fixed in the test system, no hemolysis can occur; this is a positive test. In a negative test, hemolysis is observed because no antibody was present in the patient's serum to fix complement with the antigen, leaving the complement free to be fixed later in the indicator portion of the test.

and a patient's serum or dilutions of the serum believed to contain an antibody reactive with that antigen. When the test is designed to detect syphilis, the complement fixation test is known as the Wassermann test. The serum sample is held at 56° C for 30 minutes to destroy its complement. To the antigen and the serum a predetermined amount of complement in the form of normal guinea pig serum is added, and an incubation period is allowed. If the serum does contain antibodies, they will bind both the antigen and the complement. Then, when the indicator system of sheep red blood cells and an antibody directed against these cells (hemolysin) are added, there is no complement remaining to lyse the sheep red blood cells during a second incubation period. Conversely, if the patient's serum were devoid of antibody, there could be no serologic reaction in the test system, and complement would be free to catalyze the hemolytic reaction of the indicator system. The interpretation of the complement fixation test is lysis = negative test and no lysis = positive test.

Several aspects of the complement fixation test must be kept in mind. First of all, the complement present in the patient's serum and in the hemolysin preparation must be rendered inactive. Heating is the most certain way to do this. Since hemolysin is used at very high dilutions (1:15,000 would not be unusual) no special complement-destroying procedure is required. This is because most of the complement activity of a serum will vanish when the serum is diluted 1:250. (NOTE: These dilutions apply to macrocomplement fixation procedures, not microfixation methods or other special forms of the test.) Second, the amount of guinea pig complement must be accurately determined. If a large excess were added, there would still be free complement remaining to participate in the hemolytic reaction even after binding of most of the complement in the test system. Prior complement titrations ensure that this will not be the case. A third feature is that even in negative complement fixation tests, hemagglutination is not observed. It is true that hemolysin is nothing more than a sheep red blood cell hemagglutinin renamed to describe its function with complement, but the hemolysin is used at such high dilutions that display of its agglutinating ability is precluded. Immunolytic tests invariably require less antibody than agglutination tests. Another feature of the complement fixation test, which is perhaps too obvious to be noticed, is that complement is always fixed. If it is fixed in the test system, it is a positive test; if fixed in the indicator system, it is a negative test. Still a fifth point that should be emphasized is the great versatility of complement fixation tests. By using any of a vast series of antigens, many different antibodies can be detected. By using different known antisera, an array of antigens can be detected. By using dilutions of sera, antiserum titers can be determined and have been for poliomyelitis, measles, herpes, mumps, St. Louis encephalitis, smallpox, influenza, Eastern and Western equine encephalitis, coxsackievirus, and other viruses that do not lend themselves to other common serologic tests. Complement fixation has been utilized as an aid in the diagnosis of histoplasmosis, blastomycosis, coccidioidomycosis, and most widely of all, syphilis. Because so little antibody is required for a positive fixation test, it has been appreciated as a sensitive and accurate test. However, since the positive fixation test requires several reagents and is time-consuming to perform, it is being replaced by other sensitive procedures such as passive agglutination and radioimmunoassays.

NEUTRALIZATION

The principle of neutralization tests rests on the ability of an appropriate antiserum to diminsh or abolish some biologic property of the antigen other than its antigenicity—its toxicity or infectivity for cells or laboratory animals or its enzymatic activity. Neutralization tests are usually restricted to toxins, viruses, and enzyme or enzymelike antigens but can be performed with most infectious agents.

The lethal activity of tetanus and diphtheria toxins for common laboratory animals was important in defining the etiology and the means of preventing these diseases. Conversion of these toxins to toxoids by treatment with formaldehyde and the use of the toxoids in immunization induces the formation of specific toxin-neutralizing immunoglobulins known as antitoxins. These antitoxins and those to other bacterial exotoxins can be used to identify the corresponding toxin by the capacity of the antitoxin to protect a laboratory animal against the lethal activity of that specific toxin but not of other toxins. This is infrequently required in bacteriology, but it is applied to the identification of certain viruses isolated from patients. With a stock of known viruses, antibodies in a patient's serum (acute and convalescent samples) can also be defined. The antistreptolysin test, the ASO or ASTO test, is used to detect antibodies that appear in a person's serum as the result of an antecedent infection with group A streptococci and is an important clinical laboratory procedure.

CLINICAL CORRELATION

This chapter has presented a brief discussion of more than a dozen basic reactions of immunoglobulins with antigens and haptens. By varying the antigen or hapten these tests can be applied to many different medical problems, and that aspect of these tests has been mentioned in their description. Here a few comments on the frequency of which each test is performed seems appropriate. The data in the following table are approximates, based on a 300-bed private hospital and the clinical serology laboratory performance for 1 year.

Type of test	*No./Yr.*
STS	9200
Neutralization	750
Passive agglutination	400
Fluorescent antibody	180
Miscellaneous hemagglutination	150
Fluid precipitation	100
Miscellaneous	80
Bacterial agglutination	40
Crossed immunoelectrophoresis	25
Complement titrations and complement fixation	20

The large number of STS performed is characteristic of most laboratories. All pregnant women and blood donors are routinely screened. An RPR (rapid plasma reagin) or VDRL (Venereal Disease Research Laboratories) test is performed on virtually every blood specimen in most laboratories. The second most frequent tests are not included in this chapter but are discussed in Chapter 7. These are the hemagglutination tests associated with blood grouping and cross matching of blood; they exceeded 7100 for this laboratory. The neutralization tests represent the sum of rubella hemagglutination inhibition tests and antistreptolysin tests that were performed in a ratio of about 4:1. The rubella hemagglutination inhibition test is based on the capacity of rubella virus to agglutinate chicken red blood cells. This activity of the virus is neutralized by antiviral antibody. The passive hemagglutination tests (approximately 400/year) represent the sum of tests for rheumatoid arthritis, lupus erythematosus, and C-reactive protein, although many of the latter were determined by fluid precipitation. All of the 180 fluorescent antibody tests were for the confirmation of reactive STS results. The 180 miscellaneous hemagglutination tests were for heterophil antigens (Chapter 3) and cold agglutinins (Chapter 7). The miscellaneous group encompassed immunoelectrophoresis, radial immunodiffusion, Ouchterlony immunodiffusion, and several others. It should be noted that this laboratory does not perform radioimmunoassays; when the need arises for such tests, they are sent to a specialty laboratory in a metropolitan center.

A final word of caution—the frequency of serologic tests indicated here is not presented as anything more than an illustrative example. The patient population, the size and nature of the laboratory, physician preference for certain tests due to economy or rapidity, and the development or new tests are only a few of the factors that influenced the data.

BIBLIOGRAPHY

Bennett, C. W.: Clinical serology, Springfield, Ill., 1964, Charles C Thomas, Publisher.

Chase, M. W., and Williams, C. A., eds.: Methods in immunology and immunochemistry, New York, 1967-1971, Academic Press, Inc., vols. 1 to 3.

Clausen, J.: Immunochemical techniques for the identification and estimation of macromolecules, Amsterdam, 1971, North-Holland Publishing Co.

Crowle, A. J.: Immunodiffusion, ed. 2, New York, 1973, Academic Press, Inc.

Faulk, W. P.: Recent developments in immunofluorescence, Prog. Allergy **16**:9, 1972.

Grant, G. H., and Butt, W. R.: Immunochemical methods in clinical chemistry, Adv. Clin. Chem. **13**:383, 1970.

Holborow, E. J., Brighton, W. D., Sanders, G., and Taylor, C. E. D.: Standardization in immunofluorescence; a symposium, Oxford, 1970, Blackwell Scientific Publications, Ltd.

Jaffe, B. M., and Behrman, H. R., eds.: Methods of hormone radioimmunoassay, New York, 1974, Academic Press, Inc.

Kawamura, A., ed.: Fluorescent antibody techniques and their applications, Baltimore, 1969, University Park Press.

Mule, S. J., Sunshine, I., Braude, M., and Willette, R. E., eds.: Immunoassay for drugs subject to abuse, Cleveland, 1974, CRC Press.

Nakamura, R. M.: Immunopathology. Clinical laboratory concepts and methods, Boston, 1974, Little, Brown & Co.

Newton, W. T., and Donati, R. M.: Radioassay in clinical medicine, Springfield, Ill., 1974, Charles C Thomas, Publisher.

Parker, C. W.: Radioimmunoassays, Prog. Clin. Pathol. **4**:103, 1972.

Reynoso, G.: Competitive protein binding and radioimmunoassay, Chicago, 1972, American Society of Clinical Pathologists.

Rose, N. R., and Bigazzi, P. E., eds.: Methods in immunodiagnosis, New York, 1973, John Wiley & Sons, Inc.

Sternberger, L. A.: Immunocytochemistry, Englewood Cliffs, N.J., 1974, Prentice-Hall, Inc.

Verbruggen, R.: Quantitative immunoelectrophoretic methods: a literature survey, Clin. Chem. **21**:5, 1975.

Weir, D. M., ed.: Handbook of experimental immunology, ed. 2, Oxford, 1973, Blackwell Scientific Publications, Ltd.

Case histories

CASE 1. BACTERIAL AGGLUTINATION: BRUCELLOSIS

Paul M., a 26-year-old college student, entered the hospital because of nightime chills and sweats and a general feeling of malaise. These symptoms had been occurring for over a month, during which time he had felt tired and listless and had lost about 4 pounds. At the outset of the condition his temperature had reached 102° F on at least two occasions but recently had shown only modest elevation. His medical history indicated that he had visited his wife's parents and worked on their farm during the haying season. The physical examination was not especially informative—slight hepatosplenomegaly, no significant change in white blood cell counts, and a temperature of 101.4° F. Blood was drawn for bacteriologic cultures, and serum was collected for febrile agglutinins. An agglutinin titer for *Brucella abortus* of 1:640 and for *Francisella tularensis* of 1:40 was reported.

Questions

1. What organisms are used in tests for febrile agglutinins? What cross-reactions are of concern here?
2. Explain why acute and convalescent serum samples are not needed in this instance.
3. Of what potential significance is prozone in this case?
4. What is the relative role of serologic and bacteriologic diagnosis in this disease?

Discussion

The following organisms are employed in routine analyses for febrile agglutinins—*Salmonella typhosa,* O antigen; *S. typhosa,* H antigen; *S. paratyphi* A and B, H antigens; *B. abortus; F. (Pasteurella) tularensis;* and *Proteus* strains OX-K, OX-2, and OX-19.

The utility of the *Proteus* strains is restricted to the diagnosis of certain rickettsial diseases as indicated in the following.

Rickettsial disease	*Agglutination against:* OX-K	OX-2	OX-19
Q fever	−	−	−
Scrub typhus	+	−	−
Rocky Mountain spotted fever	−	+	+
Epidemic typhus	−	−	+

The agglutination reactions with *Proteus* strains, known as Weil-Felix reactions, are the result of the presence of a heterophil antigen common to these bacteria and to the rickettsia that are the etiologic agents of these diseases. Because of the difficulty in growing rickettsia and their high infectivity and virulence, it is much simpler to use agglutinins against these *Proteus* strains rather than the rickettsia as an index to infections caused by the latter group of organisms.

F. tularensis and *B. abortus* are included in the febrile antigen set because of the difficulty in isolating and identifying these bacteria that cause tularemia and brucellosis, respectively. *F. tularensis* contains a protein antigen shared with organisms in the genus *Brucella,* but the specificity of an antiserum can be distinguished by comparative agglutination tests. Although brucellosis in man may be caused by *B. abortus, B. melitensis,* or *B. suis,* only the former is included in the febrile antigen kit because these three species share two antigens, the A and M antigens, and *B. abortus* is the most encountered species in the United States.

The antigenic formulas of the three *Salmonella* species used are as follows:

S. typhosa	9, 12, Vi	d
S. paratyphi A	1, 2, 12	a
S. paratyphi B	1, 4, 5, 12	b(1,2)

The multitudinous species of *Salmonella* that cause human disease precludes the use of a large battery of organisms in the febrile antigen set. These are used because of their incidence of disease in the United States. Cross-reactions among the *Salmonella* are extensive, cloud the diagnostic meaning of antibodies in patient sera, and depend on both somatic and flagellar antigens. Antibodies directed against the O antigens are generally accepted as of greater diagnostic significance than H agglutinins, which tend to persist longer following disease or immunization. Eventually the H antigens may be dropped from the set for this reason.

Due to the chronicity of brucellosis, antibodies are generally present in the patient's serum by the time he seeks medical attention. Suspected brucellosis is thus one example of an exception to the usual demand for acute and convalescent serum samples. The agglutinin titer of persons with brucellosis is generally high and remains high during and after the disease. Titers of 1:160 can persist for several months after the disease. Titers greater than 1:2560 are not unusual during active disease. Even higher titers are encountered (also in tularemia), and in rare instances a prozone has been known to produce negative slide tests and extend through the usual nine tubes of the dilution series for tube agglutination tests. In the face of overwhelming clinical support for the diagnosis of brucellosis and negative serology, the clinician should suggest a retest with an extended dilution series to exclude prozone phenomena. Although the inability to secure an acute serum sample hinders a satisfactory serologic diagnosis, serologic data plus a suitable medical history and clinical symptoms are used in the diagnosis of brucellosis more frequently than bacterial isolation.

Paul M. had an agglutination titer of 1:1280 with the *B. abortus* antigen, 1:160 with *F. tularensis,* and 1:20 with all other antigens. These results were considered compatible with a diagnosis of brucellosis, and proper antibiotic therapy was initiated. Health authorities in the county in which his in-laws farmed were notified of this diagnosis on the assumption that they would check cattle and workers on the farm for brucellosis.

REFERENCES

Bennett, C. W.: Clinical serology, Springfield, Ill., 1964, Charles C Thomas, Publisher.

Schroeder, S.: Interpretation of serologic tests for typhoid fever, J.A.M.A. **206**:839, 1968.

Spink, W. W.: The nature of brucellosis, Minneapolis, 1956, University of Minnesota Press.

Spink, W. W., McCullough, N. B., Hutchings, L. M., and Mingle, C. K.: Diagnostic criteria for human brucellosis, J.A.M.A. **149**:805, 1952.

CASE 2. SEROLOGIC TESTING FOR PREGNANCY

Mrs. M. D., a 30-year-old white female, arranged an appointment with her family physician to determine if she was pregnant. Two earlier pregnancies had terminated by spontaneous abortion. A urine sample was collected and the patient was informed that the results would be communicated to her the next afternoon.

Questions

1. Discuss pregnancy testing from the serologic viewpoint.
2. What are the advantages of serologic pregnancy tests?

Discussion

Serologic testing for pregnancy is based on the interference of human chorionic gonadotropin (HCG) in urine or serum with a passive agglutination test between the hormone attached to latex particles or erythrocytes and its antiserum. HCG is a hormone excreted by the placenta that appears in the blood and urine early in pregnancy. The urinary level is high enough to detect it serologically about 41 days after the onset of the last menstrual period or 10 to 14 days after the first missed menses. The hormone can be detected by its stimulation of ovulation in rabbits (Friedman's test) or in rats or mice (Aschheim-Zondek test). Such tests require pathologic examination of the animals and suffer from a 17% rate of false negative results. Since HCG has a molecular weight of 30,000 and is a protein, its antigenicity permitted the development of the more sensitive, accurate, and inexpensive serologic test.

The antigen used in the test is HCG attached to latex spherules, which are used in the slide test, or attached to erythroctyes, which are used in tube tests. The urine sample should be free of protein and not grossly contaminated with bacteria. The urine is incubated briefly with the antiserum before adding HCG-latex antigen. The urine of a pregnant woman containing HCG neutralizes the antibody, thus leaving the latex antigen unagglutinated. Urine of a nonpregnant woman produces the opposite result. This is a simple observation and can be accurately read by inexperienced technicians using either the tube or slide method. Passive agglutination tests have the required sensitivity to detect minute quantities of the hormone in urine.

False positive tests are possible if the urine contains protein or in certain neoplasms of the female reproductive system —hydatidiform mole or choriocarcinoma— that excrete HCG. Titers of HCG in urine in excess of 1:128 suggest a neoplastic condition, since normal urine titers for pregnant women seldom exceed 1:16. The test will be negative in ectopic pregnancy and will tend toward weak positive or negative reactions in the second and third trimesters of pregnancy when hormone secretion diminishes. By this time other diagnostic criteria for pregnancy are very reliable.

REFERENCES

Bennett, C. W.: Clinical serology, Springfield, Ill., 1964, Charles C Thomas, Publisher.

Olson, A. M., and Adducci, J. E.: An evaluation of the latex flocculation test for the diagnosis of pregnancy, Am. J. Clin. Pathol. **39**:589, 1963.

Raj, G. M. G., Bayron, N., Waltman, R., and Green, R.: Two-hour immunodiagnostic pregnancy tests: evaluation in 1105 cases, Curr. Ther. Res. **5**:273, 1963.

CASE 3. TOXOPLASMOSIS AND IMMUNOFLUORESCENCE

The patient, a white, unnamed, newborn male infant, had a rash, yellow pigmented skin, hydrocephaly, and chorioretinitis. No significant abnormalities were observed in the mother. The family history had not included previous hydrocephalic births or abortion. The family had a pet cat, taken into the family about 4 months before the infant's birth. A serum sample was collected from the mother and sent to the clinical serology laboratory with a request for a fluorescent antibody test for toxoplasmosis. The report was returned 2 days later as 1:256.

Questions

1. What is the nature and source of the antigen?
2. Is a direct or indirect fluorescent antibody procedure used, and what are the relative merits of each?
3. Explain why the indirect hemagglutination test was not required.
4. What is the interpretation of the results of the immunofluorescent, hemagglutination, and dye exclusion test for toxoplasmosis?
5. What is the interpretation of the fluorescent antibody test in the absence of paired serum samples?

Discussion

Toxoplasmosis is a congenital or acquired infection of mammals by *Toxoplasma gondii,* an intracellular protozoan. Close contact with cats or their waste products is a source of human infection. Infections of adults may be asymptomatic, since serologic surveys have revealed a high prevalence of toxoplasma antibodies. The most damaging effects of toxoplasmosis are fetal infections that may result in spontaneous abortion or extensive defects, including mental retardation, encephalitis, blindness, and hydrocephaly, in surviving infants.

Three serologic tests have been applied extensively to the serologic diagnosis of toxoplasmosis—the Sabin-Feldman dye exclusion test, the indirect or passive hemagglutination test, and the indirect fluorescent antibody technique, although complement fixation and skin tests have also been tried.

The Sabin-Feldman dye test is impractical. It requires the maintenance of *T. gondii* in mouse ascites fluid as a source of the viable protozoan, which is quite hazardous in addition to being expensive and time-consuming. Mixtures of antibodies and complement with the organisms makes them refractory to staining with methylene blue. Counting of the stained and unstained parasites is time-consuming and laborious. The test is sensitive but has been replaced by immunofluorescence.

The passive hemagglutination test is being evaluated by the National Center for Disease Control. At the present time only the fluorescent antibody test is performed in the routine clinical laboratory. Reagents needed for the test, which are commercially available, are *T. gondii* and a fluorescein-conjugated antihuman globulin. The parasites can be purchased as formalin-killed organisms and should be fixed to slides at a density of 50 to 100 organisms per high-power field. The antiglobulin serum can be

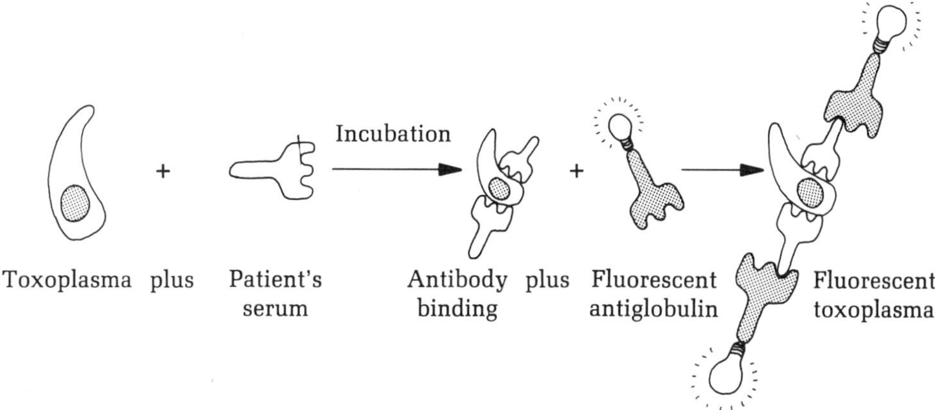

Fig. 6-9. Positive fluorescent antibody test for *Toxoplasma gondii* antibodies. The test was of the indirect type.

purchased in a lyophilized form and rehydrated when needed. Some preparations contain Evans blue, Congo red, or some other dye to serve as a counterstain and reduce autofluorescence. As this choice of reagents indicates, the test is an indirect test. It is desirable to conduct both positive as well as negative controls. Positive tests can be performed with sera saved from both high- and low-titered samples determined by previous testing or purchased from commercial sources. Fluorescent antibody titers of 1:512 are considered high; titers of 1:16 or lower are usually considered negative; and titers between 1:16 and 1:64 are of dubious importance due to the prevalence of this disease. The titer is expressed as the greatest dilution of the patient's serum that exhibits true fluorescence around the periphery of 50% of the cells. When fluorescein is the fluorochrome used, a positively stained organism will stain yellow-green, and when Evans blue is the counterstain, unstained organisms will appear red (Fig. 6-9).

Evaluation of the immunofluorescent test has proved that it is probably of slightly superior diagnostic efficiency than passive hemagglutination procedures because it will detect antibodies a little earlier in the disease; that is, it is more sensitive. Diagnostically significant titers must often be accepted from a single serum sample, and these were mentioned previously. Up to 30% of the population will have titers of less than 1:32. This may be interpreted as past exposure or recent disease and indicates the need for a retest in 7 to 14 days.

REFERENCES

Fletcher, S.: Indirect fluorescent antibody technique in the serology of *Toxoplasma gondii*, J. Clin. Pathol. **18**:193, 1965.

U.S. Department of Health, Education and Welfare: Indirect fluorescent antibody test for toxoplasmosis, Atlanta, 1970, Center for Disease Control.

Walton, B. C., Benchoff, B. M., and Brooks, W. H.: Comparison of the indirect fluorescent antibody test and the methylene blue dye test for detection of antibodies to *Toxoplasma gondii*, Am. J. Trop. Med. Hyg. **15**:149, 1966.

CASE 4. SEROLOGIC TESTING FOR SYPHILIS

H. N., a 17-year-old female, consulted her physician because of a skin rash that was generally distributed over her body. Her axillae were rather free from the rash. Since the rash was not anatomically restricted, contact dermatitis was excluded. The distribution did not correspond to poison ivy, cosmetics, antiperspirants, hair dye, etc. Further physical examination revealed enlargement of the lymph nodes and mucous patches in the mouth. Although she initially claimed sexual virginity, after an explanation of the potential dangers of untreated syphilis she admitted to sexual contact. She had never had a primary chancre to her knowledge. A blood sample was collected for STS. It was reported as RPR reactive, VDRL reactive, and FAB reactive.

Questions

1. What STS are currently recommended?
2. What is the nature of the antigen in these tests?
3. What is syphilitic reagin? How does it differ from allergic reagin?
4. What organisms share antigens with *Treponema pallidum* and how does this influence STS results?
5. What immunity, if any, develops to syphilis?

Discussion

Syphilis is caused by *T. pallidum,* which is transmitted sexually. In primary syphilis a hard chancre appears at the site of entry 10 to 30 days after contact. If unrecognized and untreated, the disease progresses to a secondary stage. This may encompass skin rash, oral mucous patches, lesions in the eye, bone, and joints, and lymphadenopathy. The original chancre has disappeared by this time. Tertiary syphilis follows, and this can assume protean forms—neurosyphilis, dermal cutaneous ulceration, visceral gummatous lesions, etc.

The antibody response to syphilis is of two types: (1) the formation of the biologically nonspecific but clinically useful reagin and (2) the formation of specific antibodies to *T. pallidum.* Syphilitic reagin, also known as the Wassermann antibody, is a macroglobulin antibody of the IgM class clearly distinct from allergic reagin, which is an IgE. It is believed that most of the reagin response is toward nonspecific antigens of mammalian tissue. Specific antitreponemal antibodies are of the IgG class.

Historically, since *T. pallidum* could not be cultivated in laboratory media, it was believed that fetuses aborted because of intrauterine syphilis would be the best available source of the antigen. Extracts of syphilitic liver were used as the antigen until it was discovered that alcoholic extracts of normal liver, heart, or other organs would serve equally well. Most antigens in present-day use begin with an alcoholic extract of beef heart (cardiolipin), which is stabilized by the addition of lecithin and cholesterol. Cardiolipin is a hapten, a diphosphatidyl glycerol, that is relatively anticomplementary; that is, it inactivates complement without combination with antibody. Supplements of lecithin neutralize this anticomplementary activity. Addition of cholesterol improves the complement fixing capacity of the cardiolipin with reagin. It has been suggested that the reagin portion of the immune response to syphilis is actually an autoimmune response to damaged tissue lipoproteins and that cardiolipin is the hapten part of the parent antigen. Another possibility is that tissue lipids combine with the spirochete to form the complete antigen. The reagin formed in response to this still uncharacterized antigen appears early in the disease, usually in the first 21 days, and 30% of the cases are positive after 1 week. Thereafter, 85% to 100% of sera from patients with syphilis will be positive at least until latency occurs and the positive percentage dwindles. Patients treated in the primary stage become STS negative about 6 months after successful treatment. Negative test results may not develop for 12 to 18 months after secondary syphilis is cured and not at all after tertiary syphilis. Loss of STS positivity is attributed largely to the loss of the IgM antibody.

False positive STS has been associated with many infectious diseases—tuberculosis, scarlet fever, malaria, smallpox, and autoimmune diseases such as lupus erythematosus. These are believed to be due to the tissue damage associated with these diseases.

STS refers to the flocculation tests or complement fixation tests with cardiolipin antigen. Presently recommended are the VDRL modification and the RPR tests. If either of these is positive, it is repeated or confirmed with the other flocculation test and with a specific treponemal antibody test.

Several forms of specific antitreponemal tests are available—agglutination lysis, immobilization, complement fixation, and immunofluorescent, with the latter being the confirmatory test of choice. It is an indirect fluorescent antibody procedure employing slides to which *T. pallidum* organisms are fixed. Since the agent of the disease is used as the antigen, it is a highly specific test. Other treponemal diseases such as yaws or pinta may cause positive results due to antigenic sharing between different treponemes. False positive test results associated with autoimmune diseases are also recognized. Once a person is positive for one of the specific tests, the positive status continues essentially for a lifetime.

Vaccines for syphilis have been of great interest due to the high incidence and national cost of syphilis. Recurrent human syphilis suggests that it will be difficult to develop a suitable vaccine, and heretofore animal experiments have been disappointing.

REFERENCES

Bennett, C. W.: Clinical serology, Springfield, Ill., 1964, Charles C Thomas, Publisher.

Harris, A., Rosenberg, A. A., and Riedel, L. M.: A microflocculation test for syphilis using cardiolipin antigen, J. Vener. Dis. Inform. **27**: 169, 1946.

U.S. Public Health Service: Serologic tests for syphilis, Washington, D.C., 1969, U.S. Government Printing Office.

Wilkenson, A. E., and Rayner, C. F. A.: Studies on the fluorescent treponemal antibody, (FTA-ABS) test, Br. J. Vener. Dis. **42**:8, 1966.

chapter 7

Immunohematology

The alloantigens of human erythrocytes are far more important on a daily medical basis than any other antigens. Hardly a patient entering a hospital or other major medical service escapes the routine blood grouping tests. Almost the entire basis of successful blood banking rests on a knowledge of immunohematology and a few blood-borne infectious diseases. Most forms of hemolytic disease of the newborn, most blood transfusion problems, and certain medicolegal situations that demand the identification of blood stains are amenable to suitable prophylaxis and therapeusis, or interpretation, when correct immunohematologic principles are applied. Erythrocyte antigens and their antibodies are of importance in tissue transplantation immunity, where they are the first line of histocompatibility checking, although erythrocyte antigens are not histocompatibility antigens per se.

ABO(H) ANTIGENS

The major human blood group, the ABO(H) blood group system (Table 7-1), is founded on the inheritance of two antigens, the A and B antigens. The immunodominant portion of the A and the B antigens is a terminal oligosaccharide located on a protein situated in the red blood cell membrane. The A and B antigens arise from a precursor substance (Fig. 7-1) that serves as a core for other erythrocyte antigens as well. In fact, there are two variations in the structure of the core, one of which is a D-galactosyl β-1,3-*N*-acetyl-D-glucosaminyl β-1,3-D-galactosyl β-1,3-*N*-acetyl-D-galactosamine. The other tetrasaccharide core substance is composed of exactly the same four sugars, but the galactose-*N*-acetylglucosamine bond is a β-1, 4 linkage rather than a 1,3 linkage. In either case the polysaccharide core is merely the immunodominant terminal portion of a large glycoprotein molecule. An additional monosaccharide is added to the core to create the pentasaccharide known as the H substance. The H substance is present on all human erythrocytes and has a fucose linked to the final D-galactose unit by an α-1,2-glycosidic bond. To form the A antigen an *N*-acetyl-D-galactosamine is attached to the same galactose via an α-1, 3 bond, and the B antigen is formed by adding a D-galactose by an α-1,3 bond to this terminal galactose. The A and B antigens are either present independent of each other (groups A and B), together (group AB), or not formed from the H substance (group O). Biochemically, a group O person can be described as lacking the requisite galactosyl transferases to form the B antigen and lacking the galactosylamino transferase needed to form the A antigen. Obviously the blood group AB person has both of these enzymes, and the A and B persons have one or the other of the transferases.

The ABO(H) antigens are structurally very similar to the Lewis (Le) blood group antigens. The Le^a antigen has a fucose attached to the core acetyl glucosamine unit by an α-1,4 bond, and the Le^b antigen has this same addition to the H substance. Special fucosyl transferases are required to form these antigens.

ABO(H) SYSTEM

Karl Landsteiner received a Nobel Prize in Medicine and Physiology in 1930 for

Precursor substance

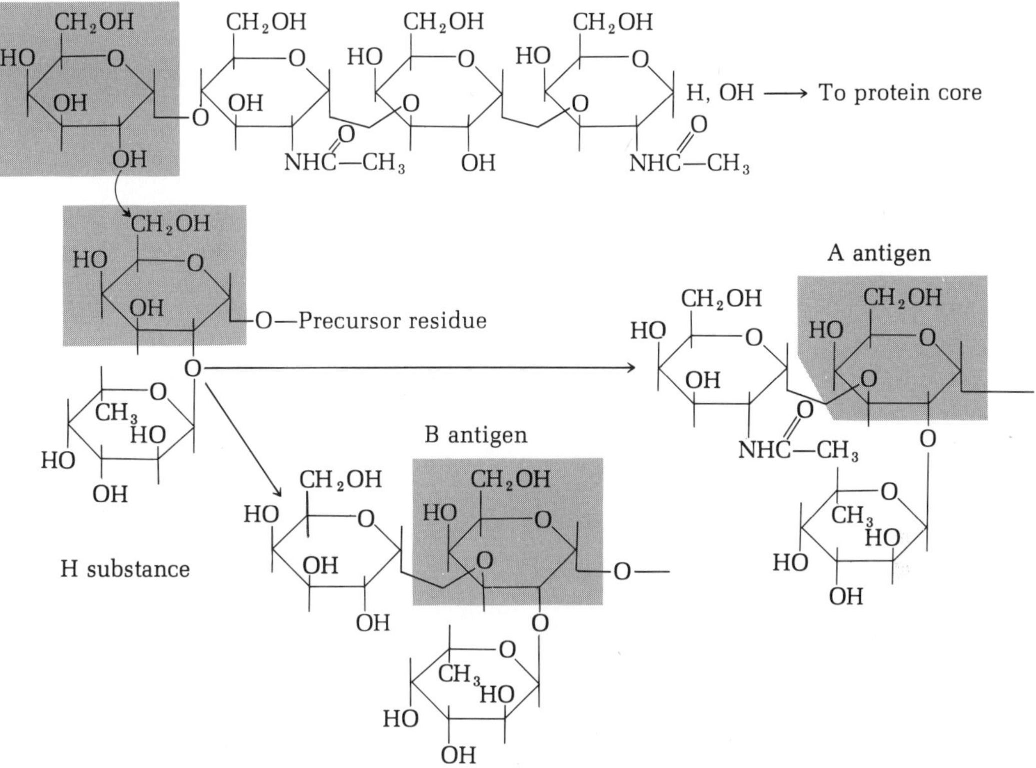

Fig. 7-1. Upper structure is the terminal or immunodominant polysaccharide portion of the ABO(H) precursor molecule. Addition of fucose to the terminal galactose of the precursor creates H substance. Addition of a galactose residue to the terminal galactose of the H substance produces the B antigen. The A antigen is produced when acetylgalactosamine is added.

Table 7-1. ABO(H) blood group system

Blood group (phenotype)	*Antigen on erythrocytes*	*Antibody in serum*	*Distribution (%)*	*Genotype*
A	A	Anti-B	42	AA or AO
B	B	Anti-A	10	BB or BO
O(H)	H	Anti-A and anti-B	45	OO
AB	A and B	Neither	3	AB

discoveries he initiated 30 years earlier in human blood group immunology. Landsteiner collected the erythrocytes and serum from the blood of several of his laboratory associates, incubated each red cell suspension with each serum, and observed these mixtures for hemagglutination. He never observed a person's serum to agglutinate his own erythrocytes, but he did observe hemagglutination in a number of the reciprocal mixtures. From these results he erected the four ABO(H) blood groups in Table 7-1. The blood group A person was described as having the antigen arbitrarily assigned the letter A on his erythrocytes, and the group B person was described as having a different antigen, given the letter B, on his erythrocytes. The sera of an individual from one of these groups would clump the red blood cells of persons in the other group, and the sera from an individual in either of these groups would clump the cells of a person in a third, the AB group. These reactions were compatible with the presence of an antibody, anti-B in group A sera and anti-A in group B sera. The AB person possesses both of the corresponding antigens on his red cells that are agglutinated by both sera. The fourth group, group O, has neither the A nor B antigen but has both anti-A and anti-B in their sera.

The distribution of the ABO(H) antigens varies from one ethnic or racial group to another, but in the United States average figures are 45% group O, 42% group A, 10% group B, and 3% group AB. American blacks are about 28% group A and 20% group B, with a similar incidence of O and AB as in the population as a whole.

Subgroups of the A, B, and O(H) antigens are known, but the frequency of the B and H variants is so rare as to be of little practical importance. The two most frequent of the A subgroups are designated as A_1 and A_2, and these are present in a ratio of about 80:20. The A_1 cells are believed to possess two antigens, A_1 and A_2, which makes them easily agglutinable by all anti-A sera. Subgroup A_2 cells are considered to possess only the A_2 antigen and hence are more feebly agglutinated by anti-A sera than are A_1 cells, since only one antibody in the antiserum can function.

It has been estimated that as many as 1,000,000 A or B antigenic sites may be present on a single red blood cell, although a figure of 500,000 is probably more realistic. The antigens appear early in fetal life as soon as the red cells are formed and may be found in a soluble form in the body fluids of approximately 78% of the population. Secretion of soluble A, B, or O(H) substances into saliva, serum, urine, gastric juice, etc. is regulated by Se, a dominant gene. The synthesis of the A, B, or O(H) antigens is also a genetic characteristic. Group O persons are homozygotic and are genotypically OO, while AB persons are genetically AB heterozygotes. Group A and B persons may be either homozygotes (AA and BB) or heterozygotes (AO or BO). Inheritance of these genes is by simple mendelian genetics, a fact that can be of considerable importance in forensic medicine.

ABO(H) ANTIBODIES

One of the uncertainties concerning the ABO(H) blood group system regards the origin of these alloantibodies. These antibodies (of the IgM class) are barely detectable in the sera of newborn infants but increase rapidly in titer in the first few months of life. This fact has been used to evaluate the maturation rate of the "bursal equivalent" in infants. Since there is a stepwise development of these antibodies, it has been suggested that inapparent immunizations in infancy and early childhood may be responsible for the production of anti-A or anti-B. It is a well-known fact that many intestinal bacteria that are a part of the normal flora *(Escherichia coli)* and certain intestinal pathogens in the genus *Salmonella* and *Shigella* have polysaccharide antigens that cross-react with the human ABO(H) antigens. According to this hypothesis, all infants are exposed to both the A and B antigens. A group A person forms only anti-B and not anti-A, because his own A antigen has conferred a specific immunologic tolerance on him in this regard. Similar logic would explain the formation of the other antibodies.

Artificial immunization with the ABO(H) antigens produces a strong IgM response that is later superseded by IgG antibodies. Such antibodies were formerly used to identify blood as belonging to a specific blood group, but the discovery that extracts of leguminous plant seeds (peas, beans, etc.)

contain substances that will agglutinate human erythrocytes has led to an inexpensive substitute for the use of immune sera. The phytohemagglutinin from the common vetch *(Vicia crassa)* is a highly specific lectin for the group A antigen. Several H-specific lectins are known, but these are of little practical importance due to the uniform distribution of this antigen. Recently a specific anti-B lectin from *Bandieraea simplicifolia* has been described that may assume significance in blood banking.

HEMAGGLUTINATION

The combination of lectins or antibodies with red blood cells of the proper antigenic constitution ordinarily results in hemagglutination, but if complement is present and the correct class of immunoglobulin is involved, hemolysis instead of hemagglutination may be observed. Unfortunately there are circumstances in which neither are observed, even when the test has been conducted under standard conditions. This is due to two separate phenomena: the prevalence of cold agglutinins and incomplete agglutinins in antierythrocyte sera. It is not uncommon for IgM hemagglutinins to display an unusual thermal requirement, functioning much better at 25° C or even 4° C than at 37° C, where they are virtually inactive. When positive hemagglutination tests performed at 4° C with these antisera are warmed to 37° C, the agglutinated cells become dispersed and the positive test becomes negative (Fig. 7-2). The laboratory technician must be aware of this behavior of cold agglutinins, which may make an important contribution to certain disease states.

IgG antibodies are less frequently cold agglutinins, but they may behave as incomplete antibodies that combine satisfactorily with their respective antigen and yet fail to continue into the aggregative phase of the serologic reaction and in this case fail to exhibit hemagglutination. The terms "incomplete" or "monovalent" antibodies have been applied to these immunoglobulins with the obvious inference that these globulins were structurally incomplete, possibly possessing only a single Fab segment, and physically unable to bridge and unify two erythrocytes. There is no evidence that this is the case; these antibodies appear to be structurally identical to complete agglutinins. Either by a failure to alter the repelling surface charge on erythrocytes or some other unknown biophysical irregularity, these antibodies attach but do not agglutinate erythrocytes. The combination of these antibodies with the red blood cell antigen is easily proved by antiglobulin tests. The British immunologist R. R. A. Coombs advanced this test in immunohematology, and his name is often

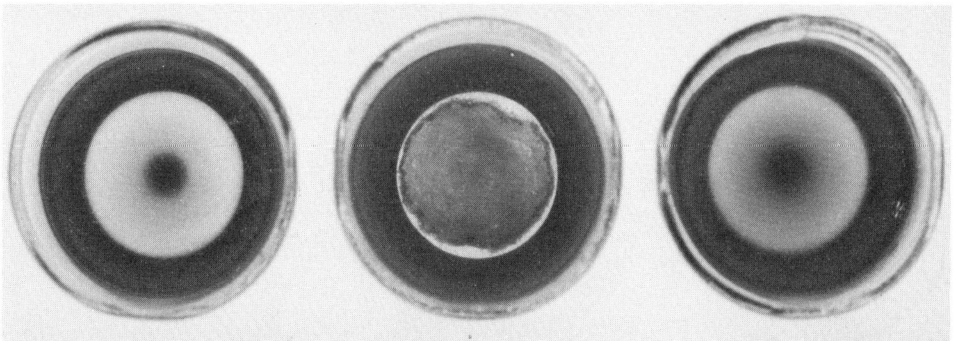

Fig. 7-2. Hemagglutination tests are often interpreted on the basis of the appearance of the cell-settling pattern. Here each end tube represents a negative test, and the center tube represents a positive test.

used to refer to the test. As described in the previous chapter, antiglobulin tests rely on the activity of a primary antibody serving in the dual capacity of an antibody and an antigen for the antiglobulin. In the Coombs test the addition of an antiglobulin to antibody-coated erythrocytes causes hemagglutination.

Rh SYSTEM

The Rh factor was originally described as an antigen common to 85% of all human erythrocytes, those of Rh-positive persons, and those of the rhesus monkey. Naturally occurring Rh alloantibodies are not present in the Rh-negative person in the sense that blood group O persons have anti-A and anti-B; so the Rh system was not discovered by cross testing human red cells and sera. The Rh system was discovered by hemagglutination testing of rabbit anti-monkey red blood cell sera with human erythrocytes, and this was not done until 40 years after the discovery of the ABO(H) system. It is now clear that there is an assembly of Rh antigens rather than one antigen. Rh antigen D, also known as Rh_0 or Rh1, is the original Rh antigen, and it still remains one of the most important (Table 7-2).

The original alphabetical designation of the Rh antigens, which used both lower- and uppercase letters C, D, E, c, d, e, etc., has fallen into disfavor. It is being replaced by the Wiener nomenclature system in which Rh in upper- or lowercase letters, supplemented by subscripts and superscripts, is employed. The move to adopt a new naming system stems in part from the fact that Wiener's hypothesis for the inheritance of the Rh antigens, which used his nomenclature, has proved to be more acceptable genetically than other hypotheses.

The chemistry of the Rh antigens is largely unknown. It is probable that the immunodominant portions are polysaccharides, and that neuraminic acid and other common saccharides are a part of their structure. The important question of how these saccharides are joined by glycosidic bonds is under investigation. These antigens are much less numerous on the red cell surface than the A and B antigens, probably being represented only 10,000 to 20,000 times.

Table 7-2. Major human blood group systems*

System	*Number of important antigens*	*Major antigens*
ABO(H)	4	A, B, H, and A subgroups
Rh	33	Rh_0 (D), hr′ (c), rh′ (C), hr″ (e), rh″ (E), etc.
MN	29	M, N, S, s, M^A, M^C, U, etc.
P	4	P_1, P_2
I	5	I, i
Kell	10	K, k
Lewis	6	Le^a, Le^b, Le^c

*Other well-known systems include Lutheran, Duffy, and Kidd.

Immunoglobulins directed against the Rh antigens do not differ significantly from antibodies against other red cell antigens. Except as mentioned, the alloantibodies arise from known immunizations and do not occur "naturally." One source of human anti-Rh antibodies is the Rh-negative person who has been immunized by a blood transfusion with Rh-positive blood. (For simplicity Rh positive in this discussion refers to the Rh_0 (D) antigen. Since all human beings possess one or another of the Rh antigens, all could be described as being Rh positive. However, the D antigen, which is one of the most potent Rh antigens, is accorded the honor of being referred to as the Rh factor.) Another route of immunization is by exposure of an Rh-negative mother to the blood of her Rh-positive child during birth. As many as 50% of the mothers in some studies were shown to have fetal erythrocytes in their circulation shortly after delivery. Abortion under similar circumstances (Rh-positive child and Rh-negative mother) could also be an immunizing experience.

Rh HEMOLYTIC DISEASE OF THE NEWBORN

When a pregnant Rh-negative woman has circulating anti-Rh_0 simultaneously with an Rh_0-positive fetus, the stage is set for the development of erythroblastosis fetalis. The Rh-positive child must be the result of its inheritance of the Rh_0 antigen from its father, since the mother is Rh negative. Such marriages are described as Rh incompatible, since only this type of mating can lead to the conception of Rh-positive children. If the father is homozygous, all children would be Rh positive, and if he is heterozygous, statistically 50% of the children would be Rh positive and at risk for erythroblastosis. Erythroblastosis is an alloimmune disease caused by the placental transmigration of maternal IgG that is specific for fetal erythrocytes. Usually this means anti-Rh_0, but hemolytic disease of the newborn due to maternal IgG specific for other erythrocyte antigens can occur. Simple ABO(H) incompatibilities seldom lead to neonatal hemolytic disease unless the mother has been hyperimmunized and has a high level of IgG. The usual ABO(H) allohemagglutinin is an IgM that cannot transgress the placental barrier.

When the maternal anti-Rh_0 IgG enters the fetal circulation and combines with the Rh-positive erythrocytes, the presence of complement ensures that lysis of the fetal erythrocytes will follow (Fig. 7-3). Imma-

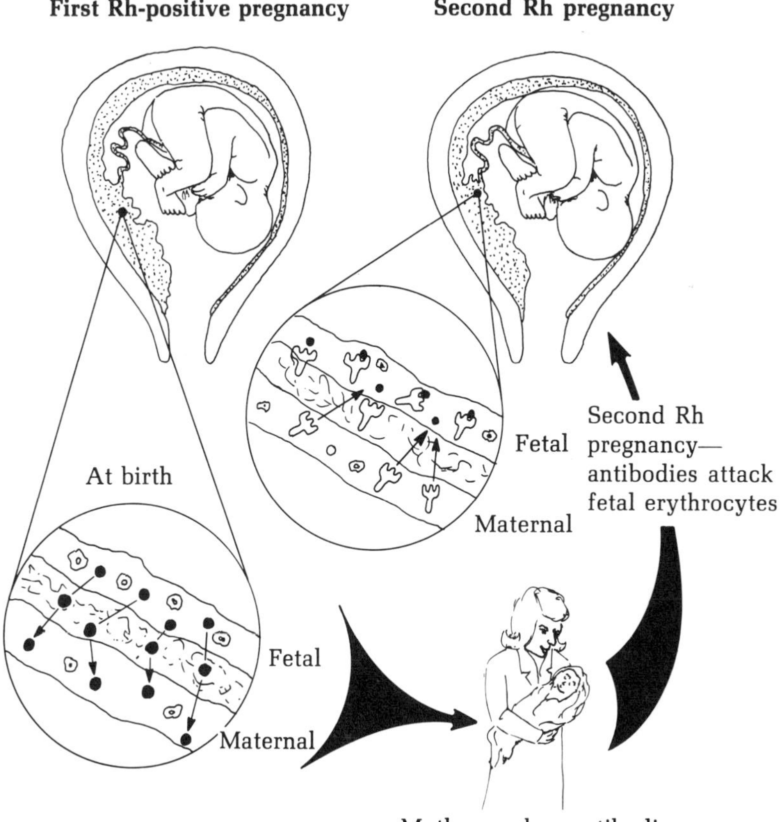

Fig. 7-3. Erythroblastosis fetalis is the result of maternal immunization to fetal erythrocytes in a first pregnancy, usually at birth, followed by the transplacental migration of these antibodies to attack fetal red blood cells in a subsequent pregnancy.

ture erythrocytes (erythroblasts) enter the circulation to compensate for the loss of the mature red blood cells, creating the condition of erythroblastosis fetalis. This may terminate the pregnancy in a stillbirth or a live abortion, or in milder cases the child may not give much evidence of the disease until the first hours after birth during its physiologic adjustment period and this may be no more serious than a mild jaundice which fades in a few days.

Coombs' testing

To determine if the mother has antibodies against Rh antigens, it is only necessary to incubate a portion of her sera with Rh-positive cells and observe for hemagglutination by complete antibodies. Since incomplete antibodies are potentially as destructive in vivo as complete antibodies, a determination for their presence in maternal sera is a must. This is accomplished by the indirect Coombs test, which requires two incubation steps. The first of these is the incubation of maternal sera with Rh-positive cells, and in the absence of agglutination at this stage, a second incubation with antihuman gamma globulin is conducted. A positive result after this second incubation is taken as proof that the mother has anti-Rh globulins that could cause erythroblastosis fetalis (Fig. 7-4).

In the case of the newborn infant who is developing jaundice or other signs of hemolytic disease the direct Coombs test is useful (Fig. 7-4). In this test, erythro-

Direct Coombs test

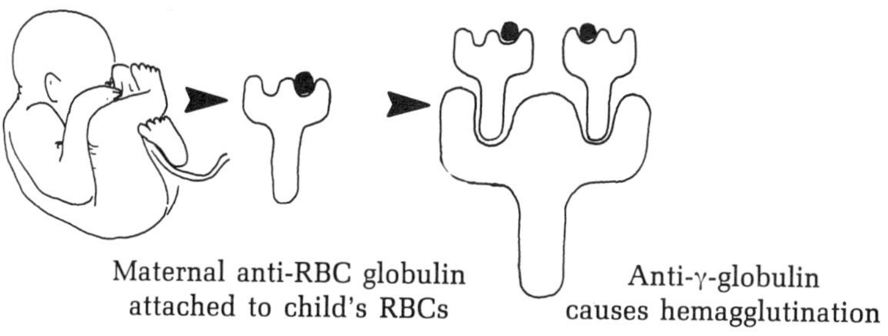

Indirect Coombs test

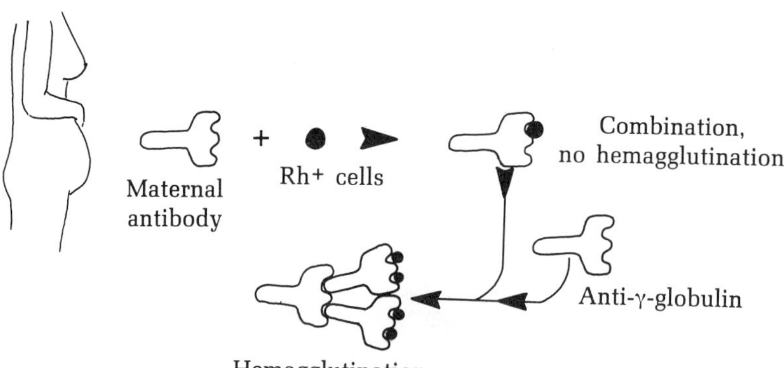

Fig. 7-4. The direct Coombs test is positive when erythrocytes precoated with a nonagglutinating antibody are incubated with an antiglobulin. In the indirect test, maternal or other sources of nonagglutinating antibody must be preincubated with the red cells prior to incubation with antiglobulin.

cytes of the neonate are exposed to antiglobulin sera and observed for hemagglutination. In this case only one incubation period is necessary, since the first incubation was performed in vivo.

Immunoprophylaxis

The problem, of course, is what medical steps to take in view of a positive indirect Coombs test. In the case of a positive direct Coombs tests an exchange transfusion may be indicated, but positive indirect tests, especially when noted early in a pregnancy, constitute a difficult medical problem. As with most situations the prevention is simpler than the cure, and the prevention of Rh immunization of women is a superb example of how basic immunologic studies have contributed to the practical solution of a serious medical situation. It will be recalled that the passive administration of an antiserum to an antigen, simultaneous with the antigen, will block the formation of antibodies to that antigen —a form of immunoglobulin-induced immunosuppression. To this knowledge was added the information that blood group O Rh-negative mothers had fewer infants with hemolytic disease than statistics would predict, and it was surmised that their maternal anti-A and anti-B combined with any A Rh-positive or B Rh-positive fetal erythrocytes and hastened their removal from the maternal circulation without antibody formation. Evidence was already accumulating that most maternal immunizations with Rh antigens were occurring at childbirth; therefore, if anti-Rh_0 were administered just after birth, it should prevent maternal immune sensitization to the antigen. This was tested and proved to be a tremendous success. In one study 173 mothers were given the antibody, and one became immunized at birth. In the control group of 176 mothers not given anti-Rh_0, 38 developed anti-Rh_0. Administration of anti-Rh_0 is now considered a regular part of perinatal care. It must be given at the first and every succeeding pregnancy; once the woman has formed the antibodies (which is also possible from mismatched blood transfusions or abortions), anti-Rh_0 gamma globulins are ineffective in preventing erythroblastosis.

OTHER HUMAN BLOOD GROUPS

MN system

More than a decade prior to the discovery of the Rh factor, the MN blood group system was recognized to be a blood group independent of the ABO(H) system; that is, the M, N, or MN antigens were present on group O cells. The MN system now consists of more than two dozen antigens given letters S, s, U, M^A, M^C, etc., which can be considered subgroups of M or N in the same sense that A_1 and A_2 are subgroups of A. The M and N antigens are inherited independently so that a person can be MM, NN, or MN, and the distribution of these individual antigens in Caucasians is 30%, 20%, and 50%, respectively.

Kell system

Although most antigens of the ABO(H) and MN systems are considerably less potent than the Rh antigens and do not contribute extensively to hemolytic disease of the newborn, this is not true of the Kell (K) system, a collection of 10 antigens of which K and k are the two originally described. K and k were detected by Coombs' tests that could not be related to the Rh system. Only 4% of Caucasians have the K antigen.

Public and private antigens

Some blood group antigens are found on nearly 100% of the red cells tested regardless of the ethnic, racial, or geographic source of the individual donor. The H substance of the ABO(H) system or the k antigen of the Kell system can be considered such an antigen, others include At^a, Co^a, Lan, Sm, and LW. The exact opposite situation occurs where antigens are apparently restricted to a few individuals in certain families. If the incidence of the antigen is 0.25% or less and meets other criteria, it can be termed a private antigen.

I antigen

The I-i blood group system, of which I can be considered a public antigen, is interesting because the human response to the I antigen is so frequently a cold agglutinin. Fetal erythrocytes do not react with anti-I but do with anti-i. During maturation the i antigen gradually disappears and is replaced with the I antigen. An autoimmune response to the I antigen that results in a hemolytic anemia can thus be explained on the basis that the antigen "matured" later than the immune response system.

MEDICAL APPLICATIONS OF BLOOD GROUPING

The relationship of blood group antigens to hemolytic anemia, just mentioned, will be discussed further in Chapter 10. Other important contributions of immunohematology include blood transfusions and the identity of blood antigens for medicolegal purposes. The latter can include uncertain parentage, baby mixing, and the identification of blood stains.

Blood transfusions

The hypothetical goal of a blood transfusion is to provide the exact antigenic type of blood for the recipient as he presently has. Naturally it is difficult to achieve this goal, but it can be very closely approached in terms of the major antigens if certain hemagglutination tests are performed, particularly the major and minor cross match (Fig. 7-5). The major cross match is performed by mixing the serum of the recipient with the red cells of the donor. If hemagglutination occurs, this blood cannot be given to the recipient for the obvious reason that he has antibodies capable, with complement and phagocytosis, of destroying the administered cells. In the minor cross match the recipient's red cells are incubated with serum of the donor and observed for agglutination. Again, when hemagglutination occurs, the donor's blood should not be given because it contains antibodies capable of attacking the recipient's erythrocytes. A positive minor

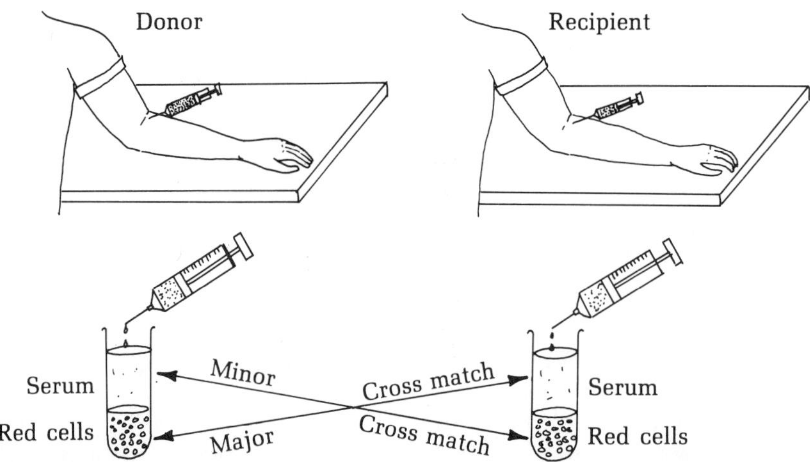

Fig. 7-5. Major cross match, also called the compatibility test, consists of a mixture of donor erythrocytes and recipient serum. When no hemagglutination occurs, the transfusion may be made successfully when the minor cross match is also negative.

cross match destroys the earlier concept that group O persons were universal donors and group AB persons were universal recipients. Group O blood contains both anti-A and anti-B and can only match with group O blood. Such blood is sometimes transfused in true emergencies on the assumption that the antibodies will be diluted beyond their reactive titer in the recipient. This is almost always an unprovable assumption. Unfortunately the minor cross match is not always used; the major cross match, renamed the compatibility test, is the only test in many laboratories. Fortunately it is supplemented by tests for incomplete antibodies in recipient sera by antiglobulin tests.

It is also desirable to determine exactly which of the major blood group antigens are on the donor's erythrocytes. For example, if the donor were Rh positive, group A, and the recipient were Rh negative, group A, the compatibility test would predict a safe transfusion. That would be true in this case, but the transfusion would hyperimmunize the person to the Rh antigen with potential disastrous results in the next transfusion or in an eventual Rh-positive pregnancy.

Forensic medicine

Disputed parentage. Medicolegal decisions associated with the identification of parents, identification of other kinships, and of potentially misidentified babies in the nursery are based on a knowledge of the inheritance of blood group antigens. These problems can only be solved by exclusion and not in a positive way. As a simple example, if a rape victim gave birth to a group O child conceived as a result of that act, an AB man cannot be implicated as the father, since he would transmit either the A or B characteristic to the child. Due to the possibility of heterozygous group A and B men as well as group O men transmitting the O gene, they are potential fathers. Statistically this would include 97% of all males. When additional antigens such as the Rh and MN antigens are identified, the possibility of exclusion approaches 50% for any male. In the case of baby mixing the same three blood groups, ABO(H), Rh, and MN, should be tested. Kinships more distant than first generation become mathematically greater challenges.

Blood stain identification. Blood stains are first confirmed as such by tests for hemoglobin and then subjected to serologic determinations for blood serum proteins by the precipitation test. This does not differentiate human blood from that of the anthropoid apes, which are cross-reactive. Fortunately dried blood stains can often be extracted to recover the alloantibodies for the A and B antigens and to recover the ABO(H) antigens. Tests for other antigens or antibodies are presently unsuitable, but the ABO(H) antigen determinations are applicable to saliva, semen, and other body fluids. Identification of the source of blood or the exclusion of a potential source of blood, is very important in homicides and other violent crimes.

BIBLIOGRAPHY

Boorman, K. E., and Dodd, B. E.: An introduction to blood group serology, ed. 4, London, 1970, J. & A. Churchill, Ltd.

Clarke, C. A.: Some immunological interactions between mother and fetus, Postgrad. Med. J. **48**:199, 1972.

Clarke, C. A.: Prevention of Rh isoimmunization, Prog. Med. Genet. **8**:169, 1972.

Clarke, C. A., and McConnell, R. B.: Prevention of Rh hemolytic disease, Springfield, Ill., 1972, Charles C Thomas, Publisher.

Erskine, A. G.: The principles and practice of blood grouping, St. Louis, 1973, The C. V. Mosby Co.

Fudenberg, H. H., Pink, J. R. L., Stites, D. P., and Wang, A. C.: Basic immunogenetics, New York, 1972, Oxford University Press.

Gold, E. R., and Butler, N. R.: ABO hemolytic disease of the newborn, Baltimore, 1972, The Williams & Wilkins Co.

Haesler, W. E., Jr.: Immunohematology, Philadelphia, 1972, Lea & Febiger.

Hakomori, S., and Kobata, A.: Blood group antigens. In Sela, M. ed.: The antigens, New York, 1974, Academic Press, Inc., vol. 2.
Hildemann, W. H.: Immunogenetics, San Francisco, 1970, Holden-Day, Inc.
McConnell, R. B., and Woodrow, J. C.: Immuno-prevention of Rh hemolytic disease of the newborn, Annu. Rev. Med. **25**:165, 1974.
Mollison, P. L.: Clinical aspects of Rh isoimmunization, Am. J. Clin. Pathol. **60**:287, 1973.
Sharon, N., and Lis, H.: Lectins: cell-agglutinating and sugar-specific proteins, Science **177**: 949, 1972.
Snyder, L. H.: Blood groups, Minneapolis, 1973, Burgess Publishing Co.
Sussman, L. N.: Medicolegal blood grouping tests (parentage exclusion tests), Prog. Clin. Pathol. **5**:143, 1973.
Zmijewski, C. M., and Fletcher, J. L.: Immunohematology, ed. 2, New York, 1972, Appleton-Century-Crofts.

Case histories

CASE 1. AN ILLEGITIMATE CHILD?

A "divorce lawyer" contacted physician R. J., a noted clinical pathologist who had consulted in several medicolegal cases, with a request to interpret blood grouping data to be used in a divorce action. The lawyer's client had reason to suspect, as a result of surgery on his youngest son and the blood grouping tests performed pertinent to subsequent blood transfusions, that this son was illegitimate. Accordingly, he was preparing to initiate divorce proceedings against his wife. The blood group data presented by the lawyer are as follows:

Person	*ABO(H)*	*MN*	*Kell*
Wife	B	M	k
Husband	O	M	k
First son (10 years old)	O	M	k
Daughter (6 years old)	B	MN	K
Second son (4 years old)	O	MN	K

Questions

1. Do the blood grouping data of the three children support or deny fatherhood by the husband?
2. What was the genotype of the wife?

Discussion

The ABO(H) blood groups of all three children are compatible with that of the husband and wife. Since the first and second son were group O, the mother would have to be genotype BO, assuming both sons to be her true children. This is supported by her daughter being group B.

The MN blood groups indicate that the husband was not the true father of the daughter or the second son. The phenotype M exists only for genotypically homozygous MM persons and obviously an MN child must have one MN or NN parent. Since this was not the case for the latter two children, in the face of genuine motherhood, the husband is not their father.

The same logic of the MN system can be applied to the Kell grouping. The daughter and second son each have antigen K, not present in the wife and husband, who are kk.

The evidence indicates that not only the second son but also the daughter are not children of the husband. The genotype of the mother is BO, MM, kk.

CASE 2.* THE CASE OF THE MISSING HEIR

When the dowager millionairess of a large pharmaceutical company executive was killed in an airplane crash, three of her four known surviving sons tried by newspaper advertisements, missing person bureaus, and other public means to locate the fourth, a prodigal son, in order to pursue an equitable division of the estate. The

*Adapted from Wiener, A. S.: Problems in immunogenetics and immunohematology, Lab. Digest **34**:7, 1970.

prodigal son had proved incorrigible as a teenager and at the age of 16 years had threatened to take up the life of a sailor and see the world. His disappearance caused no undue concern in the family because correspondence from Hong Kong, Rio de Janiero, Honolulu, etc. received by the older brothers indicated that the youngest son did indeed carry out his promise.

As a result of the missing persons search, three men of about the correct age, physical features, and with seafaring backgrounds presented themselves as the missing heir. Each of the three was asked (privately) to state his ABO(H) blood group. Two replied "group B" and the third "group A." The first two were dismissed as imposters, and the third was asked to remain for further documentation of his claim.

Question

1. What was the blood group of the two remaining brothers that they could so readily dismiss false claimants who were group B?

Discussion

There are several potentially correct solutions to this problem if the blood groups of the parents and the three known sons are all available. For example, if both parents were group O, then all four sons would have to be group O, and a reply by any putative brother of A, B, or AB would exclude him from relationship with the three remaining brothers. By similar reasoning, if the three remaining brothers were group A and the parents were either group A or O, then a group B claimant is not a true brother, since neither parent could transmit the B gene.

However, this problem makes no provision for knowledge of either parental blood type in achieving a solution. If it is assumed that one of the three true sons is group OO, then each parent had to carry the O gene. If one of the other true sons is A_1 and the other A_2, then their genotypes are A_1O and A_2O. Since each parent has one O gene, then the A_1 gene must come from one parent and the A_2 gene from the second parent again excluding the possibility of a group B son. Other possible solutions also rely on information relating to subgroups arising from separate parents.

REFERENCES

Erskine, A. G.: The principles and practice of blood grouping, St. Louis, 1973, The C. V. Mosby Co.

Issitt, P. D.: Applied blood group serology, Oxnard, Calif., 1970, Becton, Dickinson & Co.

chapter 8

Immunoglobulin-mediated hypersensitivity

As the title to this and the following chapter reveal, there are two forms of hypersensitivity, one that is mediated by immunoglobulins and one that is cell mediated. A general description of the similarities and differences of these two types of hypersensitivities or allergies will be presented in the following discussion.

IMMUNOGLOBULIN- AND CELL-MEDIATED HYPERSENSITIVITIES COMPARED

In immunology the terms "allergy" and "hypersensitvity" are customarily used as synonyms, even though allergy was originally defined simply as an altered (unexpected) response to an antigen. Obviously this could be a hyper- or hypoactivity, but since the first response was recognized to contribute to numerous human ailments, it was subject to more extensive study and was considered the most important form of allergy. Presently we recognize hyposensitivity to be an equally important immunologic phenomenon as expressed in the immunodeficiency diseases, immune tolerance, and possibly susceptibility to cancer. Anergy is also a valid term and refers to the absence of an immunologic response.

The common inciting agents for the immunoglobulin- and cell-mediated allergic reactions are antigens and haptens. The initial exposure to these substances is generally unremarkable. This may occur through natural means—by inhalation, ingestion, dermal contact, injection, or other routes. Partially because natural exposure to these allergens was often unrecognized, the allergies that followed such exposures were classified as atopic diseases (atopy = foreign). For many years little was known about the mechanism of these allergies other than an association of an antibody-like serum substance with certain allergies, the immunoglobulin-related allergies and an association of lymphocytes with others, the cell-mediated allergies. Now it is known that the immunoglobulin-mediated allergies rely almost exclusively on IgE and the cell-mediated allergies on the T lymphocyte.

After antigen exposure, regardless of its route or nature, the individual does not immediately display his hypersensitivity. There must elapse a sensitization period of approximately 1 week before this happens. After this time, a reexposure to the antigen or hapten, appropriately labeled the shocking exposure, will cause the symptoms of the allergy to appear in the sensitized person. The waiting period was essential to allow for the synthesis of the IgE and/or the development of T lymphocyte sensitivity to the antigen. When the shocking dose of antigen is given intradermally, the time course and nature of the two hypersensitivities as seen in the skin reaction are markedly different. The IgE response appears suddenly and disappears within 1 to 4 hours, whereas the T cell–dependent reaction develops slowly and does not become maximal until 48 or 72 hours after the injection of the allergen. It is because of this that the immunoglobulin-dependent hypersensitivities are identified as the immediate allergies, and the T cell–dependent hypersensitivities are known as the delayed allergies (Table 8-1). In some instances the two types of hypersensitivity are measurable in a single individual following the antigen exposure. For example, inhalant allergy to the proteolytic enzymes contained in detergents shows a marked bimodal curve—the initial response is detected in a few minutes and the delayed aspects only after 6 to 8 hours.

The major characteristics of the immediate skin reaction are a pronounced edema with wheal and erythema. Histologically an early infiltration of neutrophils is noticed, followed by a later entry of mononuclear cells into the injection site. In the delayed cutaneous skin reaction there is less edema, less pseudopodial spreading of the reaction site, and a tendency only toward erythema and the development of a thickened, leathery texture (induration) of the skin. Microscopic examination of the area will reveal that the dominant new cell in the reaction site is the mononuclear cell.

Since the immediate reaction is related to the synthesis of an antigen-specific IgE, this type of sensitivity is easily transferred to a nonallergic person by serum, plasma, or blood. This IgE functions as a cytotropic antibody for mast cells, and when antigen combines with cell-bound IgE, the mast cell degranulates, releasing several chemical compounds stored in these granules—histamine, eosinophilic chemotactic factor, serotonin, and others. Because of the pronounced pharmacologic action of these compounds on smooth muscle, the blood vessels dilate, fluid leaks into the tissue, and the symptoms of the immediate skin reaction are expressed following cutaneous

Table 8-1. Characteristics of immunoglobulin- and T lymphocyte–mediated hypersensitivities

	Immunoglobulin	*T lymphocyte*
Initiators	Antigens and injected haptens	Antigens and dermal contact with haptens
Immune reactant	IgE, possibly other immunoglobulins	T lymphocyte lymphokines
Chemical mediators	Histamine, serotonin, eosinophilic chemotatic factor of anaphylaxis, etc.	Migration inhibition factor, lymphotoxin, chemotaxins, etc.
Release of mediators after shocking dose	Within minutes, fades within hours	Gradual, maximum effect not seen for 24-72 hr
Target tissue	Smooth muscle	Monocytes, various host cells
Tissue death	Possible with IgG	Rare
Passive transfer	Yes with serum	Yes with T lymphocytes or transfer factor
Skin reaction	Erythema, edema, wheal, neutrophilic infiltrate	Erythema and induration, monocytic infiltrate
Chemotherapy	Antihistamines, catecholamines, methyl xanthines, cromolyn	Steroids (nonspecific anti-inflammatory)
Immunotherapy	Neutralization and blocking antibody formation	Usually not attempted

exposure to the antigen. On systemic exposure to the antigen the primary effect of these vasoactive compounds is noted as a contraction of smooth muscle. Antimetabolites to these vasoactive compounds competitively inhibit their function, and smooth muscle relaxants (catecholamines or adrenergic drugs) counteract their activity, providing relief to the allergic condition. It may also be possible to desensitize the person by neutralizing his cell-bound IgE with gradual doses of antigen that do not allow enough of the vasoactive agents to accumulate at one time to cause the allergic reaction.

In the case of delayed hypersensitivities no serum factor is present that can transfer the sensitivity; this can only be accomplished by lymphocyte transfers. Contact of the sensitized T lymphocyte with the antigen causes the cell to release lymphokines, some of which are chemoattractants for monocytes and some of which inhibit migration by macrophages, etc. Since no compounds other than proteins are released by these T lymphocytes, it is not possible to arrange a simple chemotherapy or chemoprophylaxis against their action, which fortunately has less of a cell-destructive component than mast cell products. Steroids and other anti-inflammatory compounds will ameliorate the delayed hypersensitive reaction, but their mechanism is based on a general antiphlogistic function and is not specifically antagonistic to the lymphokines. Antigen desensitization of the T cell is possible but is seldom practiced, again because cell-mediated allergies have little life-threatening potential.

CLASSIFICATION OF HYPERSENSITIVITIES

The traditional classification of hypersensitivities into the IgE- and T lymphocyte–dependent types, the immediate and delayed types, is useful but in the medical sciences another classification scheme is helpful in categorizing different disease states. This is the system devised by Gell and Coombs that includes four forms of hypersensitivity reactions (Table 8-2). In actuality the first of these is an IgE-dependent reaction and the last a classic T lymphocyte–related sensitivity. The middle two types include immune disease involving immunoglobulins other than IgE.

Table 8-2. Classification of hypersensitive reactions

	Type I	*Type II*	*Type III*	*Type IV*
Synonym	Anaphylactic	Cytotoxic	Immune complex	T cell type
Immunoglobulin	IgE	IgG, possibly other	IgG, IgM, etc.	None
Antigens involved	Heterologous	Autologous or hapten modified	Autologous or heterologous	Autologous or heterologous
Complement involved	No	Yes	Yes	No
Cellular involvement	Mast cells and basophils	RBC, WBC, platelets	Host tissue cells	T lymphocytes
Chemical mechanism	Mast cell products	Complement cytolysis	Immune complex blockage of tissue or vessels	Lymphokines
Examples	Anaphylaxis, hay fever, food allergy	Transfusion reactions, Rh disease, thrombocytopenia	Arthus, serum sickness, pneumonitis	Allergy of infection, contact dermatitis

In the type I reaction, described as the anaphylactic type of reaction, IgE attaches to mast cells and basophils, reacts with exogenous antigen or hapten-antigen conjugates, and prompts mast cell degranulation. The pharmacologic mediators contract smooth muscle, and the associated symptoms of the allergy are observed. Since IgE is the responsible antibody, no change in the serum complement level accompanies this reaction. Examples of this type I reaction are anaphylaxis, hay fever, and allergies to other pollens listed as inhalant allergies, food allergies, and certain drug reactions, especially to injectable antibiotics and components of the serum sickness complex.

In the cytotoxic or type II reaction, antibodies of the classic or nonreaginic type directed against host cell antigens unite with these cellular antigens to produce a cytodestructive effect. Serum complement may be involved or the antibody may contribute to cell death through its opsonic activity. Blood transfusion reactions, hemolytic disease of the newborn, certain forms of thrombocytopenia purpura, and some forms of drug allergies are classified as type II reactions.

When antigen-antibody aggregates are deposited in blood vessels or on tissue surfaces, the normal physiologic functions of the underlying cells are interrupted. Complement may be activated, and neutrophils attracted by C3a and C5a contribute to local tissue injury. Categorized as type III reactions are the Arthus reaction, immune complex pneumonitis, aspects of serum sickness reaction, and several autoimmune diseases, including lupus erythematosus and the poststreptococcal diseases (rheumatic fever and glomerulonephritis).

The type IV reaction is the T lymphocyte-mediated reaction and will be considered further in Chapter 9. Examples of the type IV reaction include contact dermatitis, allergies of infection, and autoimmune diseases such as Hashimoto's thyroiditis. The type IV reaction is also critical to tumor immunity, transplantation immunity, and immunity to many viruses and fungi.

IMMUNOGLOBULIN E

In many respects IgE, also known as reagin, is one of the most interesting of the immunoglobulins (Table 8-3). It is heat labile at 56° to 60° C for 30 to 120 minutes; it has no known protective function and is associated only with allergic conditions; it attaches to the surface of mast cells and basophils so that these cells degranulate and release their stores of vasoactive amines and peptides when the offending antigen combines with the bound antibodies.

Chemical properties

IgE shares the typical tetrapeptide structure of the other immunoglobulins in which two light (L) chains are joined by disulfide bonds to heavy (H) chains that are joined to each other by disulfide bonds. The L peptides are identical to those found in the other immunoglobulins, the κ- and λ-chains. The H chains have a molecular weight of 72,300 (of which 12% is polysaccharide) and, as they are antigenically distinct from H chains of other gamma globulins, are referred to as ϵ-chains. The greater molecular weight of the ϵ-chain, compared to the γ- and other H chains, suggests that it might be a five-domain chain with one

Table 8-3. Properties of IgE

Synonym	Reagin (homocytotropic antibody)
Molecular formula	$\epsilon_2\ \kappa_2$ or $\epsilon_2\ \lambda_2$
Molecular weight	188,000
Carbohydrate content	10.7%
S_{20} value	8.2
Serum concentration (mg/100 ml)	0.01-1.0
Heat stability	Destroyed (60° C for 30 min-4 hr)
Cytotropism	For mast cells and basophils
In vitro serologic reactions	None
Pass placenta	No
Quantitation	Total (RIST); antigen specific (RAST)

V_H unit and four C_H units, but this is not as yet established. Nevertheless, the molecular weight of IgE of either the $\epsilon_2\kappa_2$ or $\epsilon_2\lambda_2$ subclass is 188,000. The sedimentation coefficient of IgE is 8.2.

Papain digestion of IgE produces the expected two Fab-ϵ and Fc-ϵ fragments, but additional low molecular weight peptides can also be recovered. The Fc fragment has a molecular weight of 98,000. By peptic or tryptic hydrolysis of IgE the corresponding Fd and $F(ab')_2$ units are produced.

The origin of IgE is from its special class of plasma cells, where the rate of IgE synthesis, as yet not determined, is presumed to be low. The half-life of IgE is only 4.4 days, and this combined with its low synthetic rate restricts its blood concentration to 15 to 100 ng/ml. This means that IgE represents less than 1% of the total immunoglobulin content of normal blood. Consequently, it is impossible to isolate sufficient IgE from the gamma globulin fraction of normal blood to make extensive chemical studies. This became possible only when gamma ϵ-myelomas were discovered first in Sweden, then the United States, and later in other countries.

Quantitation

Two approaches to the quantitation of IgE are possible. The first of these is a determination of the amount of IgE present in a serum that will react with a specific antigen. This can often be estimated by the extent of skin reactions to the specific antigen or can be measured precisely by sophisticated radioimmunoassay techniques. Alternatively, radioimmunoassays can be applied to the quantitation of total serum IgE. The last of these will be described first.

One method of determining the total IgE content of serum is known as the radioimmunosorbent or RIST test. This procedure is dependent on the availability of a radiolabeled ϵ-myeloma protein and its antibody. The antibody is covalently bound to an insoluble carrier, and a competition is established between a known amount of radioiodinated ϵ-myeloma protein and the unknown IgE in a serum sample. Calculations of the loss of bound label in the competitive assay versus label bound in the serum-free control permit a determination of the IgE present in the serum sample. This procedure does not differ from the usual radioimmunoassay (Chapter 6).

Frequently it is important to know the amount of IgE that is specific for a certain antigen. This can be estimated by direct skin testing of the hypersensitive individual with known doses of antigens and by measuring the extent of the immediate type of skin reaction that follows. This provides only a crude estimate of the IgE directed against the antigen used. A very exact method is available in the radioallergosorbent or RAST test. In the RAST procedure the allergen is coupled to an insoluble carrier. The allergen-bound carrier is incubated with a serum sample considered to contain IgE specific for that antigen. If other classes of immunoglobulins directed against that antigen are contained in the unknown sample, it is of little consequence because the third reactant in the test is a radiolabeled anti-IgE. This antiserum will bind only to the IgE that is attached to the immunosorbent so that a measure of bound radioactivity is a measure of IgE. Of course only the IgE in the sample that is specific for the antigen used is measured. A variant of this method depends on the adsorption of the antigen onto erythrocytes. On the addition of the IgE and then anti-IgE, passive hemagglutination is observed.

The RAST method is the preferred method for measuring the serum concentration of IgE. By the use of this method it has been found that in cases of hay fever, asthma, and tropical eosinophilia due to helminth infection, serum levels of IgE as high as 6000 ng/ml may be attained. Values above 1000 ng/ml are considered pathologic.

Biologic properties

IgE, unlike most other immunoglobulins, does not complete the second phase of the serologic reaction with antigen, and for this reason the quantitation of IgE is based on antigen-binding assays rather than agglutination, precipitation, complement fixation, or other simple serologic tests. The antigen-binding activity of IgE is heat labile under the same conditions of time and temperature, 56° to 60° C for 30 minutes or more, that destroy its cytotropic ability.

Mast cell degranulation. Little is known about the in vivo activity of IgE other than its inability to pass the placental barrier and its ability to attach to mast cells and basophils. This latter function is mediated by receptors on the surface of these cells for the Fc portion of IgE, which leaves its Fab portions free to combine with antigen. When two IgE molecules on the mast cell surface are bridged with antigen, the intracellular granules of these cells disintegrate. This degranulation of mast cells can be produced by certain chemicals and by passively administering antibodies against IgE or antibodies against mast cell antigens. Mast cell degranulation is not necessarily accompanied by mast cell lysis, only by an intracellular dissolution of the granules or, in some instances, the granules are "spit out" and disintegrate extracellularly.

Mast cells are found in most tissues of the body and are especially numerous in the lungs, uterus, around blood vessels, and in connective tissue. Each ovoid-shaped mast cell is about 10 to 15 μ in diameter and is literally filled with granules measuring 0.5 to 2.0 μ in diameter (Fig. 8-1).

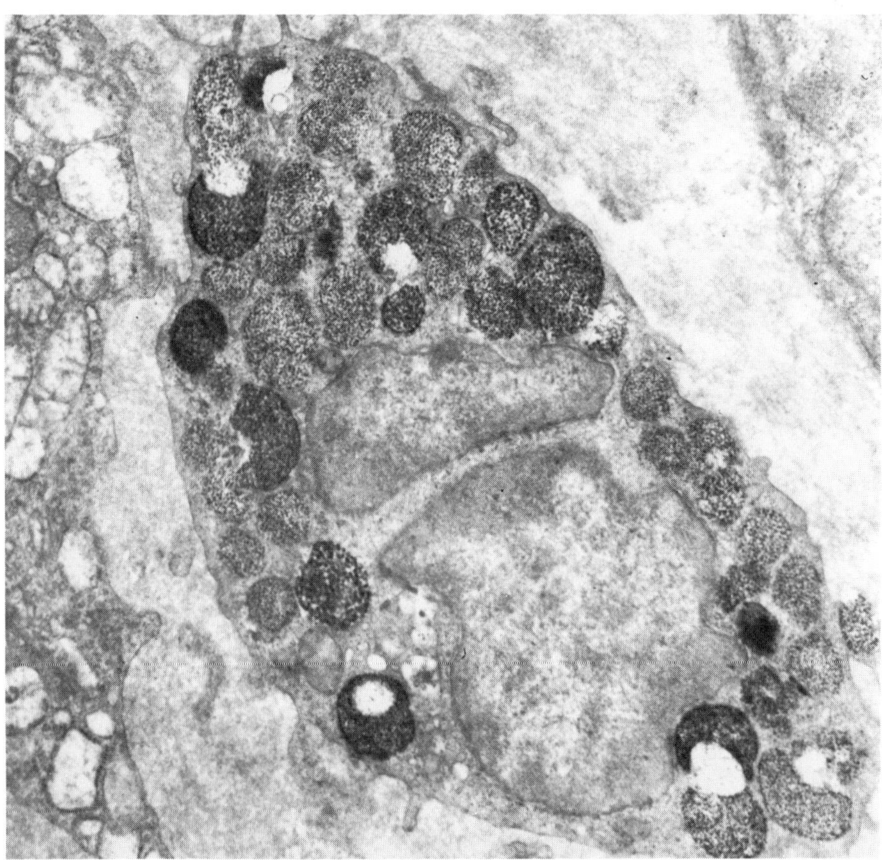

Fig. 8-1. View of a mast cell through the electron microscope. Although it gives the false impression of a binucleate cell, it indicates the extent of granulation in the mast cell cytoplasm. (Courtesy Dr. E. Adelstein.)

A single mast cell may contain as many as 500 of these granules that obscure the nucleus and stain easily with toluidine blue. The granules of the basophilic leukocyte are identical in most respects to the granules of mast cells. Both serve as storage sites for heparin and histamine, which exist as an ionically associated complex. The histamine content of 10^6 cells is about 10 to 15 μg. The stability of the mast cell granule is undoubtedly influenced by intracellular forces, but these are apparently also regulated by extracellular forces that operate at the level of the cell membrane.

Cyclic 3,5-adenosine monophosphate (cyclic AMP). Mast cells appear to fall into that class of cells that responds to an extracellular or cell membrane–bound first messenger, which operates through a cell membrane–bound second messenger. The first message comes from IgE-antigen complexes on the mast cell surface, and the second comes from adenylate (adenyl) cyclase, an enzyme that generates cyclic AMP from adenosine triphosphate (ATP). Combination of antigen with IgE inhibits adenylate cyclase, which produces a corresponding decrease in cyclic AMP. When the mast cell level of cyclic AMP is depressed to a critical level, the mast cell degranulates, releasing its heparin and histamine, reducing the clotting time of blood, and producing symptoms of the immediate-type hypersensitivities (Fig. 8-2). Compounds such as epinephrine stimulate adenylate cyclase and this inhibits the allergic

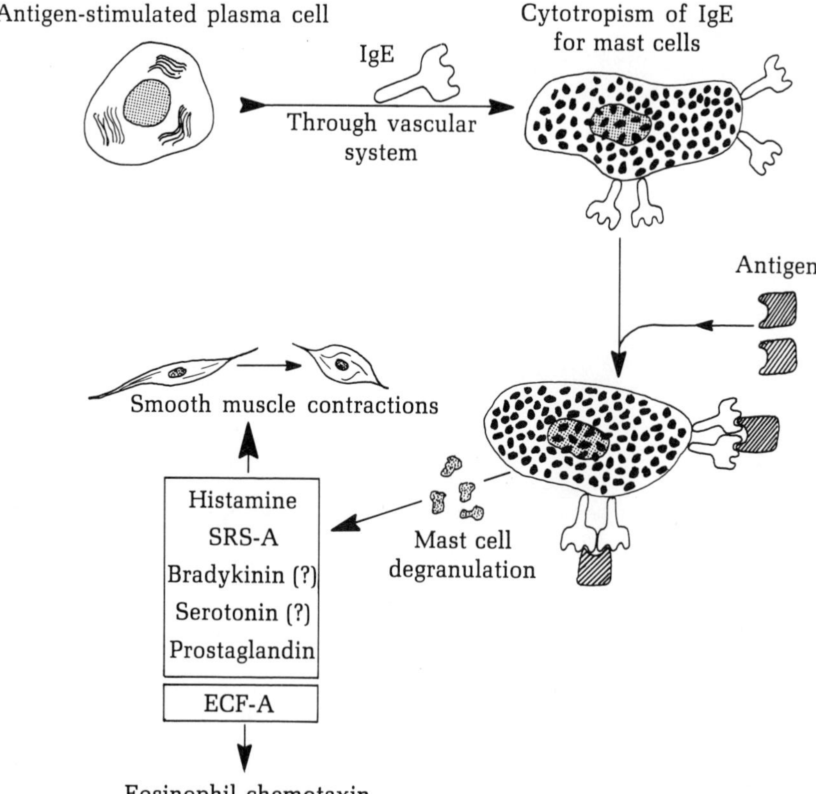

Fig. 8-2. Sequence of anaphylactic pathway indicates central role of cytotropic IgE and its combination with antigen in degranulation of mast cells. Substances from mast cells and plasma that serve as effector molecules are in boxed area at lower left.

reaction. Certain methyl xanthines block the enzyme phosphodiesterase that hydrolyzes cyclic AMP; this maintains a high intracellular pool of cyclic AMP and reduces the allergic symptoms.

Ir genes and IgE

It has been estimated that more than 30 million Americans have one form or another of atopic allergy. Of these, approximately 8,000,000 have hay fever, 3,000,000 have asthma, and 9,000,000 others are allergic to foods, animal hair, dandruff, feathers, antibiotics, house dust, insect stings, etc. For many years it has been recognized that there was a genetic basis for these conditions, and this has taken an exciting new turn with the discovery that human Ir genes regulate the responses to many allergenic substances and that these Ir genes are linked with histocompatibility antigens.

Some of the initial evidence to support the almost intuitive belief that the allergic tendency is inherited was based on clustering. When infants with eczema were reexamined 15 or more years later, it was learned that 23% had asthma and 10% had hay fever; yet a similar examination years later of what had been healthy babies indicated only 2% had asthma and 2% had hay fever. Once a person expresses one allergy he is more likely to express another later on, and this is known as clustering. Family studies have confirmed that the allergic predisposition is passed from one generation to the next. In one study of 577 patients in an allergy clinic, 58% of the patients had a family history of allergy and only 7% came from allergy-free families. In a similar study of 567 patients, 48.4% of the patients were from "allergic families" and 9.5% came from allergy-free families.

The most logical explanation of these statistics is that Ir genes exist that control the human IgE response to antigenic and haptenic determinants. These genes, like other genes, are transmissible to one's progeny. When the offspring become exposed to allergens, the allergic response is triggered and expressed as hay fever, food allergy, etc. Analysis of the human population has clearly proved this. For example, common hay fever is based on an IgE response to antigen E of the ragweed plant *Ambrosia elatior*. In the study of three generations in one family it was found that six persons were profoundly reactive to antigen E. Interestingly it was observed that four of these individuals had the histocompatibility haplotype HL-A1,8. Histocompatibility haplotype refers to the human leukocyte antigens (HL-A) that a person has on his white blood cells and other nucleated cells. These control tissue transplantation success in the sense that if a recipient of an organ transplant lacks an antigen that is present on the donated tissue, he will reject the tissue on the basis of an immune response directed against the foreign antigen. These antigens are numbered and, like the ABO(H), Rh, and other antigens, are genetically inherited. This information about the relationship of Ir gene responses to antigen E and the presence of histocompatibility antigens 1,8 indicates that histocompatibility typing would predict which family members are at risk for allergic disease. It also suggests that an allergic predisposition toward other antigens may be related to one's histocompatibility antigen makeup.

MEDIATORS OF IgE-DEPENDENT HYPERSENSITIVITIES

Although several cell types may be involved in the expression of the immediate hypersensitivities, the sensitivity of these cells to stimulation is not necessarily the same in all species of animals; thus the symptoms of the immediate hypersensitivities vary slightly from species to species. Or to state it in a different way, some species are highly resistant to certain pharmacologic agents released during the immediate hypersensitivity reaction. In addition, genetic controls may limit the capacity of some individuals to form the immunoglob-

Table 8-4. Mediators of immediate-type hypersensitivities

Mediator	*Description*	*Primary activity*	*Antagonist*
Histamine	From histidine in mast cells, mol wt 111, a heterocyclic amine	Contracts smooth muscle	Antihistamines
Serotonin	From tryptophan in mast cells, mol wt 171, an aromatic amine	Contracts smooth muscle	Methysergide
Eosinophilic chemotactic factor of anaphylaxis	From mast cells, mol wt about 500, a peptide	Attracts eosinophils	None known
Anaphylatoxins	C3a, mol wt 7500, a peptide from C3; C5a, mol wt 16,000, a peptide from C5 (neither involved in IgE-regulated reactions)	Release histamine	None known
Prostaglandins	Twenty-carbon unsaturated fatty acids, connection to allergy uncertain	Increase cyclic AMP, dose-dependent effect on histamine release, contract smooth muscle	Indomethacin
Slow-reacting substance of anaphylaxis	Fatty acid, mol wt about 400	Prolonged contraction of smooth muscle	None known
Bradykinin and related kinins	From plasma kininogens, mol wt near 1000	Contracts smooth muscle slowly	None known

ulins required for sensitization. These conditions modify the susceptibility and the expression of allergies in different species and specific individuals. In the following discussion the mediators of the human immediate sensitivities will be the focus of attention (Table 8-4).

Histamine

A role for histamine as a mediator of the inflammatory reaction received its first significant support from the studies of Lewis in the late 1920s. Lewis described the triple response of the skin to the intradermal injection of histamine. This response included an immediate edema, erythma, and wheal or spread of these effects into the surrounding tissus. It was recognized that these were the exact characteristics of the immediate hypersensitivity reaction that could be provoked in allergic individuals by the intradermal administration of the offending antigen. It was also known that during anaphylaxis a substance appeared in blood that could be injected into the skin of a normal animal and elicit the triple response. Not until 1953 was it possible to identify this activity with histamine. Even at that time it was recognized that histamine was probably not the sole mediator—that other histamine-like molecules or H substances might also participate in the immediate-type allergic response.

Chemically histamine is a simple compound with a molecular weight of 111 that is formed by the action of histidine decarboxylase on histidine with the aid of pyridoxal phosphate as a cofactor (Fig. 8-3). The required enzyme is generously available in tissue mast cells, and the histamine content of mast cells has been calculated to average between 10 to 15 μg/million cells. The human lung contains 25 μg of histamine/gram of wet weight. The mast cell histamine does not exist in solution; rather it is present in the form of an ionic complex with heparin. Heparin is a substituted polysaccharide consisting primarily of alternating units of α-D-glucuronic acid 2-sulfate in

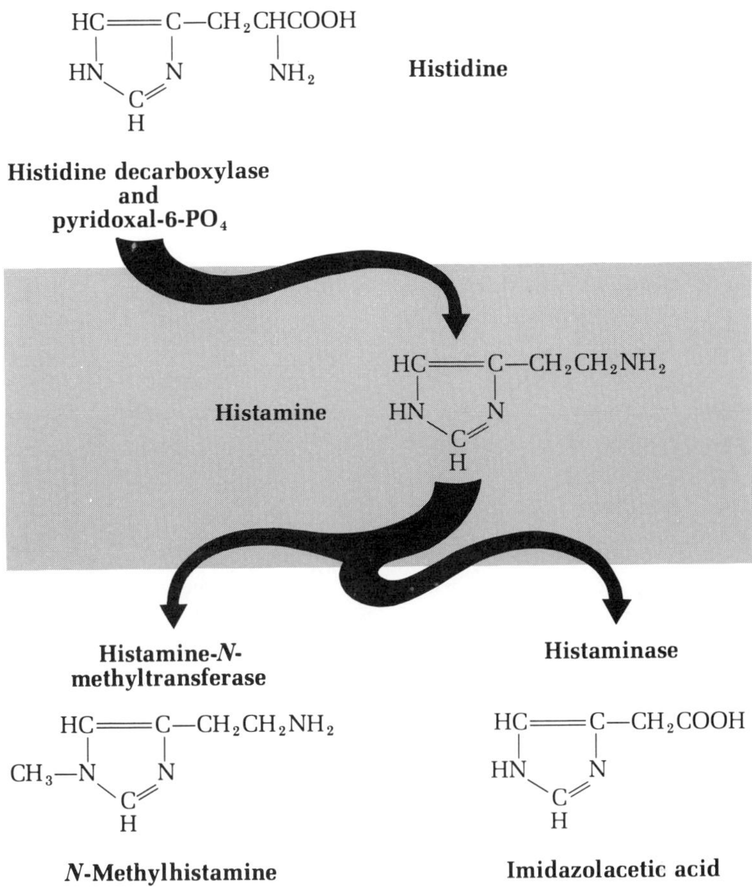

Fig. 8-3. Histamine is formed in the mast cell as indicated in upper portion of diagram. Two methods of detoxifying histamine are indicated in lower portion.

a 1,4 glycosidic linkage with α-D-glucosamine 3,6-disulfate; it has a molecular weight near 17,000. The ionized sulfate and carboxylate groups in heparin exist in an ionic complex with the protonated nitrogen atoms of histamine in a heparin:histamine weight ratio of about 6:1, that is, there are about 70 to 90 μg of heparin/million mast cells. During the immediate allergic reaction, histamine and heparin, which are collected into dense granules present in mast cells, are released through the process known as mast cell degranulation. Degranulation of mast cells is prompted by the reaction of surface-bound or cytotropic IgE with its specific antigen in the immunoglobulin-mediated allergic reactions. As a consequence, the anticoagulant activity of heparin and the potent vasodilating and muscle-contracting activity of histamine can be observed in the blood of an individual undergoing an extensive immediate hypersensitive reaction.

Circulating basophils, one type of blood cell of the granulocytic series, are considered the vascular counterparts of the tissue mast cells. The cytoplasmic granules in basophils are also storehouses for histamine and heparin, which are released during the immediate hypersensitive reaction. Basophils contain 0.5 ng of histamine/ml of packed cells.

Histamine constricts smooth muscle, and in man the musculature of the respiratory system and the smooth muscle of the venules are highly sensitive to histamine. Serious allergic reactions are accompanied by respiratory distress in which the individual takes rapid, short inhalations without an equal exhalation phase. The blood pressure may drop as the capillaries expand, a compensatory action for venule constriction. This forces fluids into the tissue bed (edema), and the accompanying capillary engorgement is observed as erythema.

These activities eventually subside as histamine is detoxified by methylation and oxidation to methylhistamine and imidazoleacetic acid, which do not have the pharmacologic activity of their precursor amine.

Serotonin

Mast cells, basophils, and platelets serve as the cellular origin of the serotonin released during immediate allergic reactions. Serotonin arises from the amino acid tryptophan as the result of two independent enzymatic transformations. The first of these is a hydroxylation at the 5 position in the indole ring by tryptophan hydroxylase, followed by a decarboxylation (Fig. 8-4). These reactions occur in the mast cells, basophils, and platelets of many species such as the rat, dog, rabbit, and guinea pig. The human mast cell is devoid of serotonin. The platelet may be the primary cell source of serotonin in most species, including man. Serotonin is also present in tissues of the central nervous system and intestinal tract.

Serotonin has basically the same pharma-

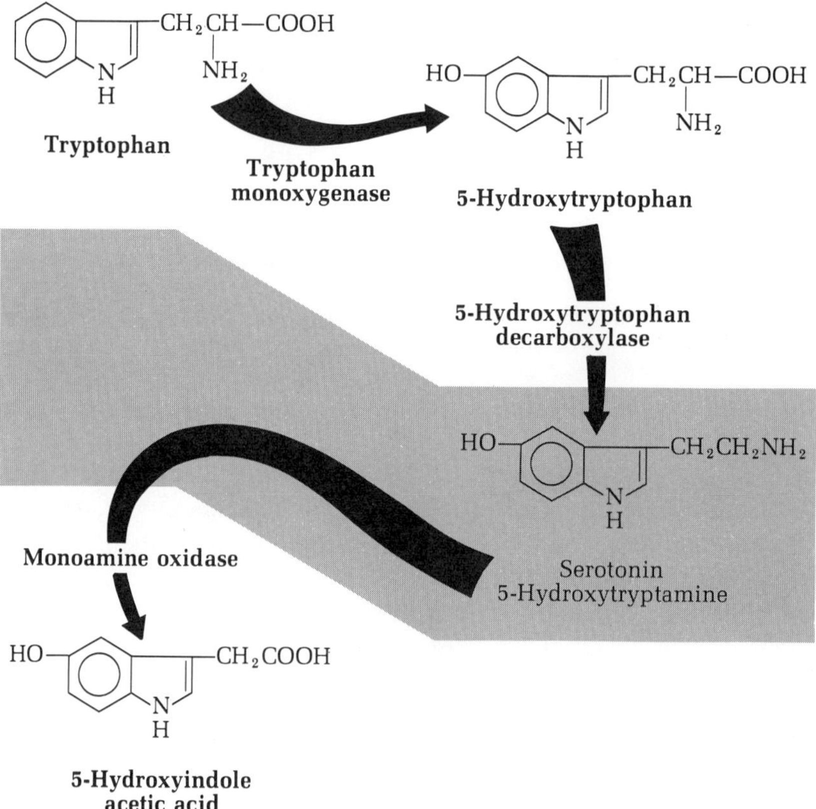

Fig. 8-4. Biochemical pathway for formation of serotonin in mast cell is indicated in upper half of diagram. Lower half illustrates how detoxification of serotonin occurs.

cologic action as histamine; it causes the rapid contraction of smooth muscles and increases vascular permeability. Rodents are especially sensitive to serotonin, and in rats there is convincing evidence that serotonin is a key mediator of anaphylactic shock. The contribution of serotonin to human immediate-type allergic reactions is of minimal significance.

Detoxification of serotonin by oxidation converts it to the pharmacologically inert indoleacetic acid.

Eosinophilic chemotactic factor of anaphylaxis

A third product of mast cells that contributes to the immediate hypersensitive response is the eosinophilic chemotactic factor of anaphylaxis (ECF-A). Human lung sensitized with IgE and then exposed in vitro to the specific antigen releases an attractant for eosinophils that, although of low molecular weight, could be easily distinguished from histamine and slow-reacting substance of anaphylaxis. ECF-A has a molecular weight near 500; it is present in mast cell granules, stable to repeated cycles of freezing and thawing, and resistant to proteolysis by trypsin and chymotrypsin. Despite the resistance of ECF-A to destruction by pancreatic proteases, its susceptibility to pronase and subtilisin suggests that it has a peptide nature. ECF-A has only recently been described and further studies of its chemical nature and pharmacologic behavior are needed. It is known to reside in mast cell granules as a preformed compound and is not synthesized during the process of the allergic reaction.

Anaphylatoxins

Anaphylatoxins are, by definition, molecules of biologic origin that can induce the release of histamine from mast cells. This definition should probably be expanded to include other mediators of the immediate allergic reaction.

Historically, anaphylatoxins were believed to originate from the antigen (or possibly also the antibody molecule) during the serologic reaction in vivo. This concept became untenable when the divergent chemical nature of antigens was recognized. Moreover, it was noted that injections of agar, starch, India ink, colloidal iron, and dyes used to determine blood volume or to aid in roentgenographic analyses could provoke anaphylactic-like reactions. These anaphylactoid reactions resulting from exposure to immunologically inert materials were also believed to depend on anaphylatoxins.

Two anaphylatoxins are known to originate from complement: C3a and C5a. In the activation of C3 two peptides are initially formed: C3a and C3b. C3a is a basic protein with a molecular weight of 7500, which in a dosage of 10^{-12} or 10^{-15} M produces edema and erythema in human skin. The vasoactive property of this molecule is dependent on a terminal arginine and is lost when this arginine is removed. Treatment of C3a with 2-mercaptoethanol also destroys its toxic activity. C5a arising with C5b during activation of C5 is also anaphylatoxic. C5a remains poorly characterized in biophysical terms. It is a peptide with a molecular weight of 16,000. C3a-like and C5a-like anaphylatoxins can also be derived from C3 and C5 by the action of tissue proteases on the parent compounds. This fact, and the knowledge that the activation of complement by nonantibody mechanisms through the properdin or alternate pathway of complement activation would release both C3a and C5a, suggests these anaphylatoxins may be very important in nonantibody-mediated immediate-type allergic reactions.

Prostaglandins

The chemical structure common to all prostaglandins, so named because they were believed to be synthesized in the prostate gland, is a 20-carbon unsaturated fatty acid that has a cyclopentane ring embodying positions C8 through 12. The prostaglandins are grouped as prostaglandins A, B, E, and F according to the position of keto or hydroxyl substitutions and unsaturated bonds in the cyclic pentane ring. Subscripts as in PGE_1 denote the position of additional double bonds in the aliphatic portion of the molecule, but the number does not refer to the carbon number of the bond—PGE_1 is unsaturated between carbons 13 and 14, PGE_2 between carbons 6 and 7, and PGE_3 between carbons 17 and 18. PGE and PGF compounds are the two best known series in terms of their biologic activity.

Prostaglandins are found in most tissues, not just the prostate. Their natural physiologic function is uncertain, and many activities have been attributed to these compounds. PGE increases the intracellular level of cyclic AMP in leukocytes, and this is associated with a restriction in the release of lysosomal enzymes. This would have an obvious effect on intraphagocytic digestion. One of the most interesting discoveries is that prostaglandins prevent the release of histamine and slow-reacting substance of anaphylaxis from sensitized cells, simultaneous with an increase in cellular cyclic AMP. Lower doses of PGE provoke the opposite response: they decrease AMP and enhance histamine release. Contrasting dose-response data of this sort have made it difficult to ascribe a precise physiologic role to the prostaglandins in allergic as well as other reactions. PGE_1 causes a lymphopenia and retards the cytotoxic activity of lymphocytes on allogenic target cells, which indicate a definite T lymphocyte sensitivity to PGE. The ability of PGE to extend graft survival may be in part through this anti-T cell effect or an alteration of B cell function, since it is known that PGE_1 inhibits the release of immunoglobulins.

Slow-reacting substance of anaphylaxis

During anaphylactic shock a substance is released into blood that has the ability to effect a prolonged contraction of smooth muscle. To distinguish this from other slow-reacting substances (SRS) that affect muscle, the SRS of anaphylaxis has been designated as SRS-A. Chemical studies have clearly distinguished SRS-A from histamine, serotonin, prostaglandins, anaphylatoxins, and the other pharmacologic agents associated with the immediate hypersensitivities. SRS-A is an unsaturated hydroxyl acid with a molecular weight near 400. It is released from sensitized human lung tissue exposed in vitro to antigen and on this basis is believed significant in the immediate-type human allergies. Mast cells serve as a source for SRS-A.

Bradykinin

Bradykinin is a peptide consisting of nine amino acids that has several of the properties of histamine (Fig. 8-5). It is a potent vasodilating agent, it causes edema by increasing the permeability of the capillary bed, and it contracts smooth muscle. Unlike histamine, bradykinin provokes a protracted contraction of muscle (*brady*, meaning slow; kinin, meaning to move), and it does not originate from mast cells. The source of bradykinin is a blood protein known as kininogen, a globulin with a molecular weight estimated to be between 50,000 and 100,000 in different studies. The discrepancy in these molecular weights may relate to the fact that there are two (possibly more) kininogens in blood. The kininogens have a central peptide core with polysaccharide situated at one or both ends. An enzyme kininogenase, also known as kallikrein, hydrolyzes this peptide to free the bradykinin peptide. There may be other kininogenases that release lysylbradykinin (kallidin) and/or methionyllyslbradykinin.

The pathway leading to the proteolysis of kininogens is complex and begins with the Hageman factor (Fig. 8-6). Hageman factor, known as factor XII in the blood clotting cascade, is a globulin with a molec-

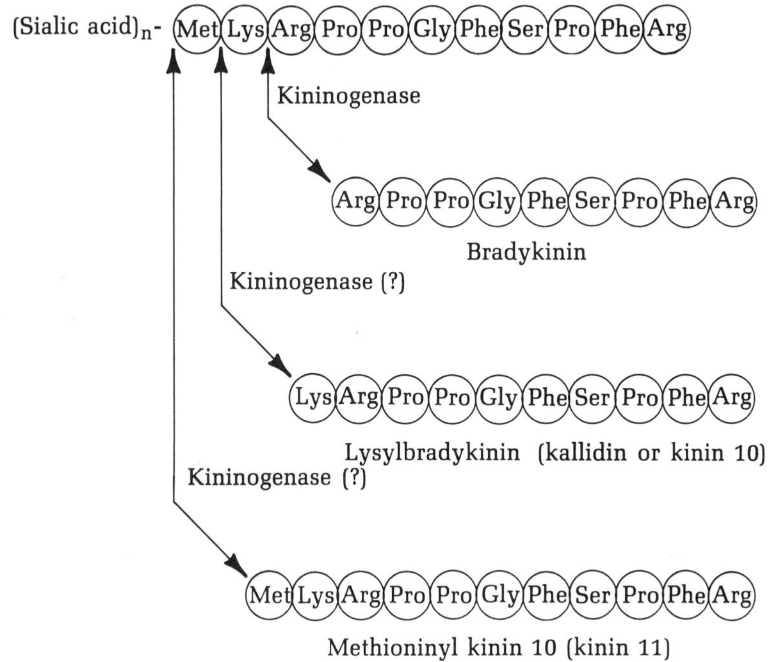

Fig. 8-5. Several kininogens and kininogenases in human tissues are known. Diagram suggests how bradykinin and its related kinins may be formed from kininogen I.

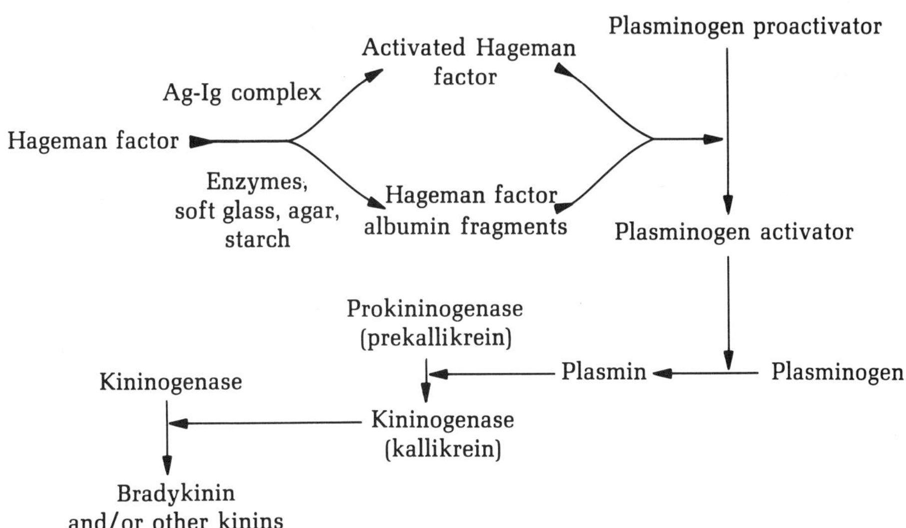

Fig. 8-6. Multistage pathway through which bradykinin and other kinins may be released by a serologic reaction or by substances that produce anaphylactoid or anaphylactic-like reactions involves at least four proenzymes.

ular weight of 110,000. Hageman factor is enzymatically inert until it is activated by contact with soft glass, colloidal silica, carbon particles, or antigen-antibody aggregates to become a proteolytic enzyme. In this activation step, fragments that resemble albumin in molecular weight and isoelectric point are liberated, and these albumin fragments are also proteolytic. Both activated Hageman factor and the Hageman factor albumin fragments can catalyze the activation of plasminogen proactivator to form the plasminogen activator. This enzyme and its proenzyme are both gamma globulins with molecular weights near 100,000. Plasminogen activator converts plasminogen, a beta globulin with a molecular weight of 80,000, into plasmin, an active proteolytic enzyme. Plasmin converts prokininogenase (prekallikrein) into kininogenase (kallikrein), which then removes bradykinin from kininogen. Thus, through the activation of four proenzymes into their respective enzymes, an antigen-antibody reaction culminates in the formation of bradykinin.

Although this complex pathway leading to bradykinin has been uncoded, there is still no certainty concerning the contribution of bradykinin to the immediate hypersensitive response. Since nonserologic reactions can terminate in bradykinin release, bradykinin may contribute to the anaphylactoid reaction.

PF/dil

The permeability factor created in serum by its simple dilution (PF/dil) has recently been identified as due to the activation of Hageman factor and ultimately to the release of kinins from blood plasma proteins.

Other mediators

Kinin from C2 could contribute to some immediate allergic reactions provided the classic complement pathway is activated by a serologic reaction or by enzymes. A platelet aggregating factor formed or released during immediate-type reactions may increase vascular permeability.

MODERATORS OF IgE-DEPENDENT HYPERSENSITIVITIES

Chemical methods

Since a variety of chemical substances may be involved in the human immediate allergic reaction and since smooth muscle is an important target organ, it is clear that antagonists of those chemicals and smooth muscle relaxants could have a combative effect in these reactions.

Antihistamines. Antihistamines are frequently substituted amines or ethanolamines that have only a vague resemblance to the structure of histamine (Fig. 8-7).

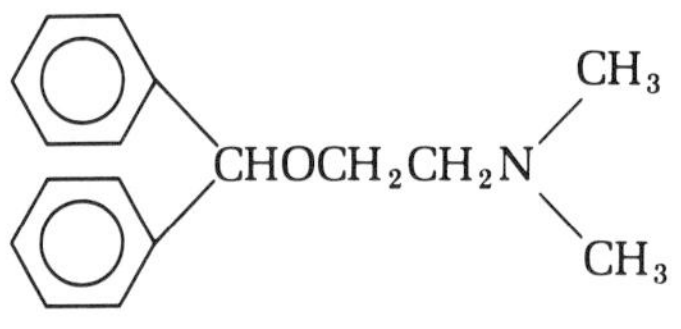

$CHOCH_2CH_2N(CH_3)_2$

Diphenhydramine

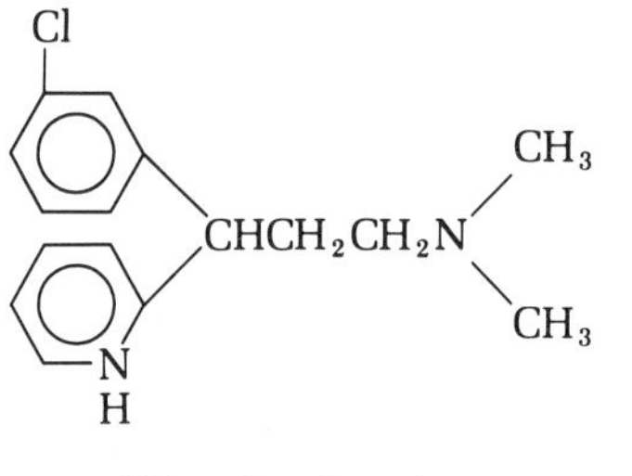

Cl

$CHCH_2CH_2N(CH_3)_2$

N H

Chlorpheniramine

CH_2

$N—CH_2CH_2N(CH_3)_2$

N H

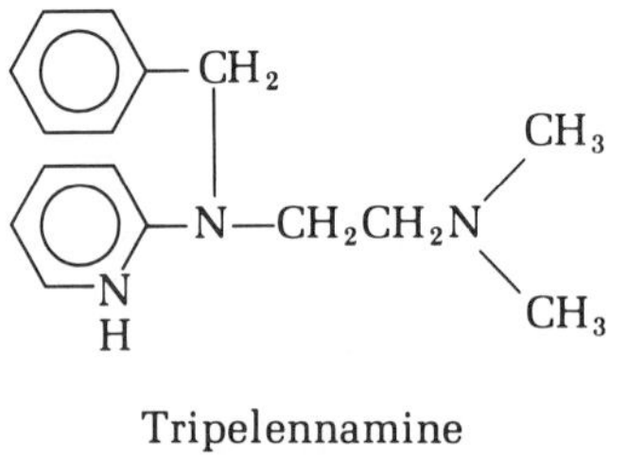

Tripelennamine

Fig. 8-7. Structures of three antihistamines. These compounds are all substituted diamines. Literally dozens of compounds with antihistaminic activity are known.

Nevertheless, these compounds plus certain substituted piperazines, phenothiazines, and hydroxyzines are considered competitive inhibitors of histamine because they block histamine receptors on nerve endings. Antihistamines have no effect on histamine release from mast cells or basophils. In man, antihistamines are effective antagonists of edema and pruritus, which are probably related to their blockage of histamine-induced increases in capillary permeability. Antihistamines are relatively less effective in man in preventing bronchoconstriction.

The competitive function of histamine analogs is best displayed when they are administered prior to the release of histamine. Since this is rarely the case in human allergies, these drugs have been thought less effective than experimental situations indicate. Drug effectiveness must always be evaluated in terms of side effects, and sedation is a major undesired effect of many antihistamines.

Antiserotonins. Inhibition of 5-hydroxytryptophan–induced constriction of smooth muscle is possible with lysergic acid derivatives, but because of the hallucinogenic activity of these compounds, they are not used extensively.

Methyl xanthines. Relaxation of smooth muscle by the methyl xanthines caffeine, theophylline, and theobromine has encouraged their use as bronchodilators. These compounds also function at the level of the mast cell by increasing the concentration of cyclic AMP and reducing mast cell degranulation. An undesirable effect of the methyl xanthines is their diuretic function.

Cromolyn sodium (disodium cromoglycate). Extracts of the seeds of the plant *Ammi visnaga* contain a complex heterocyclic compound, cromolyn sodium, that has just recently been tested for its effect in modifying allergic reactions (Fig. 8-8). The compound is absorbed poorly from the intestinal tract; it is therefore administered by inhalation. The field trial successes of its use can be attributed to its prevention of histamine and SRS-A release from mast cells, which cannot degranulate in the presence of cromolyn. Cromolyn is a prophylactic drug and is not antagonistic to SRS-A or histamine. Likewise, it is without effect on the cyclic 3,5-AMP system.

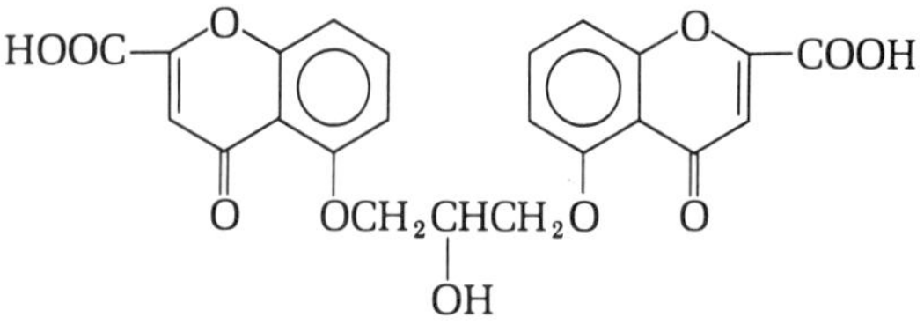

HOOC— —COOH

O OCH_2CHCH_2O O

OH

Cromolyn

Fig. 8-8. Structure of cromolyn.

Catecholamines. The terms "adrenergic drugs," "sympathomimetic drug," and "catecholamine" are used interchangeably to describe a series of substituted amines that have a potent bronchodilating and smooth muscle relaxant activity (Fig. 8-9). The physiologic response to these compounds is best explained on the basis of the concept of α- and β-receptors on the effector cells with which the catecholamines react. Attachment and blockage of the β-adrenergic receptor on mast cells allows adenylate cyclase to accumulate cyclic AMP, which in turn depresses histamine release. In this way these drugs produce a pronounced impairment of the allergic response. The β-receptors on smooth muscle of the bronchi influence muscle relaxation, and the α-receptors regulate constriction of the bronchial mucosae and influence edema. The various adrenergic drugs differ in their ability to block the α- and β-receptors, but since they may inhibit histamine release, decrease edema, and relax muscle, these compounds have both a prophylactic and therapeutic application to the immunoglobulin-dependent hypersensitivities. The best known of these compounds are adrenaline, ephedrine, propanolol, and isoproterenol.

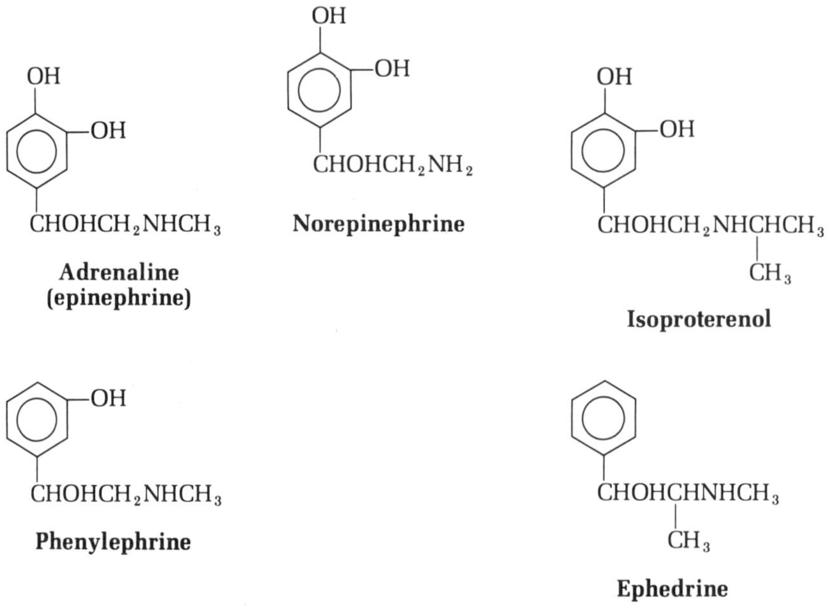

OH
OH
$CHOHCH_2NHCH_3$
Adrenaline (epinephrine)

OH
OH
$CHOHCH_2NH_2$
Norepinephrine

OH
OH
$CHOHCH_2NHCHCH_3$
CH_3
Isoproterenol

OH
$CHOHCH_2NHCH_3$
Phenylephrine

$CHOHCHNHCH_3$
CH_3
Ephedrine

Fig. 8-9. Adrenaline and several related adrenergic drugs.

Immunologic methods

Neutralization. When skin tests reveal that an intended recipient is allergic to an antigenic injectable or inhalant allergen, the existing cell-bound IgE can be neutralized. This can be accomplished and yet avoid the life-threatening hazard of a massive release of histamine if minute and increasing doses of the antigen are injected over the space of a few hours. The first small amounts of antigen provoke only a minimal amount of histamine release, and this is rapidly converted to the inert imidazoleacetic acid. When any symptoms of histamine shock have disappeared, another dose of antigen is given, and this is continued until the individual can tolerate the therapeutic dose of the injectable or further desensitizing doses of the allergen.

Before IgE neutralization is attempted it is prudent to administer antihistamines and to have adrenaline ready to reverse any accidental severe shock. This desensitization is temporary and in fact consists of booster exposures to the antigen. A week or so after neutralization has been completed the production of IgE may place the individual in a state of heightened hypersensitivity.

Blocking antibody. It does not necessarily follow that repeated exposure to an allergen will accentuate the hypersensitivity. Specific desensitization procedures are based on booster injections of antigen spaced over periods of weeks rather than hours to prompt the formation of blocking antibodies. It had previously been assumed that blocking antibodies were circulating IgG antibodies that combined with the antigen in the vascular system and prevented antigen diffusion into the tissues where IgE-coated mast cells resided. This mechanism of action for blocking antibodies is still favored, but it has been difficult to identify such antibodies as IgG.

REAGIN-REGULATED ALLERGIC DISEASE

Heat-labile antibodies or reagin certainly plays a much greater role in immunoglobulin-mediated allergic diseases than heat-stable antibodies. Heat-stable antibodies may contribute to these reactions, but this is apparently of modest significance and needs further clarification.

Anaphylaxis

Systemic anaphylaxis is a life-threatening expression of an IgE-based sensitivity to an antigen in which the shocking dose of the antigen is administered in such a way as to favor a massive release of histamine (and other vasoactive compounds) at one instant. This generally implies that the antigen be injected in the form of a solution, because cellular or particulate antigens cannot escape from the vascular system and enter the tissue bed where the mast cells reside until the time-consuming process of their conversion to a solution condition is completed. Anaphylaxis is easily demonstrated when the antigen is given intravenously, but due to the ease of rupturing small blood vessels while performing intramuscular, subcutaneous, or other injections, a high risk of provoking an anaphylactic reaction also accompanies these injections. Even insect stings, ophthalmic drops, and other seemingly superficial exposures to allergens can incite a lethal anaphylactic reaction in a highly sensitized person.

The Nobel Prize winning discovery of anaphylaxis (*ana,* meaning without; *phylaxis,* meaning protection) by Portier and Richet dates to 1902. They found that known nonlethal injections of sea anemone toxins into dogs were resisted as expected; however, when subsequent injections of the same amount of toxin were given to the dogs after the expiration of the immunologic waiting period, the dogs developed the convulsive canine form of systemic anaphylaxis. Symptoms of anaphylaxis in the dog include vomiting, diarrhea, urination, pruritus, restlessness, and accelerated pulse and respiratory rates. The vomitus may take on a fecal characteristic, and the diarrhea may be bloody. Although collapse occurs within a few minutes, death may not come for several hours.

Fatal anaphylaxis is more sudden in the guinea pig where the early symptoms include a bristling of the hair on the nape of the neck, pawing at the nose, sneezing, gasping for air, cyanosis, urination, defecation, and collapse, all within 5 minutes. The pulse may continue for several minutes after collapse. Death is due to asphyxiation.

Fatal anaphylaxis in man is related to contraction of the bronchiolar smooth muscle, asphyxiation, and edema of the central nervous system. This follows a tingling sensation in the throat, warm flashes, shortness of breath, pharyngeal edema, and collapse. The primary cause of death, which may transpire within 5 or 10 minutes after the shocking dose of antigen, is due, as in the guinea pig, to the inability to expire used gases from the lungs. Since inspiration can still occur, the lungs are fully inflated but devoid of oxygen.

The anaphylactic experience need not terminate fatally. The individual may not be lethally sensitized by the previous antigen exposure or the shocking dose may not reach enough sensitized mast cells at one time. However, it must be recognized that minute doses of antigen or autocoupling haptens, doses consisting of as little as 0.001 mg of protein, have been known to sensitize and lethally shock a person.

Awareness of a potential previous sensitization demands the application of two important precautions. The first of these is a skin test or a substitute test such as an ophthalmic test to determine if the sensitivity does in fact exist. When the immediate-type skin reaction is seen, then the intended injection should not be given—a substitute therapeutic should be chosen. Whenever any potential for anaphylactic shock exists and the offending substance must be given, the person should be pretreated with antihistamines and a syringe prefilled with adrenaline should be available. It may be possible to desensitize the person by fractional doses of the antigen administered over a period of a few hours.

When the individual escapes the fatal outcome of anaphylaxis, he is temporarily desensitized. His mast cells have given up their histamine, and it takes a few days to replenish this supply. When this has been completed, the individual may be even more sensitive than before, because the shocking dose serves as a booster. All forms of desensitization for both the immediate and delayed hypersensitivities are but temporary events and sensitization will recur.

The major cause of anaphylaxis in modern medicine is the injection of therapeutic drugs, and a well-studied offender is penicillin. More precisely it is not penicillin that is the offender; it is a degradation product of penicillin that conjugates with tissue proteins to form neoantigens. Several compounds with potential autocoupling activity arise in the in vivo degradation pathway of penicillin. Sulfhydryl exchange reactions are possible at each of these stages with the sulfur atom in the thiazolidine ring, and although some hypersensitive reactions may be directed against —S—S— conjugates of penicillenic acid or penicillamine, penicilloic acid-protein complexes are more frequent sensitizers. These penicilloyl conjugates are formed by an opening of the unstable oxazole ring of penicillenic acid during its coupling to free amino groups in proteins. It cannot always be determined which proteins in vivo serve as carriers, but it is known that the degradation products from penicillin can attach to most serum proteins.

Detection of hypersensitivity to haptens such as penicillin is not always possible by simple skin tests with the hapten. It is believed that although 10,000 to 40,000 IgE molecules may be attached to the surface of a mast cell, they cannot cause the cell to discharge its granules unless two IgE molecules are joined by an antigen or antigen-hapten bridge. Since haptens are monovalent, they cannot link two IgE molecules and cannot cause histamine release. Artificial conjugates of the hapten are required for this, and to avoid sensitization to the carrier, a weakly antigenic or nonantigenic carrier is obviously preferred. In the case of penicillin a penicilloyl polylysine is commercially available for skin testing, and it has proved itself to be decidedly superior to penicillin for this purpose.

Serum sickness

Although it is true that autocoupling haptens are often responsible for anaphylaxis today, in the earlier era of medicine the primary incident leading to anaphylaxis was the injection of foreign serum used in immunotherapy for its content of antitoxin. If the person was fortunate enough to escape an anaphylactic experience, accelerated or primary serum sickness remained distinct possibilities. As with anaphylaxis, serum sickness is presently less frequently caused by injections of serum than by injections of haptenic compounds.

Primary serum sickness is evidenced by extensive edema about the face, neck, and joints with joint pain, hives, fever, malaise, and eosinophilia—symptoms that usually occur 7 to 10 days subsequent to the injection of a large quantity of an antigen or an autocoupling hapten. These symptoms, which are consistent with a picture of histamine poisoning, develop gradually. For this reason serum sickness has been called protracted anaphylaxis. The reason for its insidious onset is that it takes 5 to 10 days after the antigen injection before the requisite cytotropic antibodies are formed and begin to attach to mast cells. As a result of the injection of a substantial quantity of antigen, antigen will still be available for combination with the cell-bound antibodies as soon as they attach to the mast cells. Thus it is the kinetics of the situation that causes a gradual but steady release of histamine so that a life-threatening concentration is never achieved. As heat-stable immunoglobulins are formed, they complex with the antigen in the circulation and are removed in the kidney, where they contribute to the immune complex nephritis so common to serum sickness.

An accelerated form of serum sickness is noted whenever a person has had a significant interlude, usually measured in years, between the sensitizing exposure to antigen and its reinjection. Even if this second injection is performed at a time when the cytotropic antibody level is essentially nil, the IgE anamnestic response will abbreviate the time needed to accumulate IgE-coated cells as compared to primary serum sickness, and the symptoms of serum sickness are seen within 2 to 5 days.

There has been a surprising reluctance to classify serum sickness as an immediate hypersensitivity, apparently because the symptoms are not manifest until a few days after the antigen injection. However, all the hallmarks of the immediate hypersensitivities are seen in serum sickness—a dependence on IgE (and other antibodies), mast cell degranulation, histamine release, protection with antihistamine, therapy with adrenergic drugs, etc. Serum sickness is unique only in that the sensitizing and shocking doses of antigen are one and the same because of the magnitude of the antigen (or autocoupling hapten) dose given.

Inhalant allergy

Common inhalant allergens are as follows:

Seasonal

Pollens
- Trees
  - Elm, oak, maple, ash, birch, hickory (early spring in southern states; late spring in northern states)
- Grasses
  - Bluegrass, orchard grass, timothy, red top (spring and summer)
- Weeds
  - Ragweed, amaranth, plantain, thistle (midsummer to early autumn)

Nonseasonal

House dust
- *Dermatophagoides* mites

Danders and feather
- Dog, cat, horse, other domestic pets, chicken

Mold
- *Mucor, Aspergillus, Penicillium,* etc.

Occupational airborne allergens
- Plant seeds, cereal grains and flour, detergent enzymes

Hay fever. The form of inhalant allergy that affects the mucosae of the upper respiratory tract and eyes and is characterized by sneezing, itching, and/or burning of the nose and eyes with associated tears, nasal discharge, and swollen mucosae is defined as hay fever. It is an atopic allergy related to specific IgE responses to airborne seasonal or perennial allergens. Seasonal allergies, especially in summer during the haying season, have given the name hay fever to these conditions even though hay is rarely an offending antigen.

Hay fever of springtime is often misconstrued as a head cold and is due to pollens of trees and early spring grasses. Summer hay fever is due to pollens of grasses and weeds, with species of *Ambrosia* (ragweed) being a common offender (Fig. 8-10). Nonseasonal hay fever is an allergic

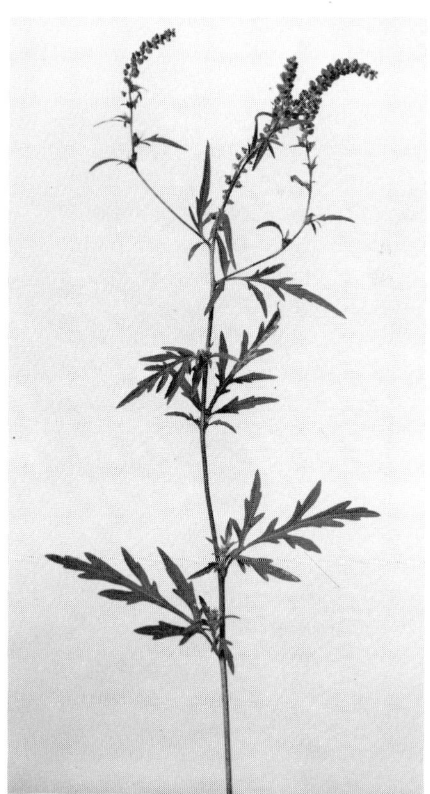

Fig. 8-10. Photograph of ragweed plant showing uppermost pollen-bearing spines.

response due to animal dander, cereal dusts, house dust, house mites, and other sources of antigens in a regular, airborne association with the victim.

It is not possible to discuss the chemistry of the multitudinous antigens associated with hay fever, since this would include the spores of virtually all fungi, the pollens of hundreds of plants—ragweed, timothy grass, elm, oak, pine trees, etc.—flour dusts, cereal grains, etc. One of these antigens, antigen E from the dwarf ragweed plant *Ambrosia elatior,* is responsible for naming reagin IgE. It has been extensively purified and represents about 6% of the total protein in ragweed pollen. It has a molecular weight of 38,000 and apparently exists as a pair of noncovalently linked peptides of 16,000 and 22,000 daltons. It is a far more potent stimulator of IgE formation than the ragweed antigens K, Ra3, or Ra5, although K has about one-half the activity of E.

Contact with inhalant allergens is unavoidable. Reexposure of the mucous membranes of the eye, nose, pharynx, etc. to antigens after specific IgE has coated mast cells results in mast cell degranulation. Because of the mode of contact with the antigen and its insoluble state, hay fever can be thought of as a mild local form of anaphylaxis.

Treatment of hay fever has traditionally included antihistamines and similar drugs, geographic dislocation to a more allergen-free environment, and hyposensitization. Hay fever acquired in childhood is often less severe after puberty for reasons that remain unknown.

Asthma. It is virtually impossible to define asthma, although most clinicians recognize it as an inhalant allergy characterized by marked wheezing. This stressed breathing is aggravated by climatic changes such as humidity and cool night air. Asthma following and clearly related to an upper respiratory infection is also well known.

Exactly why asthmatics respond in their peculiar way to inhalant allergens as compared to those with regular hay fever is unknown. Both groups show immediate-type skin reactions, IgE is clearly associated with both conditions, and antihistamines are of some benefit although asthmatics as a group rely heavily on adrenaline inhalants or vaporizers to open their airways to permit easier breathing. It may be that other immunoglobulins contribute to asthma or some aspect of cell-mediated hypersensitivity may be involved. Asthma is a serious disease that can assume a chronicity that can contribute to other forms of lung disease.

Food allergy

Allergies to food are frequently identified by the eruption of urticarial splotches on the skin following ingestion of the incitant food. Other symptoms may include oral inflammation, erythema and edema of and around the lips, gastrointestinal cramping, nausea, gaseous distention, and even diarrhea. Respiratory symptoms may also be noted if dry foods that ensure respiratory contact are involved. Studies of allergic children reveal that the following foods are the dominant allergens: codfish, strawberries, oranges, wheat and wheat products, cow's milk, and chocolate. Other highly allergenic foods include peanuts and other nuts, rye and other cereal grains, eggs, and tomatoes. Avoidance of these foods is the most practical route to prevent a recurrence of these IgE-mediated allergies.

TYPE II OR CYTOTOXIC IgG ALLERGIES

Type II allergies are often considered synonymous with the precipitin allergies, so named because of the ease with which precipitating antibodies could be demonstrated in the sera of the involved persons. IgG and IgM appear to dominate the cytotoxic response, which appears to rely less on IgA and IgD.

Arthus reaction

Although the Arthus reaction has been described as a form of local anaphylaxis, it is an absolutely unrelated entity and should not be compared to anaphylaxis. The Arthus reaction is entirely dependent on the presence of a high level of circulating antibody that precipitates with antigen in the vascular system to block local blood vessels and produce necrosis. The Arthus reaction is best developed by a series of one-a-day intradermal injections of antigen, although any immunizing schedule that results in a potent precipitating antiserum is satisfactory. When this has been achieved, a subsequent injection of antigen into the skin will produce some local erythema and edema, but shortly thereafter a bluish purple zone under the injection site will develop. This will progress to a purple-black necrotic area that will continue to form a dry eschar over the succeeding 2 to 5 days. Eventually healing beneath the eschar will cause it to slough.

This reaction is caused by a diffusion of antigen primarily into the venules, where precipitation and thrombosis develop. Deprivation of normal gas exchange, adequate waste elimination, and cell nutrition results in death of cells near the thrombus. Tissue destruction is further favored by the participation of complement, the attraction of neutrophils, neutrophilic death, and the release of lysosomal enzymes.

Immune complex pneumonitis

Immune complex pneumonitis is discussed in case 2 at the end of this chapter.

Shwartzman reaction

The dermal Shwartzman reaction is a nonimmunologic mimic of the Arthus reaction. A disseminated form of the Shwartzman reaction is also known. To provoke this reaction the skin is first sensitized by an intradermal dose of a culture filtrate of a gram-negative bacterium known to contain a generous content of bacterial endotoxin (lipopolysaccharide). Cultures of *Escherichia coli,* the cholera vibrio, the typhoid bacillus, and many other bacteria are equally suitable. Twenty-four hours later an intravenous injection of the same filtrate causes a hemorrhagic necrosis to develop at the initial skin site. The intravenous injection can consist of a dilute solution of agar, starch, or other nonantigenic material that clearly illustrates that the Shwartzman reaction is not an immunologic reaction. Instead, this reaction relies on a primary sensitization of tissues by endotoxin, which causes local vascular coagulation, fibrin deposition, and cell necrosis that is supplemented by a second set of fibrin deposits following the second injection.

• • •

Refer to Itkin (1973) and Swineford (1971) for further discussion of problems in the diagnosis and management of allergic disease.

BIBLIOGRAPHY

Aas, K.: The radioallergosorbant test (RAST): diagnostic and clinical significance, Ann. Allergy **33**:251, 1974.

Austen, K. F., and Becker, E. L., eds.: Biochemistry of the acute allergic reactions, ed. 2, Philadelphia, 1971, F. A. Davis Co.

Baer, H.: In vitro methods in allergy, Med. Clin. North Am. **58**:85, 1974.

Becker, E. L.: Nature and classification of immediate type allergic reactions, Adv. Immunol. **13**:267, 1971.

Bennich, H., and Johansson, S. G. O.: Structure and function of human immunoglobulin E, Adv. Immunol. **13**:1, 1971.

Berrens, L.: The chemistry of atopic allergens, Basel, 1971, S. Karger, A.G.

Blumstein, G. L.: Drug treatment of allergies. I. The pathophysiologic basis of allergy, Semin. Drug Treat. **2**:353, 1973.

Braun, W., Lichtenstein, L. M., and Parker, C. W., eds.: Cyclic AMP, cell growth, and the immune response, New York, 1974, Springer-Verlag New York, Inc.

Brostoff, J., ed.: Clinical immunology-allergy in

pediatric medicine, Oxford, 1973, Blackwell Scientific Publications, Ltd.

Cohen, C.: Genetic aspects of allergy, Med. Clin. North Am. **58**:25, 1974.

Eisner, J. W.: Drugs used in allergic states and their mode of action, Semin. Drug Treat. **2**: 367, 1973.

Flick, J. A.: Human reagins: appraisal of the properties of the antibody of immediate-type hypersensitivity, Bacteriol. Rev. **36**:311, 1972.

Gell, P. G. H., Coombs, R. A., and Lachmann, P., eds.: Clinical aspects of immunology, ed. 3, Oxford, 1974, Blackwell Scientific Publications, Ltd.

Goodfriend, L., Sehon, A. H., and Orange, R. P., eds.: Mechanisms in allergy. Reagin-mediated hypersensitivity, New York, 1973, Marcel Dekker, Inc.

Hyde, H. A.: Atmospheric pollen grains and spores in relation to allergy, Clin. Allergy **3**: 109, 1973.

Itkin, I. H.: Allergy case studies; 65 case histories related to allergy, Flushing, N.Y., 1973, Medical Examination Publishing Co., Inc.

Kirkpatrick, C. H.: Steroid therapy of allergic diseases, Med. Clin. North Am. **57**:1309, 1973.

Kreithen, H.: Allergy in adverse drug reactions, Semin. Drug Treat. **2**:431, 1973.

Lepow, I. H., and Ward, P. A., eds.: Inflammation, mechanism and control, New York, 1972, Academic Press, Inc.

Lichtenstein, L. M.: Allergy, Clin. Immunobiol. **1**:243, 1972.

Patterson, R., ed.: Allergic disease, Philadelphia, 1972, J. B. Lippincott Co.

Patterson, R.: Rhinitis, Med. Clin. North Am. **58**:43, 1974.

Pepys, J.: Types of allergic reactions, Clin. Allergy **3**(suppl.):491, 1973.

Samter, M., ed.: Immunological diseases, ed. 2, Boston, 1971, Little, Brown & Co.

Sanders, G. E., and Huggins, C. G.: Vasoactive peptides, Annu. Rev. Pharmacol. **12**:227, 1972.

Stanworth, D. R.: IgE and hypersensitivity in man, Scientific Basis of Medicine: Annual Reviews p. 33, 1972.

Stanworth, D. R.: Immediate hypersensitivity, Amsterdam, 1973, North-Holland Publishing Co.

Stewart, G. T., and McGovern, J. P., eds.: Penicillin allergy: clinical and immunological aspects, Springfield, Ill., 1970, Charles C Thomas, Publisher.

Swineford, O.: Asthma and hay fever, Springfield, Ill., 1973, Charles C Thomas, Publisher.

Turk, J. L.: Immunology in clinical medicine, London, 1973, William Heinemann, Ltd.

Wide, L.: Clinical significance of measurement of reaginic (IgE) antibody by RAST, Clin. Allergy **3**(suppl.):583, 1973.

Zwiefach, B. W., Grant, L., and McCluskey, R. T., eds: The inflammatory process, ed. 2, New York, 1973, Academic Press, Inc.

Case histories

CASE 1. PENICILLIN HYPERSENSITIVITY

Ruth L., a 25-year-old female with a history of asthma and eczema since early childhood, came from a family with a history of atopy. She had a sore throat for about 1 day, and her physician husband gave her an injection of 300,000 units of penicillin. Previous exposure to penicillin had been without incident. Since no improvement had occurred and she still had difficulty in swallowing, that evening she was given a second injection of penicillin. Within 5 minutes she developed laryngeal constriction, became cyanotic and dyspneic, and collapsed. Her husband immediately administered 0.25 ml of 1:1000 epinephrine intramuscularly. Very little improvement was noticed and he called an ambulance. An emergency tracheotomy and additional epinephrine prevented what was almost certain to be a fatal outcome. Within a few days complete recovery ensued and the tracheotomy was closed.

Questions

1. Why do allergic reactions to penicillin develop in the presence of a past history of acceptance of penicillin?

2. What is the antigenic basis of penicillin hypersensitivity?
3. What is the status of skin testing for penicillin allergy?
4. Are penicillin reactions always of the immediate type?
5. Is hyposensitization to penicillin practical?

Discussion

Allergic reactions to penicillin injections are difficult to predetermine. Serious allergic reactions have occurred following the first exposure and have been attributed to unknown hypersensitization to penicillin, allergy to contaminants in the antibiotic preparation, or cross-sensitivity resulting from hypersensitivity to related antibioties such as cephalosporin. Prior uneventful exposures to penicillin are not a reliable index to continued freedom from an allergic reaction, as this case illustrates. Human variation in response to antigens and haptens is so great that only the generality that the greater the exposure the greater the probability of developing an allergic reaction is acceptable.

Hypersensitization to penicillin resides in the ability of penicillenic acid to combine with tissue and/or blood proteins to form penicilloyl-protein conjugates. The immunoglobulin response, of which the IgE response is the most important, is directed almost exclusively against the penicillin-haptenic portion of the complex; hence the allergy does not persist when the penicillin moiety is eliminated from the body. At one time it was felt this could be accelerated safely with injections of penicillinase that hydrolyze the lactam ring of the antibiotic molecule, but this only added the complication of penicillinase hypersensitivity to the already significant population, estimated at 10% to 20%, that is sensitive to penicillin. All penicillin hypersensitivity is not of the anaphylactic type—the serum sickness type of reaction and delayed type hypersensitivity may also develop.

Diagnosis of penicillin hypersensitivity by skin testing with penicillin, although possible, will reveal only a limited number of those individuals who will display an allergic reaction after the injection of penicillin. A synthetic polylysine molecule to which penicilloyl groups have been attached is a much safer reagent and will identify approximately 75% of those with a penicillin hypersensitivity. In practice this product is not extensively used and neither is desensitization. When knowledge of penicillin hypersensitivity is revealed, the physician selects another antigenically unrelated antibiotic.

REFERENCES

Levine, B. D.: Immunochemical mechanisms of drug allegry, Annu. Rev. Med. **17**:23, 1966.

Levine, B. D., and Zolov, D. M.: Prediction of penicillin allergy by immunological tests, J. Allergy **43**:321, 1969.

Tuft, L., Gregory, D. C., and Gregory, J.: Evaluation of skin testing methods employed in the diagnosis of penicillin allergy, Am. J. Med. Sci. **230**:370, 1955.

CASE 2. FARMER'S LUNG

J. B., a 37-year-old farmer, on admission to the hospital complained of shortness of breath that had begun in the middle of the winter. To his knowledge he had not had a cold all winter, although he did have a slight fever and cough associated with his dyspnea. He was a nonsmoker and not known to be allergic to animal hair or dander, grain dust, or other potential sensitizers in his environment such as grass or weed pollens. The PPD test was negative. X-ray films revealed a diffuse reticulonodular infiltrate of the lungs. Lung cultures were negative for mycotic and bacterial pathogens. It was suggested that he had farmer's lung, and after a brief description of the disease, J. B. recalled that he had experienced a mild form of his present illness the previous winter.

Questions

1. What is the etiology of farmer's lung?
2. How is farmer's lung classified as an allergic disease?

Discussion

Farmer's lung is only one of several respiratory ailments (Table I) that share many common features. All are lung diseases developing in persons who work or play in a dusty environment. Moldy hay, grain dust, compost, wood bark dust, bird droppings, etc. all initiate a rather singular form of disease. In several instances the important if not sole antigen involved is the spore of a mold.

The mold grows in the moist, rich medium that the hay, wood bark, or cotton provides, and the growth cycle ends in sporulation. Fungal spores, most of which are less than 10 μ in diameter, are inhaled as the laborer or hobbiest works with the spore-bearing material. The respiratory route is a very satisfactory immunizing avenue as the variety of organisms involved in these diseases testify.

To immunologists the problem of defining the exact cause of these diseases was greatly dependent on the work of Pepys. It had been noted that even in the acute forms of these diseases there were rarely any reactions that could be classified as of the anaphylactic or life-threatening type. In fact, the affected persons seemed to suffer most from their illness a few hours after contact with the allergen, suggesting a cell-mediated mechanism for the illness. However IgG antibodies specific for the organisms listed for each disease in Table I have been identified in the sera of these patients. Moreover, IgG precipitates in lung tissue biopsies have been noted. The histopathology of the lung lesion is completely compatible with that of an Arthus-type reaction since IgG precipitates are noted, platelets and fibrin deposits are seen, and neutrophilic infiltration of the alveolar capillary walls is observed. The present and rather firm opinion is that these forms of extrinsic allergic pneumonitis are naturally induced reactions. In every instance removing the source of exposure terminates the disease.

REFERENCES

Pepys, J.: Hypersensitivity diseases of the lungs due to fungi and organic dusts, Basel, 1969, S. Karger, A.G.

Reed, C. E.: Hypersensitivity pneumonitis, Postgrad Med. **51**:120, 1972.

Table I. Immune complex pneumonitis

Disease	*Source of antigen*	*Antigen*
Farmer's lung	Moldy hay	*Thermoactinomyces vulgaris*
Mushroom worker's lung	Compost	Thermophilic actinomycetes
Bird fancier's lung	Dry bird droppings	Avian proteins
Laundry worker's lung	Detergent	Enzymes of *Bacillus subtilis*
Pigeon breeder's lung	Pigeon dander or droppings	Pigeon proteins
Bagassosis	Moldy bagasse	Thermophilic actinomycetes
Maple bark pneumonitis	Maple bark dust	*Cryptostoma corticale*
Malt worker's lung	Moldy barley	*Aspergillus clavatus*
Wheat weevil disease	Infested flour	*Sitophilus granarius*
Sequoiosis	Moldy sawdust	*Graphium* species

Salvaggio, J. E., Seabury, J. H., Beuchner, H. A., and Kundur, V. G.: Bagassosis: demonstration of precipitins against extracts of thermophilic *Actinomycetes* in the sera of affected individuals, J. Allergy **39**:106, 1967.

CASE 3. RESPIRATORY ALLERGY

N. B., a 20-year-old female was seen in the allergy clinic. The following history was taken. She was born and lived in Colorado until last year when she married a young college student in June and moved to Missouri. In August of this year she began to work in the used-book section of the university book store. Within a few days she developed swollen, itching red eyes and periodic sneezing while at work. Her discomfort was severe enough for her to take extra time from work and remain at home, where her condition persisted in a mild but extensive enough form to seek medical attention.

Questions

1. What does the patient's relocation to Missouri and her employment have to do with her allergic rhinitis?
2. What skin testing reagents should be included in the allergy workup?
3. What desensitization process, if any, is to be recommended?

Discussion

The appearance of rhinitis in the autumn, especially in persons who have moved to the central states within the past few years, often signals that the etiology of the rhinitis is due to ragweed pollen. In this instance the first summer's residence in Missouri undoubtedly served as the sensitization period. During the following winter, spring, and summer no discomfort was noted because the antigen was not present in sufficient quantity. The ragweed season usually begins in Missouri in August, its severity depending on climatic conditions during the summer and in August, being favored by a good growth season followed by dryness and light breezes. After the first frost the pollen count usually falls drastically, providing relief until the next pollen season.

This woman was skin tested by the scratch method for autumn pollens with the following results:

Ragweed pollen	2+ (0.8 cm wheal, marked areola)
Amaranth	–
Hemp	–
Chenopod	–
Russian thistle	–
House dust	2+

The patient was treated with ephedrine sulfate, 25 mg every 4 hours, and an antihistamine, chlorpheniramine maleate, 8 mg every 4 hours. This provided sufficient relief that the patient could return to work. Her employer transferred her to the new book section, a relatively dust-free environment.

After the first of December the patient entered a hyposensitization program for house dust and on the first of April for ragweed—both have been successful. In the meantime the patient developed a contact allergy to eye shadow and lipstick. This was eliminated by removing them from her cosmetic preparations and substituting hypoallergenic cosmetics with the warning that such cosmetics are only relatively hypoallergenic and that she must terminate their use at the first indication of an allergic response.

There is still considerable debate about the exact dosage and schedule of pollen injections to be used in desensitization programs. The arbitrary dilutions previously recommended have been improved by labeling of pollen and other allergen extracts with their protein nitrogen content. It has been shown that pollen collected in 1 year may contain less protein than that in other years, and simple dilution did not account for their differences in potency. Patients are often classed as very sensitive, moderately sensitive, weakly sensitive, and relatively insensitive, with the first class receiving the lowest allergen dose. Progressive increases in allergen dose are regulated by patient tolerance of previous doses. Desensitization is recommended not only for the relief it may provide to the existing hay fever but because it is believed to deter progression to an asthmatic state.

REFERENCES

Lieberman, P., and Patterson, R.: Immunotherapy for atopic disease, Adv. Intern. Med. **19**:391, 1974.

Sherman, W. B.: Hypersensitivity: mechanisms and management, Philadelphia, 1968, W. B. Saunders Co.

Tuft, L.: Allergy management in clinical practice, St. Louis, 1973, The C. V. Mosby Co.

chapter 9

Lymphokine-mediated hypersensitivity

Cell-mediated hypersensitivity as a synonym for T lymphokine–mediated hypersensitivity is a misnomer; it is no more cell dependent than immunoglobulin-mediated hypersensitivity. The term arose because it was felt that T lymphocytes had to be in direct physical contact with the antigens to which they responded. This has now proved to be untrue, and the identification of several lymphokines has provided a realization that T cells, like B cells, excrete peptides responsible for their specific hypersensitive and immune reactions. Unlike the immunoglobulins produced by B cells, the lymphokines never achieve concentrations in blood of several milligrams per 100 ml. Consequently, the transfer of T cell hypersensitivity to a normal recipient could not be accomplished with serum but required living T cells, and this further supported the concept of cell-mediated hypersensitivity. It is now possible to effect successful transfers with concentrates of culture fluids in which T cells were exposed to mitogens or antigens. This experiment conclusively demonstrates that T cells function through their cell products rather than by direct contact.

The term "cell-mediated hypersensitivity" is also misapplied when used in synonymy with cell-mediated immunity. The latter should be used only to refer to protective functions of T lymphocytes and the former to untoward effects of these cells.

CLASSIFICATION

The characteristics of the cell-mediated allergies were compared with those of the immunoglobulin-mediated allergies in Chapter 8 (Tables 8-1 and 8-2). Briefly, these include a protracted emergence of the hypersensitive reaction after the shocking exposure to antigen, the absence of any specific shock organ in systemic reactions, erythema and induration with relatively little edema in dermal reactions, and a monocytic infiltration of these reaction sites. This hypersensitivity is dependent on lymphokines excreted by T lymphocytes. Since all lymphokines are large polypeptides, no simple therapeutic combatants are available to modify these reactions, and the precise chemical mechanisms underlying these lymphokine functions are not known. Palliative anti-inflammatory compounds are the only useful therapeutic agents. The T lymphokine–mediated hypersensitivities or delayed hypersensitivities represent the type IV reactions in the classification scheme of Gell and Coombs.

ALLERGY OF INFECTION

Two main routes of exposure account for essentially all T lymphocyte–mediated allergic reactions encountered in the human being, and these are microbial infections and dermal contact.

Koch is credited with the discovery of delayed hypersensitivity during his studies of tuberculosis in guinea pigs. Koch found that the intradermal injection of concentrated culture filtrates of *Mycobacterium tuberculosis* into tuberculous guinea pigs caused a gradual reddening and thickening around the injection site that reached its peak between 48 and 96 hours and then gradually disappeared. Similar injections into normal guinea pigs were innocuous. This reaction is the tuberculin skin reaction that can be produced by injecting old tuberculin (OT) or purified protein derivative (PPD) into the skin of an animal that presently has or previously had tuberculosis.

OT is prepared from the culture medium in which *M. tuberculosis* has grown for several weeks. The bacteria are heat killed and removed by filtration. The culture fluid is then evaporated to one-tenth its original volume, reclarified, tested for potency, and used as OT. The active factor in OT is a peptide with a molecular weight of only 2000 that can be precipitated with trichloroacetic acid. After being returned to solution and passing potency tests it is used as PPD (Fig. 9-1). Other peptides contained in OT may also have some activity in eliciting the delayed cutaneous reaction. OT and PPD are quite stable during storage, but some decay in activity is unavoidable. This may cause minimal reactions in highly allergic individuals. The percentage of false negative reactions and the strength of positive reactions are more accurately determined with the PPD preparations now commercially available.

Tuberculin skin testing procedures are numerous. The intradermal injection of PPD is known as the Mantoux test; the multiple puncture or Tine test is a refinement of the earlier method used by von Pirquet in which tuberculin was rubbed into scarified skin. The Vollmer patch test is popular, especially in pediatric practice, because no injection is required. For the Vollmer patch test, PPD is impregnated onto a paper square that is held against the skin with a piece of adhesive tape. One benefit of the Vollmer patch test is its incorporation of a normal bacterial growth medium control. Positive tests are much like those described initially by Koch—erythema and induration with small vesicle formation in highly reactive individuals (Fig. 9-2).

There are many infections that induce a delayed type of dermal hypersensitivity, and these span the range from viruses to animal parasites (Table 9-1). Mumps, lymphogranuloma venereum, and smallpox can

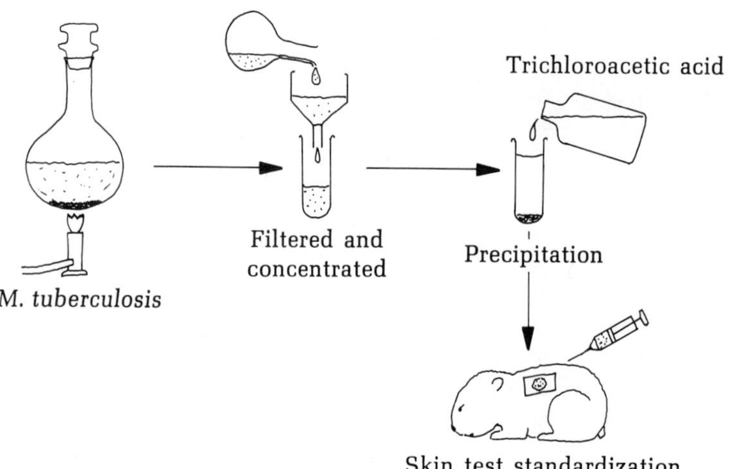

Fig. 9-1. Important stages in the preparation of purified protein derivative.

A

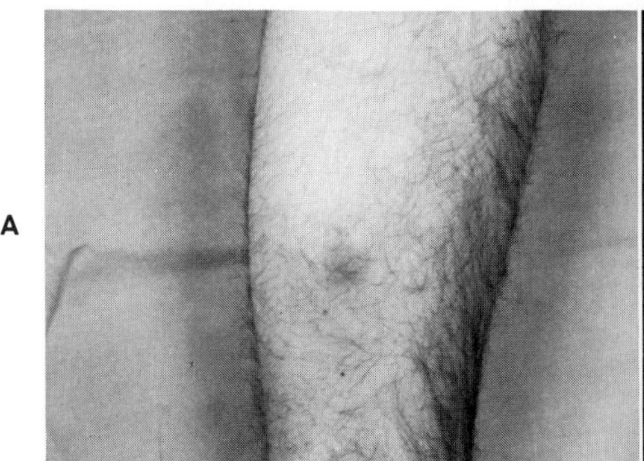

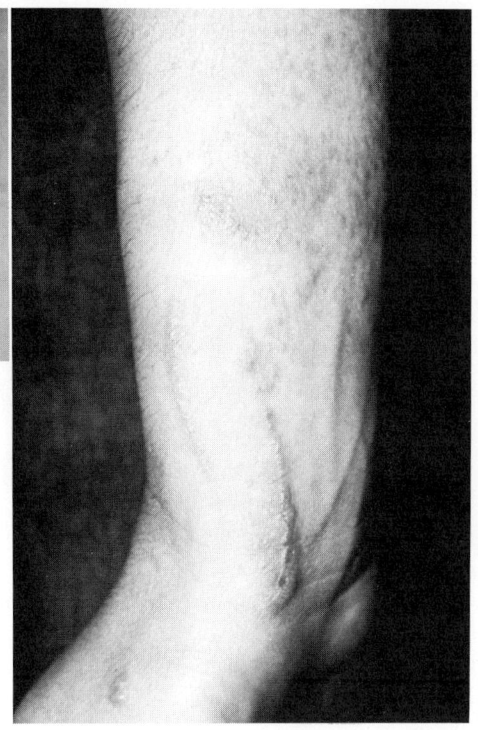

B

Fig. 9-2. **A,** Positive skin test for an allergy to infection is demonstrated by erythematous but not edematous response. **B,** In contrast, poison ivy rash demonstrates obvious vesicle formation and edema. This is probably due to the presence of some anti-urushiol IgE.

Table 9-1. Delayed-type hypersensitive skin tests for allergies of infection

Disease	*Name of skin test*	*Reagent used*
Bacterial		
Tuberculosis	Mantoux, Vollmer, etc. according to method	OT or PPD
Leprosy	Lepromin (Mitsuda)	Extract of lepromatous tissue (lepromin)
Diphtheria	Moloney	Diphtheria toxoid
Brucellosis	Brucellergen	Heat-killed organism
Tularemia	Foshay	Bacterial protein antigen
Streptococcal infection	—	Streptokinase-streptodornase
Viral		
Lymphogranuloma venereum	Frei	Inactive virus
Smallpox		Vaccinia virus
Mumps		Mumps virus vaccine
Fungal		
Histoplasmosis	Histoplasmin	Concentrate of culture filtrate (histoplasmin)
Coccidioidomycosis	Coccidioidin	Concentrate of culture filtrate (coccidioidin)
Blastomycosis	Blastomycin	Concentrate of culture filtrate

be listed in the viral group. Bacterial infections that result in cell-mediated allergy include tuberculosis, leprosy, brucellosis, diphtheria, salmonellosis, and streptococcal infections. The fungal diseases histoplasmosis, blastomycosis, and coccidioidomycosis produce a pronounced delayed hypersensitivity. Allergies of infection persist throughout life and remain positive long after the infection has been halted. For this reason such tests are seldom diagnostic for an existing disease, with the obvious exception being in the early pediatric age group, where the possibility of a diagnostic application of these tests is very real due to the brief time span within which these children could have become infected.

The use of skin testing reagents for allergies of infection, except for OT or PPD, has recently been curtailed because of the uncertain effect they may have on antibody titers. Particularly in the case of the systemic fungal diseases it is suspected that the skin testing reagents may be antigenic. Skin tested subjects would thus become seropositive, and since serologic tests are used as a supportive criterion for clinical diagnosis of these diseases, skin testing reagents would contribute to erroneous diagnoses. The low molecular weight peptides in PPD have not yet been incriminated, apparently because they are too small to be antigenic. Moreover, serologic tests are not used in the diagnosis of tuberculosis.

CONTACT DERMATITIS

Intermittent or constant dermal contact with a wide selection of chemicals will induce a lymphokine-mediated hypersensitivity (Table 9-2). Such chemicals are present in leather, rubber or other elastic products, cosmetics, hair dyes, detergents, insecticides, and many compounds encountered occupationally—photographic chemicals, dyes, plastic and rubber industrial products, etc. These products often cause a skin rash, usually seen as a dry, thickened, erythematous, sometimes scaly area at the place of contact with the incitant chemical—under leather or metal belts or jewelry such as rings, bracelets, or necklaces; over the facial area where cosmetics are applied; on the scalp in cases of hair dye, hair spray, or shampoo allergy; on the hands in instances of allergy to detergent additives, etc. The anatomic distribution of the rash is often helpful in eliminating other diagnoses (skin infections, for example). Specific chemicals responsible for these reactions include formaldehyde, mercury, or other metals in insecticides; nickel and copper in watchbands, earrings, metal buckles, other jewelry, and coins; potassium dichromate in yellow-dyed leather goods; paraphenylenediamine in black-, brown-, and blue-dyed cloth, leather, and animal pelts or hair; and phenyl-β-naphthylamine in rubber. A complete listing of chemicals involved is not possible simply because of

***Table* 9-2.** Sources of contact dermatitis and the allergens involved

Object	*Sources*	*Compounds involved*
Metal	Jewelry, belt buckles, watches, watchbands, scissors, thimbles, cosmetics	Nickel, chromium, iron, cobalt, copper, mercury
Clothing		Animal and plant fibers; anthraquinone and other dyes; vinyl, acrylate, glycol, and other permanent press agents; formaldehyde
Rubber	Swim wear, garters, shoes, condoms	Hydroquinone and other antioxidants; benzothiazole and other accelerators
Cosmetics	Rouge, lipstick, eye shadow, hair dye, depilatories, perfumes, lotions, sprays	Iron and cobalt dyes; sulfide depilatories, phenylenediamine, and other dyes; balsam
Leather	Belts, shoes, leather watchbands	Potassium dichromate, dyes
Plants	Poison ivy, oak, sumac, etc.	Catechols

the magnitude. Theoretically, few chemicals or natural products could be excluded from the list.

Contact-type allergies to poison ivy, poison oak, sumac, primrose, and other plants are attributable to low molecular weight chemicals present on the leaves and other parts of these plants. Poison ivy is a delayed hypersensitivity to substituted urushiols, which are substituted aromatic halogen or hydroxyl compounds. This allows a direct coupling of the compounds with skin or tissue proteins to form neoantigens. The hypersensitivity develops to these neoantigens; there is nothing intrinsically toxic in these compounds, which produce no reaction in skin exposed to the chemical for the first time. It is interesting that the application of a complete antigen to healthy skin rarely produces contact dermatitis, and yet if a new antigen is created in the skin, it is often effective in inducing a delayed hypersensitivity.

IMMUNOCHEMISTRY

The antigens and haptens that induce the delayed type of hypersensitivity have few special qualities that endow them with the capacity to induce that type of response. Indeed, simultaneous with the T lymphocyte–mediated allergies, immunoglobulin-induced allergies may also be evoked by these same antigens. And yet there are differences in the B lymphocyte and T lymphocyte responses. The latter appears to be favored by dermal contact with the incitant when it is an autocoupling hapten. The use of certain mycobacterium-containing adjuvants such as Freund's complete adjuvant favors the development of delayed hypersensitivities if the antigen is given by injection. The T lymphocyte tends to respond more strongly to the antigen carrier of hapten-antigen conjugates than does the B lymphocyte, which exhibits a stronger response to the hapten portion. There appears to be very little difference in the size of the antigenic determinants that activate T and B cells.

Immunosuppression of T cells differs in some respects from that of B cells. The same chemical immunosuppressants applied to B lymphocytes are used to suppress T lymphocytes—corticosteroids, alkylating agents, purine, pyrimidine, and folic acid analogs, and a variety of ungrouped agents. Certainly the steroids are widely used to modify skin reactions of the contact type, but this takes place after sensitization and the use here is therapeutic, not as an immunosuppressant. Methotrexate and certain T cell–suppressing antibiotics such as vincristine are often chosen for the latter purpose. Irradiation is often combined with these chemical treatments and antilymphocyte globulin (ALG) for the maximum benefits.

The condition of immune tolerance was early recognized in studies of T lymphocyte–mediated contact dermatitis when ingestion was found to impair the emergence of sensitivity to neoarsphenamines and picryl chloride. Oral preparations are commercially available to prevent the development of sensitivity to the urushiols. These are also used as desensitizers, but their efficacy needs to be evaluated by the newer methods available to study delayed hypersensitivities. Antilymphocyte serum (ALS or ALG), since it is customarily prepared by immunizing animals with circulating lymphocytes (dominantly T cells), is usually quite effective as an immunosuppressant of delayed hypersensitivities (Fig. 9-3).

Neonatal thymectomy effectively prevents the development of any T lymphocyte–dependent responses, since the immature T cell must be modified in the thymus before it becomes fully active. This compares functionally with the impairment or prevention of immunoglobulin synthesis by bursectomy. Congenital failure to form a lymphoid thymus gland totally precludes the development of T lymphocyte–related functions in the affected individual. Thymosin and transfer factor therapy can benefit those persons with vestigial lymphoid tissue in an abnormally developed thymus.

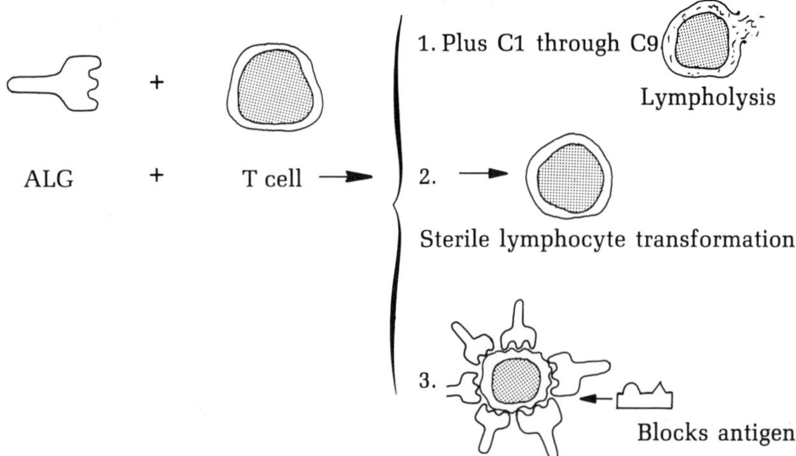

Fig. 9-3. Three methods by which ALG may act as an immunosuppressant: through lympholysis, lymphocyte transformation, or as an antigen-blocking antibody.

Table 9-3. T cell effector molecules involved in delayed-type hypersensitivities

Name	*Nature*	*Activity*
Transfer factor	Low molecular weight polynucleotide-polypeptide	Activates inert T cells
RNA	High molecular weight RNA	Activates inert T cells
Migration inhibition factor	Protein, prealbumin, mol wt near 25,000	Impedes macrophage motion
Chemotactic factor	Protein, albumin, heat stable, mol wt near 25,000	Attracts monocytes
Lymphotoxin	Protein, beta globulin, mol wt over 35,000	Destroys target cells
Blastogenic factor	Protein (?), nondialyzable, heat labile	Recruits T cells for transformation

T CELL EFFECTOR MOLECULES

Delayed hypersensitivity in man is transferable to unsensitized persons with extracts of the lymphocytes of the sensitized donor. These extracts contain a nonantigenic polynucleotide-polypeptide substance in the molecular weight range of 700 to 4000 known as transfer factor (TF). An RNA with a molecular weight greater than 10^6 daltons that will also transfer delayed hypersensitivity has been described. TF and the large molecular weight RNA do not exist in unsensitized cells; they are synthesized as a result of the sensitization. These nucleotides, in some fashion not ascertained as yet, enter T lymphocytes and stimulate them to produce their lymphokines. Neither TF nor the larger RNA molecules are antigenic, which makes it possible to use them therapeutically without the development of antibody-based resistance (Table 9-3).

The chemistry of the lymphokines and some aspects of their biologic activity were presented in Chapter 2. Briefly, all lymphokines appear to be polypeptides with molecular weights of less than 55,000 that act on a second host cell. Macrophage migration inhibition factor (MIF), chemotactic factor, lymphotoxin, blastogenic factor, and interferon are among the best known lymphokines. Chemotactic factor, MIF, and blastogenic factor could all be expected to contribute to the delayed-type skin reaction. The T lymphocyte chemotaxin is specific for monocytes, which are drawn from the blood into solid tissues where they transform into macrophages. MIF prevents the emigration of these cells and holds the macrophages near the lymphocyte. This accounts for the infiltration and persistence of macrophages in allergic skin reactions of the delayed type. The macrophage population in these reaction sites may also be dependent on specific chemoattractants excreted by neutrophils that precede the macrophage into the area where the antigen or hapten has been deposited. The blastogenic factor stimulates noncommitted T lymphocytes to begin lymphocyte transformation, which increases the concentration of lymphokines in the area where the initial lymphocyte-antigen interaction began. Lymphotoxin does not act on normal host cells, although it may be responsible for the destruction of oncogenic cells. The primary target of lymphotoxin is foreign cells such as fungal, parasitic, and grafted tissue that are caused to lyse on exposure to the toxin. Some T cells apparently cooperate with antibody in these cell-destroying activities as a second mechanism of protection.

PREVENTION AND CONTROL

There is little one can do to prevent the development of the cell-mediated allergic reactions that arise atopically. Since most infectious microbes and many substances in leather, rubber, plastic, metal, animal fibers, etc. with which we come into almost daily contact possess at least a modicum of allergenicity, there is simply no way to totally avoid exposure. Fortunately the development of these sensitivities is regulated by Ir genes, and exposure does not necessarily lead to allergy. Hyperallergic parents naturally must take a more conservative attitude concerning the possible exposure of their children to environmental allergens, but total protection against exposure is probably impossible. Certain occupations in the rubber, photographic, dye, and other chemical industries are known for the high incidence of contact dermatitis.

When an allergy of the delayed type has been detected, there may be no need to take any unusual action other than avoidance of the allergen. These delayed allergic reactions are painful and discomforting, but since they are not life threatening there is no need to attempt antigen-specific desensitization. Avoidance of "poisonous" plants and allergenic chemicals or chemically impregnated articles of apparel is usually sufficient to markedly restrict the reactions to these substances. It should be recognized, however, that the term "hypoallergenic" as applied to cosmetics and lotions is a relative term, and these substances may contain allergenic substances also.

Treatment of reactions of the dermal type is largely restricted to the use of corticosteroids applied topically. These drugs are beneficial through their general anti-inflammatory effect.

CUTANEOUS BASOPHILIC HYPERSENSITIVITY

A skin reaction described earlier by Jones and Mote that bore their name for years is now generally referred to as cutaneous basophilic hypersensitivity. Although this skin reaction is not identical with the delayed dermal skin reaction, it does share some of its features. The reaction is erythematous but is relatively free of edema and does not progress to a necrotic state. This reaction reaches its maximum at 24 hours and fades. The reaction is transitory in another sense too—a few weeks after the development of the sensitive state, the reaction can no longer be elicited. This is a distinguishing feature from delayed dermal sensitivity, which rarely disappears once the hypersensitivity is acquired. But like delayed hypersensitivities, the cutaneous basophilic reaction can be elicited in persons with agammaglobulinemia and is dependent on T lymphocytes. Histologically, the skin reaction is dominated by a basophilic and lymphocytic infiltrate rather than that of macrophages and lymphocytes as in the delayed skin reaction. The medical importance of the cutaneous basophilic hypersensitive response has not yet been established.

BIBLIOGRAPHY

Benacerraf, B., and Green, I.: Cellular hypersensitivity, Annu. Rev. Med. **20**:141, 1969.

Bloom, B. R.: In vitro approaches to the mechanism of cell-mediated immune reactions, Adv. Immunol. **13**:102, 1971.

Bloom, B. R., and Glade, R. R., eds.: In vitro methods in cell-mediated immunity, New York, 1971, Academic Press, Inc.

Dash, C. H., and Jones, H. E. H.: Mechanisms in drug allergy, Edinburgh, 1972, Churchill Livingstone.

David, J. R.: Lymphocyte mediators and cellular hypersensitivity, N. Engl. J. Med. **288**: 143, 1973.

David, J. R., and David, R. A.: Cellular hypersensitivity and immunity; inhibition of macrophage migration and the lymphocyte mediators, Prog. Allergy **16**:300, 1972.

Fisher, A. A.: Contact dermatitis, ed. 2, Philadelphia, 1973, Lea & Febiger.

Gell, P. G. H., Coombs, R. R. A., and Lachman, P., eds.: Clinical aspects of immunology, ed. 3, Oxford, 1974, Blackwell Scientific Publications, Inc.

Granger, G. A.: Lymphokines—the mediators of cellular immunity, Ser. Haematol. **5**:8, 1972.

Lawrence, H. S.: Cellular immunity, Clin. Immunobiol. **1**:48, 1972.

Lowenthal, D. T.: Tissue sensitivity to drugs in disease states, Med. Clin. North Am. **58**: 1111, 1974.

Maddison, S. E.: Delayed hypersensitivity and cell-mediated immunity. A survey of current insights into these responses of the body to antigens, Clin. Pediatr. **12**:529, 1973.

McCluskey, R. T., and Cohen, S.: Mechanisms of delayed hypersensitivity, Pathobiol. Annu. **2**:111, 1972.

McCluskey, R. T., and Cohen, S.: Mechanisms of cell-mediated immunity, New York, 1974, John Wiley & Sons, Inc.

Polak, L., Turk, J. L., and Frey, J. R.: Studies on contact hypersensitivity to chromium compounds, Prog. Allergy **17**:146, 1973.

Rajka, G.: Atopic dermatitis, London, 1975, W. B. Saunders Co., Ltd.

Remold, H. G.: Purification and characterization of lymphocyte mediators in cellular immunity, Transplant Rev. **10**:152, 1972.

Russell, A. S., and Lessof, M. H.: Hypersensitivity to drugs, Clin. Allergy **1**:179, 1971.

Salvin, S. B.: Roles of haptens and carriers in delayed allergies, Adv. Biol. Skin **11**:95, 1971.

Samter, M., ed.: Immunological diseases, ed. 2, Boston, 1971, Little, Brown & Co.

Samter, M., and Parker, C. W., ed.: Hypersensitivity to drugs, New York, 1972, Pergamon Press, Inc.

Turk, J. L.: Immunology in clinical medicine, London, 1973, William Heinemann, Ltd.

Valentine, F. T., and Lawrence, H. S.: Cell-mediated immunity, Adv. Intern. Med. **17**: 51, 1971.

Wilkinson, R. D., and Rose, B.: Drug reactions in man: expressions and diagnosis, Adv. Biol. Skin **11**:141, 1971.

Case histories

CASE 1. POISON IVY DERMATITIS

J. P., a 26-year-old male employee of the forestry division of the state department of conservation, sought medical attention for what he recognized as a poison ivy rash. Numerous vesicles, some 2 to 3 mm in diameter, surrounded by erythema were present on the back of both hands, between the fingers, and on the lower arms and right cheek. Some edema was also noted about the eyes. The patient complained of severe itching around the rash and of the eyes. Since becoming employed by the forestry division 4 years ago, the patient had developed poison ivy dermatitis three times (each summer), but this was the most severe episode. Because of the nature of his work, the patient asked about the possibility of desensitization.

Questions

1. What is the antigenic basis of poison ivy dermatitis?
2. How successful is specific desensitization in preventing poison ivy?
3. What treatment regimens for poison ivy have an immunologic basis?

Discussion

Poison ivy and poison oak present the most important examples of contact dermatitis in the rural United States. *Rhus radicans* (the poison ivy plant), *Rhus toxicodendron* (poison sumac), and *Rhus diversiloba* (poison oak) cause contact dermatitis because of the common catechols present in the plant sap and on the surface of bruised leaves. Urushiol is the name given to the mixture of four catechols found in the poison ivy plant. These catechols differ from each other only in the degree of saturation of their pentadecyl side chain. The fully saturated compound is 3n-pentadecylcatechol; the compound that is singly unsaturated has a double bond at position 8-9; the doubly unsaturated compound has a double bond at positions 8-9 and 11-12; and the trienyl compound has a double bond at positions 8-9, 11-12, and 14-15 (Fig. 9-4). These compounds exist in urushiol in the ratio of 3, 15, 60, and 22, respectively; thus it is not surprising that patients show more strongly positive allergic reaction to the latter two than to the former two compounds.

Catechols are haptenic and can couple to tissue proteins by virtue of their ready oxidation to quinones, the sensitizing form of these compounds. Blocking quinone formation by substituting the hydroxyl groups renders the catechols inert. When applied to skin, only 44% of pentadecylcatechol re-

OH
OH
3n-Pentadecylcatechol

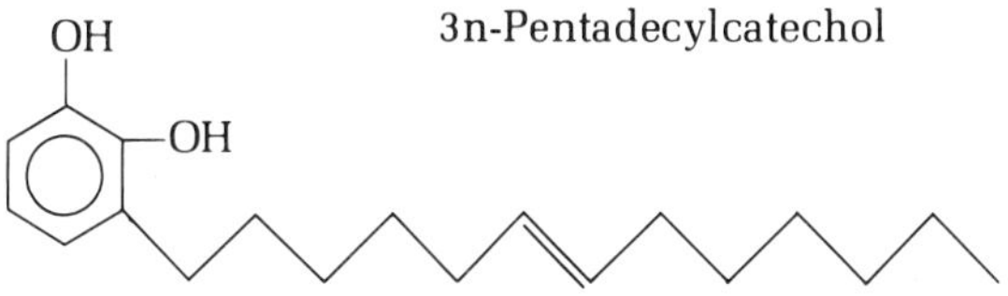

OH
OH
3n-Pentadecenylcatechol

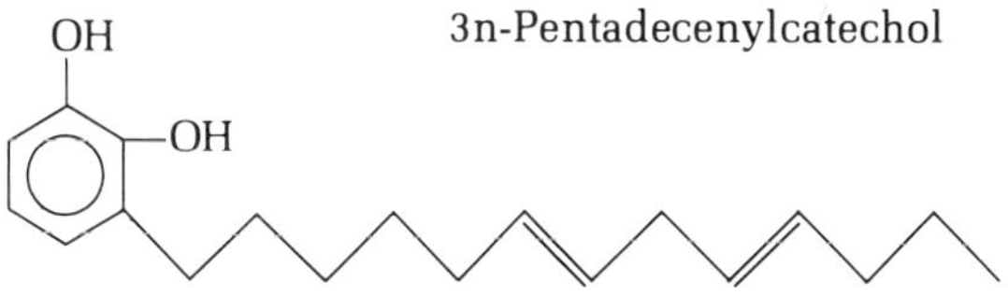

OH
OH
3n-Pentadecadienylcatechol

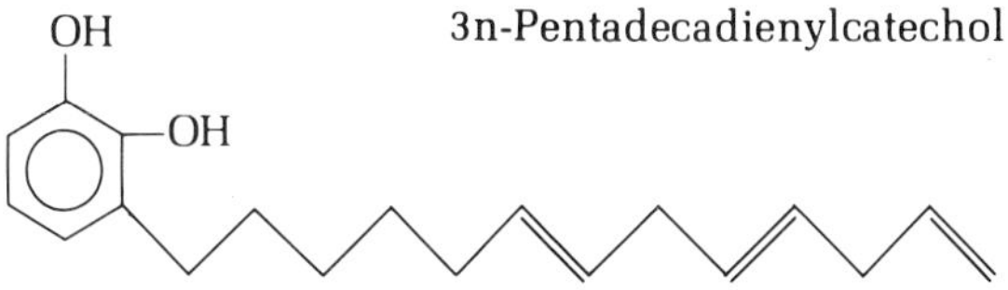

OH
OH
3n-Pentadecatrienylcatechol

Fig. 9-4. Urushiols found in poison ivy.

mains at the site of application; the remainder is recoverable from feces, urine, lymph nodes, and internal organs. The exact form of the catechol-protein conjugate and the identity of specifically involved proteins is not known.

In 1934 it was discovered that injection of poison ivy extracts into human beings did not hypersensitize, whereas topical application did. Since that time, specific desensitization by injection or oral exposure to urushiol has been attempted with various pharmaceutical products. Generally, only partial desensitization is accomplished, but this may be recommended for those who are inevitably exposed to *Rhus*, that is, telephone repairmen, farmers, foresters, etc. Hyposensitization consists of the daily oral intake of poison ivy urushiols for a period of 4 months, although hyposensitization by injection is also possible. Relief is incomplete and temporary.

Mild poison ivy dermatitis treatment is palliative; calamine lotion or other topical treatment is generally adequate. Severe poison ivy dermatitis, as in the case described here, may require, in addition, topical steroid ointment or even oral steroids (prednisone, 10 mg, 1 to 5 times daily) to arrest the inflammatory response. An antihistamine may also be recommended, not so much for its antiallergic activity, since histamine release is not extensive in the case of contact dermatitis, but for its sedative effect (50 mg diphenhydramine hydrochloride at bedtime).

REFERENCES

Godfrey, H. P., Baer, H., and Watkins, R. C.: Delayed hypersensitivity to catechols. V. Absorption and distribution of substances related to poison ivy extracts and their relation to the induction of sensitization and tolerance, J. Immunol. **106**:91, 1971.

Johnson, R. A., Baer, H., Kirkpatrick, C. H., Dawson, C. R., and Khurana, R. G.: Comparison of the contact allergenicity of the four pentadecylcatechols derived from poison ivy urushiol in human subjects, J. Allergy Clin. Immunol. **49**:27, 1972.

Kligman, A. M.: Hyposensitization against Rhus dermatitis, Arch. Dermatol. **78**:47, 1958.

CASE 2. ANTIPERSPIRANT ALLERGY

D. H., a 45-year-old male business executive, contacted his physician about an itch under both axillae on his return from an extended vacation in Europe. On examination an eczematous rash was apparent. The patient's history was very revealing. The rash began approximately 10 days after arrival in southern Spain and was more bothersome in that warm climate than at home, although it had continued on his return. The patient feared he had some kind of "crabs." A pubic rash was not seen. On further questioning it was revealed that the patient had failed to pack his usual toilet articles and had been forced to buy new supplies while on vacation.

Questions

1. What "underarm" applications are apt to lead to dermatitis?
2. What treatment is suggested for contact dermatitis?

Discussion

In the absence of any convincing sign of arthropod infestation of other hairy parts of the body, axillary rashes are most apt to be due to depilatory preparations in females or to antiperspirants in either sex. The efficacy of most antiperspirants on the market in the United States is based on the activity of aluminum salts—aluminum chloride, most commonly—which are not considered effective sensitizers. Formaldehyde, which is in widespread use in European antiperspirants, and glutaraldehyde are active sensitizers. Formaldehyde may not appear as such on the label of the product, since it may be incorporated in a condensed form with other compounds as in methenamine. Formaldehyde products are sometimes used as accelerators in rubber products and may be released from the valves of pressurized atomizer dispensers, thereby causing the sensitization.

Most patients with axillary dermatitis recognize the source of their sensitivity as an antiperspirant and discontinue use of the product. In this instance the patient was inclined to think of other causes of his condition. When he returned to the use of a formaldehyde-free product, his symptoms disappeared.

REFERENCES

Fisher, A. A.: Contact dermatitis, Philadelphia, 1973, Lea & Febiger.

Shelley, W. B., and Hurley, H. J.: Allergic origin of zirconium deodorant granulomas, Br. J. Dermatol. **70**:75, 1958.

chapter 10

Autoimmune disease

AUTOANTIGENS

The existence of autoimmune disease in no way repudiates the concept of horror autotoxicus that Ehrlich postulated to explain the inability of an individual to marshal an immune response against his own proteins and polysaccharides that met all other criteria of antigenicity except foreignness. According to the postulate of horror autotoxicus, an individual does not mount an immune response against "self-antigens" that are normally present in his circulatory system, and this definition is not inconsistent with the concept of autoimmunity. In fact, there are at least five escapes from a conflict between autoimmunity and horror autotoxicus and these involve neoantigen, sequestered antigen, maturation antigen, cross-reactive antigen, and mutation.

Neoantigen

A neoantigen is a new antigen in the sense that it is an altered form of some previously existing antigen. Here the concern is with existing structures of the body that become altered by complex formation with haptens or by physical rearrangement caused by heat, cold, ultraviolet light, pressure, or chemicals so that new antigenic determinants are created or exposed in the conjugated form of the molecule. The immune response is directed against the altered form of the antigen and, when this is expressed as a type II cytotoxic response, is clearly disease associated. When the altered antigen is removed or destroyed, the symptoms of the autoimmune disease are alleviated.

Sequestered antigen

A second possibility for the development of an autoimmune condition is based on an immune response to a sequestered or hidden antigen that does not normally reach the circulation. Certain proteins such as proteins in the lens of the eye are biochemically quite inert; there is little in the way of new synthesis or degradation of these proteins once the lens is formed. The lens is situated in a relatively avascular location. These features suggest that lens proteins do not normally exist in the circulation, and any immune response directed against them would not abrogate the principles forwarded by Ehrlich. Naturally it is difficult to prove that such antigens never enter the circulation; failure to detect them may mean that the method used was too insensitive or an improper assay time was chosen. Despite these loopholes the concept of sequestered antigens is a well-accepted theory.

Maturation antigen

Closely related to the concept of sequestered antigens is that of maturation antigens. A maturation antigen is one that develops after the maturation of the immune response. It is generally believed from the experiments of Burnet and Medawar that our customary failure to invoke a self-directed immune response is due to the fact that these antigens were formed early in fetal life and through the process of immune tolerance suppressed any immature immunocytes possessing a specificity to them. During immunologic maturation at or near the birth of the animal, further development of these lymphocytes was not possible, thus creating self-tolerance. However, antigens that were formed after that time, such as those of sperm and spermatic fluid as well as female reproductive antigens and milk casein, could stimulate cells with their specificity to function and to contribute to autoimmune disease.

Cross-reactive antigen

An autoimmune response may be directed against a foreign antigen and contribute to an autoimmune disease through a cross-reaction with normal antigens (Fig. 10-1). This cross-reactive antigen hypothesis has received strong support from two poststreptococcal diseases, glomerulonephritis and rheumatic fever. In each instance it has been possible to identify antigens in the streptococci that are similar to antigens in the affected tissues (kidney and heart) of the person with the autoimmune disease. The entire chemistry of these antigens is yet to be determined, and the precise structures responsible for their cross-reactivity have, accordingly, escaped definition.

Mutation

The last possibility—that of an altered immune response—refers to a mutation or to some other type of creation or release of suppressed immunologic information to allow a response to a self-antigen. Mutation is a universally accepted method for a cell to express or acquire new activities, and there is no reason to exclude B or T lymphocytes from such a possibility. It has been suggested, on the basis of their relatively greater sensitivity to irradiation than other cells, that lymphocytes should be susceptible to a fairly high mutation rate.

WITEBSKY'S POSTULATES

Many diseases have an autoimmune component, but it is not always an etiologic part of the disease complex. It is quite possible that self-directed immune responses, although present, may have little or nothing to do with the disease state. When the original inducing antigen is no longer present or is no longer released from cells, the immunoglobulins or sensitized T cells activated in response to the antigen are obviously no longer able to react with it.

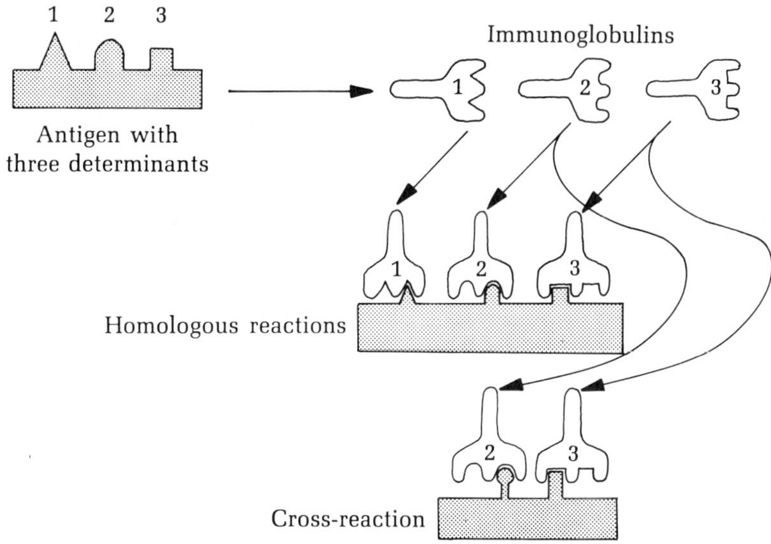

Fig. 10-1. Schematic representation showing how cross-reactive antigen theory may function in autoimmune diseases when first antigen is foreign and second one is a self-antigen.

These immunoglobulins and cells simply remain as vestiges of an antigen exposure but are not contributory to the disease state.

Witebsky proposed criteria to analyze a disease and establish its autoimmune etiology, and these have become known as Witebsky's postulates in the same sense that Koch's postulates are used to establish the etiology of infectious disease. Witebsky's postulates are the following:

1. An autoimmune component must be regularly associated with the disease.
2. A model of the disease must be duplicated in laboratory animals.
3. The experimental and the natural sample of the disease must exhibit parallels of immunopathology.
4. The disease must be produced by the transfer of immunoglobulins or lymphoid cells from the afflicted individual to a normal recipient.

In addition to these criteria for establishing a disease as an autoimmune disease, other features may support an autoimmune etiology of a specific disease. Among these can be listed a general hypergammaglobulinemia, a hypocomplementemia, and increase in complement-dependent activities as further suggestive evidence that an antibody response followed by complement consumption and expression of complement-associated activities is in progress. A therapeutic response to immunosuppressant drugs or those with anticomplementary activity would be further support for an immunoglobulin association with the disease. It is often more difficult to detect and evaluate self-directed T lymphocyte responses, and since transfer of these cells must be made into syngeneic or otherwise histocompatible recipients, it is not always easy to fulfill Witebsky's fourth criterion even when all other evidence is harmonious with an autoimmune etiology of the condition (Table 10-1).

IMMUNOGLOBULIN-ASSOCIATED DISEASES

Hemolytic disease

Anemia is not necessarily severe in hemolytic disease of autoimmune origin.

Table 10-1. Human diseases expressing autoimmune phenomena

Disease	*Antigen(s)*	*Ig and/or T cell response*
Autoimmune hemolytic disease	I, Rh, and others on surface of RBCs	IgM and IgG
Thrombocytopenic purpura	Hapten-platelet or hapten-adsorbed antigen complex	IgG
Rheumatic fever	Streptococcal and heart	IgG and IgM; cross-reactive
Glomerulonephritis	Streptococcal and kidney	IgG and IgM; cross-reactive
Rheumatoid arthritis	IgG	IgM to Fc(γ)
Systemic lupus erythematosus	DNA, nucleoprotein, RNA, etc.	IgG
Myasthenia gravis	Myosin	IgG
Hashimoto's disease	Thyroglobulin	IgG and T cell
Postvaccinal and postinfectious encephalomyelitis	Myelin	T cell
Graves' disease		Long-acting thyroid stimulator (LATS)
Aspermatogenesis	Sperm	T cell
Sympathetic ophthalmia	Uvea	T cell

When anemia is present, it may be transient as in paroxysmal cold hemoglobinuria in which the hemolytic episodes are correlated with exposure to cold and the presence of cold agglutinins. Cold agglutinins tend to be antierythrocyte globulins of the IgM class that are active at 4° C and room temperature but only feebly active at normal body temperature. When the afflicted individual is exposed to cold, the hemoglobinuria follows. This may be associated with necrosis of the earlobes, fingertips, end of the nose, or other chilled areas where intravascular hemagglutination destroyed the patency of the capillary bed. Since the IgM antibodies are good complement fixers, red cell lysis follows. Blood cells taken from these patients are Coombs' test positive because of the IgM on their surface; they also result in positive tests with anticomplement (usually anti-C3) sera. Cold agglutinins of the IgG class are also known. The antigen involved is often the I antigen, the maturation antigen that is progressively more apparent on red cells following birth. It is unknown what sparks the immune system to attack this antigen and produce hemolysis.

Ordinary "warm" antibodies are also associated with autoimmune hemolytic disease. These antibodies seldom cause much hemolysis, although there are exceptions. These are usually IgG antibodies that fix complement but are apparently so distributed on the surface of the red cell as to minimize lysis. About one third of these cases are associated with an Rh antigen. Autoimmune hemolytic disease can be associated with drug therapy when the drug combines with the erythrocyte to present a novel hapten-antigen determinant.

Thrombocytopenic purpura

Alloimmune thrombocytopenic purpura (lowered platelet count associated with petechial hemorrhages) can be noted in a restricted number of infants whose maternal IgG antiplatelet globulin has passed the placental barrier, entered the fetal circulation, and contributed to the destruction of these platelets. Loss of platelets generally is associated with hemorrhage due to their role in the blood clotting cascade.

Autoimmune thrombocytopenic purpura is seen almost exclusively in adults who have some attending illness for which they are being treated with a chemotherapeutic agent. These patients may be taking aspirin, digitoxin, or any of a number of tranquilizers, antibiotics, antihistamines, antimalarials, sulfonamides, etc. Their thrombocytopenia invariably emerged during the course of the drug treatment and will subside when the drug is withdrawn from the treatment regimen. Reinitiation of the drug therapy causes an exacerbation of this iatrogenic disease. These features signal that a hapten-antigen complex, in which the dominant region of the antigenic determinant is in the hapten, is the incitant. One theory suggests that the antigen is some protein or polysaccharide of the platelet itself (Fig. 10-2), whereas an alternative suggestion is that a serum protein binds the hapten and then the complex adsorbs to the platelets. In this theory the platelet is lysed as a bystander cell by the antigen-antibody-complement complex and is not itself a part of the antigen. This is merely an immunologic distinction because the end result is the same in either system. The dominance of the hapten is illustrated by the fact that passive immunization conveys the disease to a normal individual only if he also receives the offending drug. In vitro mixtures of patient sera with platelets are inert until the drug is added and then lysis occurs (when complement is also present).

Poststreptococcal glomerulonephritis

Glomerulonephritis can be easily produced by immunologic methods and also exists as an autoimmune disease. Experimental nephritis of the heteroimmune type, known as Masugi nephritis, can be pro-

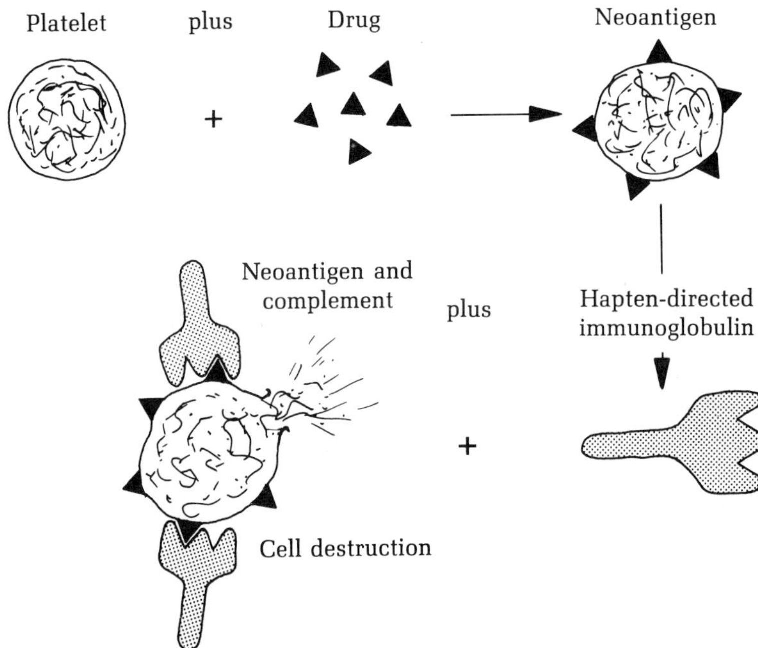

Fig. 10-2. Drug-induced autoimmune thrombocytopenia may be the result of reactions shown. Alternatively, hapten could couple with a protein that adsorbs nonspecifically to thrombocyte surface.

duced by the passive administration of nephrotoxic serum into an animal. The initial experiments of Masugi were conducted in rats that received injections of rabbit antirat kidney serum, and this experiment has been duplicated in several species of animals since the original example was described. Masugi glomerulonephritis is important as a model of autoimmune disease, although the pathology of the renal lesions differs somewhat from species to species. Alloimmune glomerulonephritis is produced by preparing kidney homogenates with adjuvants and using these preparations to immunize animals of the same species as the kidney donor. Freund's adjuvant is the adjuvant of choice and has replaced streptococcal toxins or bacteria that were used earlier. The interest in using streptococcal-derived preparations as the adjuvant stemmed from a desire to more clearly define human glomerulonephritis. Two early findings concerning human glomerulonephritis, which were ultimately woven into a common theory, were that many of these patients had autoantibodies that would react with human kidney and had also experienced a previous infection with streptococci. One supposition was that exotoxins of the streptococci were damaging kidney tissue and creating neoantigens that initiated the autoimmune disease.

Although many different serologic types of β-hemolytic streptococci produce these exotoxins, only certain types, predominantly types 12, 4, 3, 5, and 25 of group A, seemed to be associated with prenephritic infections in these patients; moreover, the symptoms of glomerulonephritis customarily appeared 10 or 15 days after recovery from the streptococcal infection and at a time when the population of the microbes and the concentration of their toxins was very low. After considerable further epidemiologic and laboratory research, it became possible to erect a hypothesis for human autoimmune glomerulonephritis compatible with the aforementioned conditions. The evidence indicates that certain types of group A β-hemolytic streptococci contain antigens that are cross-reactive with human kidney. Rabbit or human antisera prepared against these streptococci—or a lipoprotein of 120,000 molecular weight that is extractable from their cytoplasmic membrane—will localize on the human glomerulus. Human biopsy specimens frequently contain IgG and complement attached to the glomerular basement membrane. Poststreptococcal glomerulonephritis is now believed to be caused by these antibodies.

Another type of heteroimmune glomerulonephritis is the immune complex type associated especially with serum sickness. When soluble antigen-antibody complexes of the correct antigen-antibody ratio are formed in vivo, these, when filtered through the kidney, become deposited along the capillary basement membrane of the kidney in irregular lumpy deposits when viewed with fluorescent antibody techniques. Immune-complex glomerulonephritis contributes to the chronic phase of disease in Masugi nephritis, since the injected animals make antibodies against the serum proteins with which they have been infused.

Rheumatic fever

Much of the immunologic data used to support a cross-reactive antigen hypothesis for glomerulonephritis can be applied to rheumatic fever. Patients with rheumatic fever often have high antistreptolysin O titers, antistreptococcal hyaluronidase, and NADase titers that support a recent previous infection with group A β-hemolytic streptococci. Identification of the serologic types of the antecedent streptococci, unlike the situation in glomerulonephritis, resulted in the discovery that over 50 different types caused infections that preceded the development of rheumatic fever. Fluorescent antisera prepared against these bacteria localize on the sarcolemma and cardiac myofibers with little if any staining of the voluntary muscle. Heart muscle tissue from patients with rheumatic fever reveals a deposition of IgG with less IgM and IgA but with complement in the sarcolemma. Again, antistreptococcal globulins that cross-react with human tissue appear to be responsible for parts of the rheumatic fever syndrome.

The streptococcal antigen responsible for the development of these autoreactive immunoglobulins is unknown. Conceivably it could be a type of lipoprotein, since lipoproteins are involved in the cell membrane structure of many different types of cells.

Rheumatoid arthritis

In adult-type rheumatoid arthritis, the etiology of which is still obscure, tests for rheumatoid factor (RF) can be very useful in establishing the diagnosis. RF is not specific for rheumatoid arthritis and has been found in the sera of patients with other types of autoimmune connective tissue disorders, including lupus erythematosus, polyarteritis, and scleroderma. RF is a 19S IgM with a potential to combine with the Fc portion of IgG. This reaction is not restricted to the patient's own IgG, and RF was first described as a substance in rheumatoid sera that would expand the hemagglutination titer of rabbit antisera to sheep erythrocytes. The induction of RF synthesis has been assumed to progress through a multistage sequence in which some infectious or chemical insult to the synovial membranes of the joints initiates an emigration of inflammatory cells into the synovial fluid. Antibodies also enter the synovial fluid if the initial incident is due to an antigenic agent, and by the immunoglobulin-antigen activation of complement and the attending release of chemotaxins, these antibodies increase the inflammatory cell infiltrate. This combination, possibly through the action of lysosomal enzymes re-

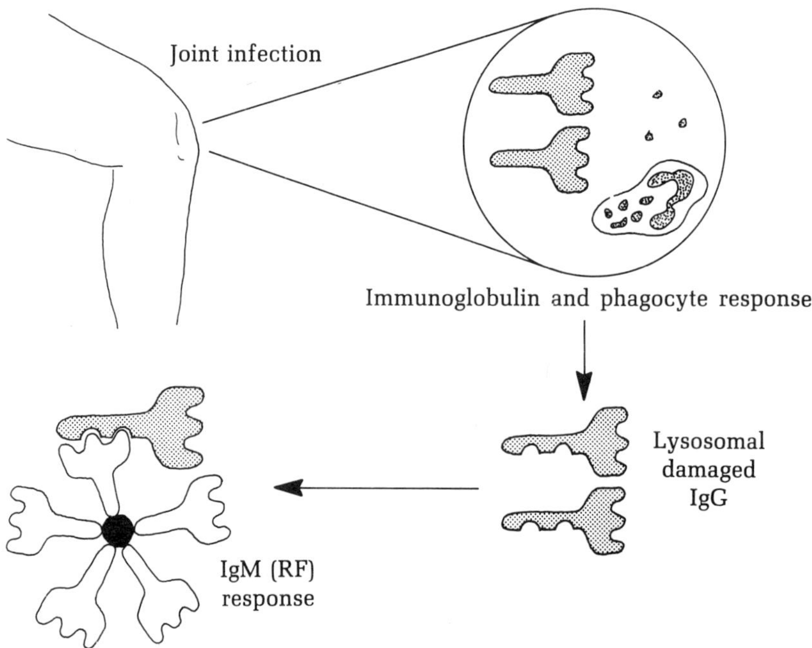

Fig. 10-3. One hypothesis for the origin of rheumatoid factor is related to formation of damaged IgG in infectious joint disease. Rheumatoid factor attaches to the Fc section of IgG molecule.

leased from the PMNs or synovium itself, causes a derangement in the IgG molecule, which then expresses new antigenic determinants in its Fc portion (Fig. 10-3). Because of the broad specificity of RF and the fact that most RF molecules are of the IgM class, it is believed that these new determinants include a part of the polysaccharides in the Fc region.

Several aspects of this hypothesis are open to criticism. Although lymphocytes and plasma cells are detectable in the synovium of patients with rheumatoid arthritis, it is unknown if they are responding to foreign antigens or to the altered IgG. Thus a cellular support for the hypothesis is not yet established. Also it is known that RF has little to do with the disease itself—it is not present in all instances, its concentration is not necessarily related to the severity of the disease, and a blood transfusion made with seropositive blood does not cause rheumatoid arthritis in the recipient. It has also been demonstrated that some RF molecules are IgG and others IgA. Many RF sera are specific for the Gm allotype of the IgG of the host, the Gm allotypes being dependent on the specific amino acid sequence of the Fc fragment and not its polysaccharide structure. RF is a molecule associated with rheumatoid arthritis, but one whose role has not yet been defined.

Systemic lupus erythematosus

The discovery of the lupus erythematosus or LE cell by Hargraves in 1948 stimulated a new direction of immunologic research into a serious disease characterized by a facial rash across the nose and cheeks and serious internal lesions in the kidney, heart, and blood vessels as well as in the white blood cells where the LE cell was recognized.

The LE cell can be described as a phagocyte, usually a neutrophil, that has engulfed the nuclear mass released from other

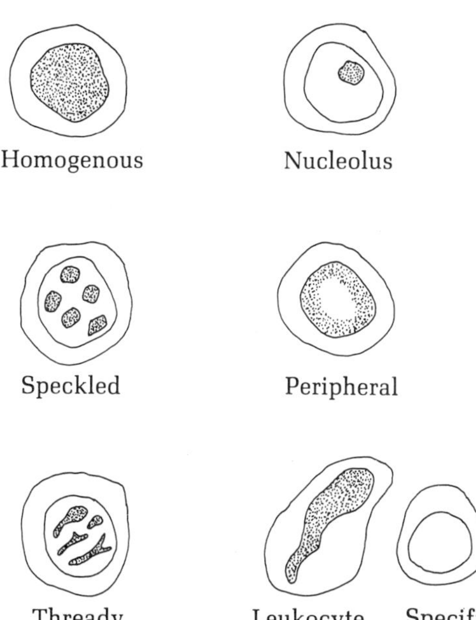

Fig. 10-4. Fluorescent antinucleic acid (FANA) tests for autoimmune collagen diseases present results varying from total nuclear fluorescence to that in which only nucleolus is stained. Each staining pattern can be associated with a specific condition and prognosis. Peripheral fluorescence is associated with severe lupus erythematosus; speckled pattern is rare in lupus erythematosus; thready pattern may be seen in lupus erythematosus but not rheumatoid arthritis; leukocyte-specific staining is characteristic of lupus erythematosus and rheumatoid arthritis, whereas nucleolar pattern is rare in these two diseases.

white blood cells (Fig. 10-4). Artificial preparations of LE cells can be prepared by incubating sera from LE patients with whole blood or the buffy coat of the blood from a normal donor. Time-lapse cinemicrography will record the disintegration of the nucleus of certain white blood cells. Since all cells do not exhibit this nuclear sensitivity, it is believed that the susceptible cells are previously damaged or injured in some way. Surviving PMNs approach and engulf the nuclear mass of the damaged cell after stripping away its cytoplasmic remnant. Occasionally competition of several viable neutrophils for the nuclear morsel can be observed. Stains made of the preparation will reveal either the diffuse nuclear body inside the successful LE cell or a nuclear body surrounded by a rosette of the competing neutrophils. These configurations are also seen in whole blood from the LE patient, particularly when the blood has been incubated for a time in vitro; however, these LE preparations are an unreliable diagnostic aid, since they are positive in less than 75% of active cases. LE cells may also be associated with rheumatoid arthritis, hepatitis, and drug sensitivities.

The cytotoxic activity in LE sera that is responsible for LE cell formation probably consists of several autoantibodies with a nuclear specificity. One of these is an antinucleoprotein of the IgG class, or less often of the IgM class, that attaches to the DNA-histone complex of the nucleus. Other antibodies are believed specific for the DNA portion, which presumably arose in response to a haptenic role played by the DNA in an unidentified complete antigen. These antinuclear antibodies are identified in LE sera by indirect fluorescent antibody procedures using antihuman gamma globulin conjugated with fluorescein to stain the patient's globulins that have attached to a preparation of DNA. This can consist of crushed cells, yeast cells, or extracted nucleic acids. When whole cells are utilized, the pattern of staining will be distinctive from one patient to another. Staining of the perimeter of the nucleus indicates the serum is dominated by an anti-DNA antibody. A homogeneous staining of the nucleus indicates nucleoprotein staining. Fluorescence in the nucleolus indicates an antibody specificity for RNA and a speckled pattern reflects the presence of an antibody to an extractable nuclear antigen (ENA), which is RNA-like. Patients with the latter staining pattern tend to have a better prognosis. These antibodies are believed to function in vivo and cause some of the symptoms of SLE, since immunosuppressive therapy will lower the titer of these antibodies and elevate the patient's complement level simultaneous with recovery.

Several diseases exist that have associated tissue and serologic alterations much like SLE. These changes include LE cells, antinuclear antibodies, hypergammaglobulinemia, and antiglobulin factors similar to RF. Chronic lupoid hepatitis, drug-induced lupus, a disease with an etiology much like thrombocytopenic purpura, polymyositis (dermatomyositis), mixed connective tissue disease, polyarteritis, and possibly scleroderma and the viral hepatitis-arthritis syndrome are all included in this category.

Myasthenia gravis

The progressing muscle weakness seen in patients with myasthenia gravis is a striking clinical symptom. These patients, to the extent of about a 15% incidence, also have thymomas, which early led to the possibility that disturbances in the immunologic system were associated with the etiology of the disease. This view was strengthened by the recognition that germinal centers could be detected in the thymus tissue of these patients, whereas normal thymus is otherwise well recognized to be deficient in germinal center formation unless antigen is inoculated directly into the gland. A myoid-specific antibody has been recognized in as many as 65% of the patients in some studies. This antibody may be an aftermath of the primary disease, since muscle fiber necrosis does occur during the illness. The myoid antibody characteristically attaches to the A bands of the myofibrils with some binding to the I bands, the latter of which is a prominent finding in normal sera as well. One of the important antigens may be myosin, which is a contractile protein localized in the A bands. Much further study is needed to clarify the immunologic aspects of myasthenia gravis.

Other diseases

Antibodies to tissue antigens have been recognized in a long list of human ailments, including Addison's disease (adrenal), Sjögren's syndrome (keratoconjunctivitis), Felty's syndrome (a characteristic type of leukopenia), Hashimoto's disease (thyroiditis), Graves' disease (hyperthyroiditis), pernicious anemia, celiac disease, diabetes, and cirrhosis of the liver. In certain of these diseases (for example, Hashimoto's disease) it is suspected, as in myasthenia gravis, that autoantibodies serve as a convenient diagnostic support when present but do not reflect any role of the autoantibody in the origin or continuation of the disease. For most of these conditions it is simply not possible to make any conclusions other than stating that autoantibodies are often associated with the disease.

T LYMPHOCYTE–ASSOCIATED DISEASES

Postvaccinal encephalomyelitis

The use of the Pasteur type of rabies vaccine customarily prepared by treating the emulsified spinal cord of rabid rabbits with phenol is recognized to provoke an autoimmune encephalomyelitis in about 1 in every 4000 to 5000 recipients. The vaccine is administered as a series of daily inoculations given intracutaneously or subcutaneously in the abdomen for a period of 2 weeks. Near the end of the second week, symptoms of encephalomyelitis expressed as backache, headache, muscle weakness, and loss of reflex responses develop in those few unfortunate individuals whose T lymphocytes have been activated to produce an autoimmune response. A well-established opinion is that the strongly basic myelin proteins present in the vaccine, which contains a myriad of neural system antigens, is the key antigen. Collagen-like proteins, proteolipids, and lipid haptens are believed less capable of provoking the disease.

The recognition of the role of myelins as

the encephalitogenic factor stems from studies of experimental allergic encephalomyelitis (EAE) in laboratory rats, guinea pigs (Fig. 10-5), and other animals. In certain strains of these animals the injection of homogenized spinal cord in Freund's adjuvant will induce EAE with a frequency approaching 95%. Purification of spinal cord homogenates has permitted the identification of encephalitogenic myelin-derived proteins from various species that have molecular weights near 20,000 and between 135 and 180 amino acid residues. The bovine and rabbit proteins contain a peptide core of approximately 4700 daltons, which is the primary encephalitogenic portion of the molecule. The amino acid composition of this peptide is very similar, if not identical, for the two species and suggests that when it activates T cells, those cells would be unable to distinguish host from foreign neural tissue, which would then result in the autoimmune disease.

The evidence is quite good that it is the T lymphocyte and not immunoglobulin that is associated with the disease. Transfer of sera between animals with EAE and normal animals does not cause disease, but the transfer of T lymphocytes (between congeneic animals) will. Animals with EAE do not necessarily succumb from the ascending flacid paralysis so typical of the disease, nor do human victims of postvaccinal encephalomyelitis often die. The suggestion has been forwarded that coexistent autoantibodies formed against the myelin antigen may function as blocking antibodies and accelerate recovery from the acute neurologic symptoms.

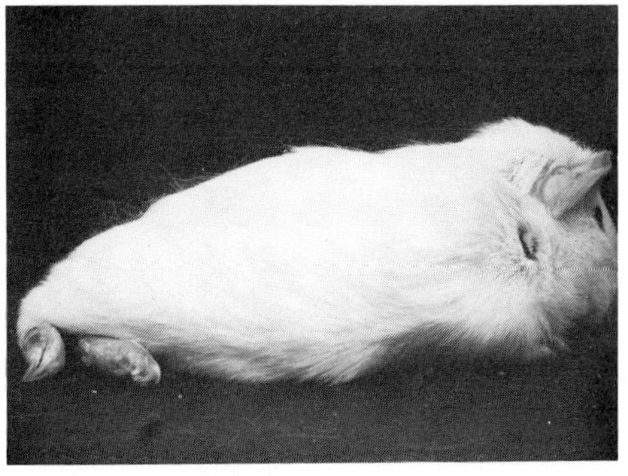

Fig. 10-5. Ascending flaccid paralysis is characteristic of experimental allergic encephalomyelitis in the guinea pig. (Courtesy Dr. W. Purdy.)

Postvaccinal encephalomyelitis is also possible following immunizations with vaccines devoid of neural tissues and containing active attenuated viruses of smallpox, rubella, measles, mumps, and probably with the newer chickenpox vaccines. Infectious encephalitis may be a better name for these incidents, since the diseases are based on the infectious capacity of the viruses; this form of autoimmune encephalomyelitis is discussed in the following section.

Postinfectious encephalomyelitis

In all respects, except for its inciting cause, postinfectious encephalomyelitis closely parallels the postvaccinal form of the disease. The postinfectious form of this disease has been known to follow measles, rubella, mumps, chickenpox, herpes simplex, herpes zoster, influenza, and smallpox or immunization with attenuated strains of these and other viruses. In several instances it has been demonstrated that these viruses cause the emergence of new antigens on the tissue cells that they infect. These novel cell-membrane antigens, if formed in vivo —just as those in tumor cells or grafted tissue—would incite a potent T lymphocyte response. These activated T cells would logically attempt to destroy the "foreign" cells in a typical rejection fashion. Because of the pantropism of many of the viruses involved, cells of the central nervous system are induced to form these antigens and thus become susceptible to T cell attack in a suicide-like fashion. Postinfectious encephalomyelitis is noticed just at the time that recovery from the true viral phase of the illness has passed—usually after 1 to 2 weeks—and just at the time that T cells with a specificity for these neoantigens would be expected to emerge. Again, this type of encephalomyelitis is not necessarily fatal, but persistent neural deficiencies associated with these viruses, of which the resulting autoimmune response is a part, can occur. Since these are more frequently sequelae to natural infections with fully virulent wild viruses, this has encouraged the development of attenuated vaccines.

Hashimoto's disease

A histologically unique form of hypothyroiditis characterized by infiltration of lymphocytes and plasma cells into the thyroid gland, loss of thyroid colloid from the gland (Fig. 10-6), thyroid hormone insufficiency, and a very high frequency (99.7% in one study) of thyroglobulin antibody is known as Hashimoto's thyroiditis. The hypergammaglobulinemia seen in about 60% of these patients can be related to their antithyroid globulin, which can be detected by gel immunodiffusion, passive agglutination, complement fixation, immunofluorescence, or other serologic tests.

Hashimoto's disease is of historical interest because it was the first to meet the criteria established by Witebsky. The findings just mentioned, the immunologic features

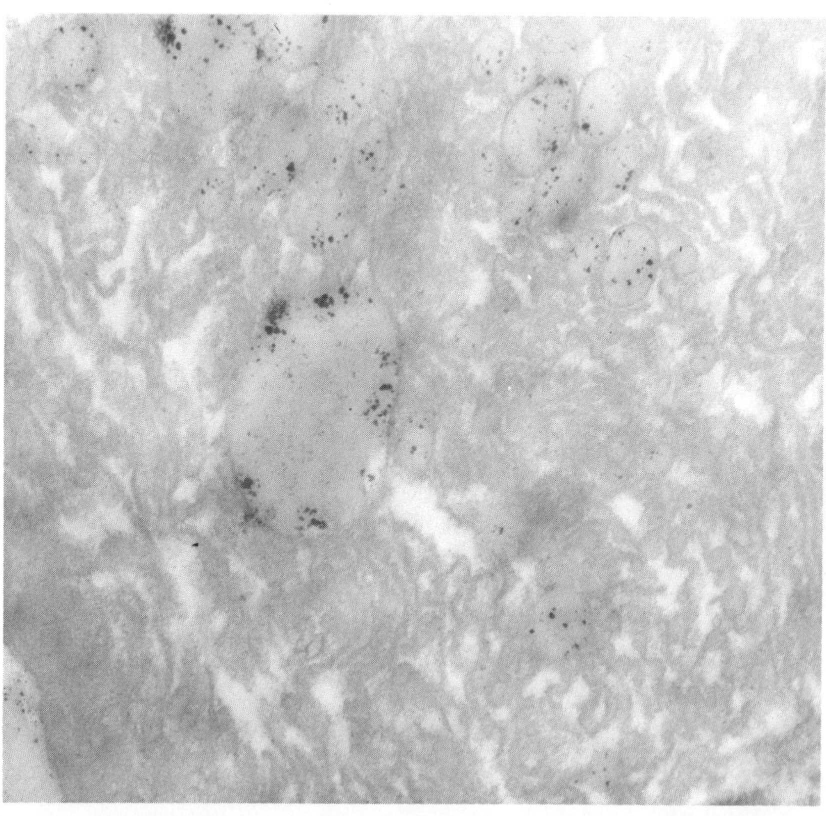

Fig. 10-6. Colloid-filled spaces of normal thyroid gland are scarce in this electron micrograph of thyroid gland from patient with Hashimoto's disease. Dark granules around colloid indicate point of ferritin-labeled antithyroglobulin attachment. (Courtesy Dr. E. Adelstein.)

associated with the disease, established the first criterion. Experimental disease can be produced in the rabbit by surgically removing one lobe of the thyroid gland and using it in the form of a homogenate with Freund's adjuvant to immunize the donor animal. When the rabbit shows evidence of hypothyroidism and circulating autoantibody, histologic examination of the remaining thyroid lobe will reveal exactly the same changes as in the human form of the disease, thus fulfilling criteria two and three. The fourth criterion has actually been met by transferring the disease with T lymphocyte and/or hyperimmune sera from affected donor animals. Most investigators have had greater success in transferring the disease with sensitized T lymphocytes than with sera, and for this reason the disease is more often classified as a T lymphocyte–mediated disease. What causes the thyroglobulin to acquire autoantigenicity is unknown, but autoantibodies to other thyroid antigens are much less frequently observed in Hashimoto's disease.

Graves' disease

More common than Hashimoto's disease is Graves' disease, a type of hyperthyroidism, which is an immunoglobulin disorder but is included here for comparison with Hashimoto's disease. The evidence, accumulated at a rapid pace after 1956, indicates that the hyperthyroidism associated with Graves' disease is caused by a long-acting thyroid stimulator (LATS) found in nearly 85% of all patients and present in the gamma globulin fraction of their sera. Purified IgG that contains this LATS activity has been further analyzed with the discovery that the Fc, Fab, and $F(ab)_2$ portions of the molecule contain the LATS activity. The LATS autoantibody is a type of enhancing antibody. This autoantibody operates at the cellular level, much like the thyroid stimulatory hormone does, to stimulate thyroid hormone release and thyrotoxicosis.

Aspermatogenesis

Autoimmune aspermatogenesis is easily induced in the rat, guinea pig, and other laboratory animals by immunizing the animal with one testis emulsified in Freund's adjuvant. The remaining testis gradually becomes less able to replace preformed sperm lost in the ejaculate, and the male becomes aspermatogenic after about 3 weeks. There is little generalized tissue damage even when whole testis is used as the antigen, but spermatic fluid or sperm can substitute for the gonad as the antigen. The aspermatogenic condition is temporary, and after 3 to 6 months, regeneration of spermatogenesis can be observed but this may not return to normal for a year.

The aspermia is accompanied by circulating sperm-immobilizing globulins and anaphylactic sensitivity to spermatic fluid, but the condition is not transferrable with immune serum, only with viable T lymphocytes. The condition is thus caused by sperm-sensitized T lymphocytes.

The ease by which aspermatogenesis can be induced with injections of sperm or spermatic fluid and the temporary state of the condition once stirred excitement relative to immune birth control procedures, but surgical and chemical methods have been so successful that population control by immunologic methods is now discounted as unfeasible.

BIBLIOGRAPHY

Allison, A. C.: The roles of T and B lymphocytes in self-tolerance and autoimmunity, Contemp. Top. Immunobiol. **3**:227,1974.

Burnet, M.: Autoimmunity and autoimmune disease, Philadelphia, 1972, F. A. Davis Co.

Cochrane, C. G., and Koffler, D.: Immune complex disease in experimental animals and man, Adv. Immunol. **16**:186, 1973.

Doniach, D.: Autoimmunity in liver disease, Prog. Clin. Immunol. **1**:45, 1972.

Gell, P. G. H., and Coombs, R. R. A., eds.: Clinical aspects of immunology, ed. 3, Oxford, 1974, Blackwell Scientific Publications, Ltd.

Koffler, D.: Immunopathogenesis of systemic lupus erythematosus, Annu. Rev. Med. **25**: 149, 1974.
Lyampert, I. M., and Davilova, T. A.: Immunological phenomena associated with cross-reactive antigens of micro-organisms and mammalian tissues, Prog. Allergy **18**:423, 1975.
Osler, A. G., and Siraganian, R. P.: Immunologic mechanisms of platelet damage, Prog. Allergy **16**:450, 1972.
Parish, W. E.: General concepts of autosensitivity in disease, Adv. Biol. Skin **11**:233, 1971.
Roelcke, D.: Cold agglutination, antibodies and antigens, Clin. Immunol. Immunopathol. **2**: 266, 1974.
Rowlands, L. P., ed.: Immunological disorders of the nervous system, Baltimore, 1971, The Williams & Wilkins Co.
Roy, L. P., Fish, A. J., Michael, A. F., and Vernier, R. L.: Etiologic agents of immune deposit disease, Prog. Clin. Immunol. **1**:1, 1972.
Samter, M., ed.: Immunological diseases, ed. 2, Boston, 1971, Little, Brown & Co.
Shulman, S.: Thyroid antigens and autoimmunity, Adv. Immunol. **14**:85, 1971.
Shulman, S.: Tissue specificity and autoimmunity, Berlin, 1974, Springer Verlag.
Stiller, C. R., Russell, A. S., and Dossetor, J. B.: Autoimmunity: present concepts, Ann. Intern. Med. **82**:405, 1975.
Taylor, G.: Immunology in medical practice, London, 1975, W. B. Saunders Co., Ltd.
Turk, J. L.: Immunology in clinical medicine, ed. 2, New York, 1972, Appleton-Century-Crofts.
Vischer, T. L.: Immunological aspects of chronic hepatitis, Prog. Allergy **15**:268, 1971.
Weigle, W. O.: Experimental autoimmune thyroiditis, Pathol. Annu. **8**:329, 1973.
Whittingham, S.: Serological methods in autoimmune disease in man, Res. Immunochem. Immunobiol. **1**:123, 1972.
Yu, D. T.: Cellular immunological aspects of rheumatoid arthritis, Semin. Arthritis Rheum. **4**:25, 1974.
Ziff, M., ed.: Models for the study and therapy of rheumatoid arthritis, Fed. Proc. **32**:131, 1973.
Zvaifler, N. J.: The immunopathology of joint inflammation in rheumatoid arthritis, Adv. Immunol. **16**:265, 1973.

Case histories

CASE 1. SYSTEMIC LUPUS ERYTHEMATOSUS

J. L., a 28-year-old female employee of a local boutique, first contacted a dermatologist because of a rash that developed over the bridge of her nose and across her upper cheeks while she was on vacation in Florida. She had masked the rash with cosmetics. However, the rash persisted, and when she began to develop other vague symptoms of illness—fever, malaise, and a slight weight loss—she contacted her dermatologist. A laboratory workup revealed a slight normochromic anemia and leukopenia (9.8 gm hemoglobulin/100 ml and 3600 WBC/mm^3). Serum protein analysis revealed a slight hypergammaglobulinemia, a low C3 component of complement, and a positive RF test. A second serum sample was subjected to antinuclear antibodies (ANA) and found to be positive. Her condition was diagnosed as SLE, and she was placed on prednisolone and azathioprine. Her condition deteriorated and then, surprisingly, improved when therapy was halted.

Questions

1. What is the general immunopathology of SLE?
2. What is the ANA test?
3. Is the ANA test the most reliable serologic test for SLE?
4. What was the basis for the initiation and removal of immunosuppressant therapy in this case?

Discussion

SLE is more frequently a disease of young females by a ratio of nearly 9:1 with males. The etiology of the disease is unknown, but sunburn or extensive exposure to sun or ultraviolet light often seems associated with flare of the facial rash. A genetic predisposition to SLE has been suggested, and this is based on studies of New Zealand mice that have a tendency to develop several connective tissue disorders with associated autoimmune phenomena.

SLE has had a vacillating history in terms of trying to establish a firm immunologic basis for the disease. The rather early recognition of ANA suggested an autoimmunoglobulin basis for the disease. This suggestion fell into disfavor because it was agreed that only white blood cells would be permeable to the antibodies, which could thus contribute little to the arthritis, the renal involvement (proteinuria, hematuria), the facial rash, or the neurologic symptoms of the disease. Moreover, it was also agreed that drug-induced SLE, an antibody-related form of SLE in man or experimental animals, was a similar but significantly different phenomenon. Drug-induced SLE created by therapy with hydralazine, procainamide, isoniazid, *p*-aminosalicylic acid, etc. is an antibody-mediated disease in which the chemically altered DNA of white cell nuclei served as the antigen. This readily explained the 70% incidence of positive ANA tests in patients who received these drugs. However, when little evidence for a T cell–mediated association with the disease emerged, a reevaluation of SLE as an immunoglobulin-based disease was necessary. Now SLE is accepted as having a strong immune-complex component. A nucleic acid–antigen complex with ANA immunoglobulins and complement has been identified in the renal lesions. These deposits are trapped in the glomerular basement membranes and contribute to the glomerulonephritis seen in SLE patients. These immune complexes do not cause serious kidney disease in all patients because the complex must be at the proper antigen/antibody ratio to provoke tissue damage.

One of the most useful drugs in SLE therapy is prednisone. When complement levels begin to return to normal, the prognosis is, at least temporarily, favorable. Either whole hemolytic complement or C3 measured by the Mancini test may be used for estimation of complement, with the latter being favored. LE cell preparations are relatively insensitive and should not be relied on as a sole diagnostic or prognostic aid. ANA tests performed by indirect immunofluorescence require less antibody and are preferred for measuring circulating antibody. Cyclophosphamide and azathioprine are also being used with variable success. An occasional patient will continue to decline in health even when the dosage of these drugs is carefully monitored to prevent their well-known side effects. The reason for this is not known, but it is believed that the immunosuppressive action of these drugs reduces the ANA titer and forces the ANA-antigen complex into a ratio that favors immune-complex glomerulonephritis. When the therapy is halted, the antibody titer rises; the immune aggregates are dominated by their antibody content and produce less kidney disturbance. This may be the sequence of events in this case.

REFERENCES

Koffler, D., Schur, P. H., and Kunkel, H. G.: Immunological studies concerning the nephritis of systemic lupus erythematosus, J. Exp. Med. **126**:607, 1967.

Schur, P. H., and Sandson, J.: Immunological factors and clinical activity in systemic lupus erythematosus, N. Engl. J. Med. **278**:533, 1968.

Sharp, G. C.: Autoantibodies and complement in SLE: a reexamination, Hosp. Prac. **6**(11): 109, 1971.

CASE 2. RHEUMATOID ARTHRITIS

F. B., a 53-year-old pastry worker in a small homestyle bakery, contacted his physician because of pain in his wrists and thumbs. Morning stiffness in these joints was also a chief complaint, and some swelling and warmth in the wrist area was noticed. This condition had developed slowly over the past year or more, eventually causing enough distress to necessitate medical attention. The patient was informed that there was a good possibility that he was developing rheumatoid arthritis, although other diagnoses were possible. Blood was collected for serologic and hematologic studies and x-ray films were taken of the affected joints. The findings confirmed rheumatoid arthritis, and aspirin was prescribed.

Questions

1. What serologic tests are used to aid in the diagnosis of rheumatoid arthritis?
2. What is the immunopathology of this disease?
3. What is the status of immunosuppressant therapy of rheumatoid arthritis?

Discussion

The laboratory findings in rheumatoid arthritis often include a normocytic anemia, an elevated erythrocyte sedimentation rate, low albumin/globulin ratio associated with an elevated gamma globulin level, and positive RF tests. Increases in IgG, IgM, or IgA are not diagnostic. The RF test is positive in about 80% of all patients with classic rheumatoid arthritis when the latex agglutination test is used. In this test, pooled human gamma globulin is adsorbed onto latex particles and used as the antigen in passive agglutination tests. The patient's serum containing RF has the antiglobulin, most frequently an IgM but it may also be either an IgG or IgA, that fixes to the globulin on the latex particle, thus causing agglutination. The latex test or its alternatives (the sensitized sheep cell, sensitized human cell, or bentonite test), each of which is a passive agglutination test, is a poor index of IgG or IgA antiglobulins but is acceptable for the detection of IgM antiglobulins.

Positive RF tests are not diagnostic of rheumatoid arthritis, since such tests are positive in many connective tissue diseases, including lupus erythematosus, scleroderma, Sjögren's syndrome, viral hepatitis-arthritis, polyarteritis, cirrhosis, and polymyositis. Many infectious diseases also lead to false positive RF tests, of which leprosy, syphilis, tuberculosis, viral hepatitis, and even influenza can be mentioned. The titer of RF even in frank rheumatoid arthritis does not correlate with the intensity of the disease. As a consequence, positive RF tests must be interpreted cautiously; clinical and radiologic findings are probably more important in the diagnosis of rheumatoid arthritis.

Other tests that are positive in rheumatoid arthritis include ANA (incidence of 20% to 60%) and positive LE preparations (incidence of 10% to 20%).

The immunopathology of the disease is unproved but is possibly based on an infectious joint disease, followed by an outpouring of IgG and inflammatory cells into the synovial fluid. IgG molecules become altered, expose new antigenic determinants, and stimulate IgM formation. Hypocomplementemia is rare, but complexes of complement with IgM and IgG may occur in synovial fluid or blood.

Treatment with aspirin or other anti-inflammatory agents remains the dominant therapy for rheumatoid arthritis. Steroids are generally a second line of therapy when salicylates, chloroquine derivatives, or gold salts no longer provide relief. Large immunosuppressant doses of corticosteroids are usually not recommended, and dosages at the anti-inflammatory level are preferred. Cytotoxic drugs such as azathioprine, methotrexate, 6-mercaptopurine, and cyclophosphamide are now being used on an experimental basis. The short-term results (6 to 8 months) have been promising, but the benefits of long-term therapy are yet to be evaluated.

REFERENCES

American Rheumatism Association Expert Committee: A controlled trial of cyclophosphamide in rheumatoid arthritis, N. Engl. J. Med. **283:** 883, 1970.

Ruddy, S., and Austen, K. F.: The complement system in rheumatoid synovitis, Arthritis Rheum. **13**:713, 1970.

Stage, D. E., and Mannik, M.: Rheumatoid factors in rheumatoid arthritis, Bull. Rheum. Dis. **23**:720, 1973.

Zvaifler, N. J., and Robinson, C. A.: Rheumatoid arthritis, Disease-A-Month, p. 1, May, 1974.

chapter 11

Transplantation and tumor immunology

The most perplexing immunologic aspect of tumor formation and growth is that oncogenic tissues contain new antigens with which the host has had no previous experience, antigens that can be considered as foreign; and yet the host fails to mount an adequate rejection system to destroy the tumor cells carrying these antigens. It is true that in many instances the immune surveillance system may function perfectly to prevent the growth of cancerous cells, but since this is observed simply as good health, it goes unnoticed. As the prevalence of cancer indicates, the surveillance system also fails with a disappointing frequency. Tissue transplantation immunologists are faced with the diametrically opposite problem. When tissues are transplanted between two genetically unrelated individuals, the tissue (in the absence of supportive treatment) is rejected. There is overwhelming evidence that this rejection, in the presence of faultless surgical technique, is due to a host response against the foreign antigens present in the grafted tissue. Why foreign tissue antigens are destroyed so effectively in the case of organ or tissue transplants and not when the tissue is oncogenic is the dilemma that immunologists are trying to solve and reverse.

TRANSPLANTATION IMMUNOLOGY

Graft rejection

When tissue is transferred from a donor to an unrelated recipient, rejection of the graft will follow one of three possible sequences. These are known as the hyperacute, first set, and second set reactions. Immunologic phenomena of different types and to different degrees are involved in these three reactions.

Hyperacute rejection. In the hyperacute graft rejection sequence there is never a moment when the grafted tissue appears to be accepted by its new host. As soon as the vascular connection of a deep-seated organ destined for hyperacute rejection is completed, it will become engorged with blood, the blood may fail to pass through the organ and even clot, and the tissue will assume that bluish purple cast that signifies that it is anoxic. The surgeon will remove the organ immediately in one and the same operation as the transplantation itself, because it is obviously nonfunctional and in the process of destruction by the host. In hyperacute rejection of skin the transferred tissue never becomes revascularized and remains as a "white graft" that soon dries and is sloughed (Fig. 11-1).

The hyperacute rejection sequence develops under two circumstances, both of which involve immunoglobulins with a specificity for antigens in the donated tissue. The first of these is related to grafts made across the ABO(H) blood group barrier such that the recipient has naturally present isohemagglutinins that combine with the corresponding antigens on the surface of cells of the grafted tissue. The other situation exists

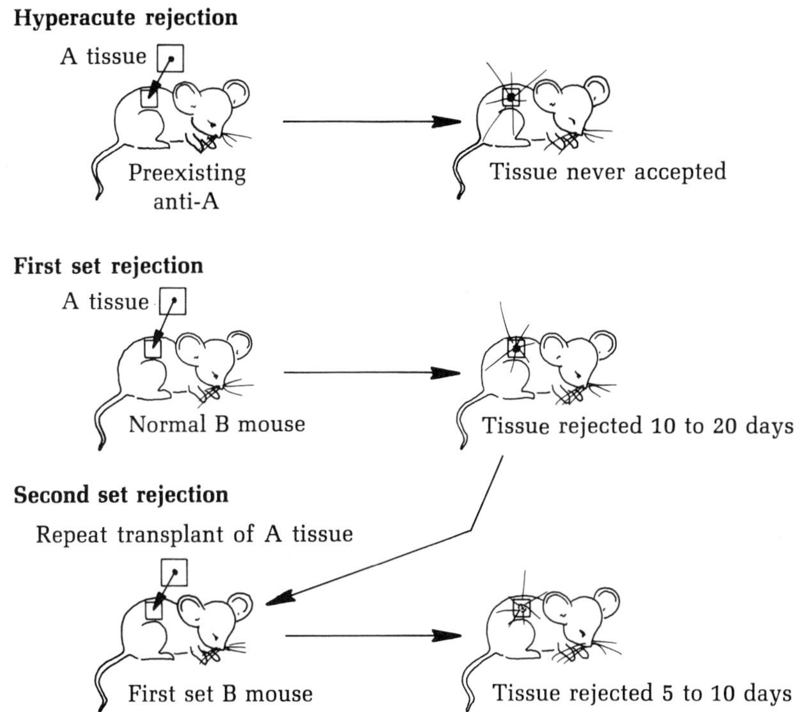

Fig. 11-1. Hyperacute rejection results from placement of tissue in an animal already possessing antibodies to antigens of grafted tissue. Second set rejection is an accelerated first set reaction and is seen in animals that have already rejected tissue at least once.

when by blood transfusions, childbirth, or other means the recipient has antibodies directed against other blood group antigens represented on donor cells. Matching of blood groups between the donor and recipient is clearly an essential first step in ensuring a successful transplant.

First set rejection. Even when major and minor blood grouping cross matches prove satisfactory, the first or second set reaction may result in elimination of the transplanted tissue. In the first set rejection sequence the initial events belie the fact that the graft will be rejected. The tissue becomes revascularized normally and assumes its normal hue, a feature easily observed in the case of skin grafts. In the case of organ transplants the organ will quickly resume its physiologic function—the excretion of urine by the kidney, the pumping of blood by the heart, the production of hormones by the pancreas, etc. But these events are short-lived. Within 5 to 10 days the organ will diminish in effectiveness. Skin grafts will acquire a deep purple hue that steadily progresses in the following days to a black necrotic patch. The patient will usually develop malaise and fever if large areas of skin or a visceral organ are involved in the rejection. Depending on the circumstances the first set rejection sequence will be complete between the eleventh and seventeenth day when the transplantation becomes an obvious failure (Fig. 11-1).

A histologic examination of tissues involved in first set rejection reveals that the tissue gradually becomes infiltrated with macrophages, lymphocytes, and plasma cells—cells that signify that rejection of the tissue is founded on immunologic grounds.

Fibrin deposition and a loss of vascular patency are also seen. These features obviously indicate that the grafted tissue was no longer able to receive nutrients from the host, to effect a proper gas exchange, or to dissipate its waste products, factors that ultimately terminate in its death. The immunologic findings suggest that it is largely the T lymphocyte that is responsible for graft destruction. In the first few days of the graft's existence in the recipient, T cell sensitization to donor antigens develops, and in the latter days the sensitized cells express their newly developed powers through their lymphokines and force a rejection of the graft.

Second set rejection. If a retransplant of tissue from the same or antigenically related donor is made to the victim of a first set reaction, the sequence of the first set reaction follows but at an accelerated pace. At first the graft again appears successful, but within 5 to 10 days it will cease functioning and be eliminated. In this second set reaction, immunoglobulins directed against donor antigens plus presensitized T cells contribute to rejection of the graft. This combination hastens graft rejection compared to the first set reaction (Fig. 11-1).

Terminology

The events of the hyperacute, first, and second set rejection of transplanted tissue apply when the tissue transfer is made between antigenically disparate individuals within a single species. Such a transplant is now referred to as an allograft, although the older term, "homograft," is still sometimes used (Table 11-1). The tissue itself is described as allogeneic and contains alloantigens. A syngraft is a graft between two antigenically identical individuals, and in human medicine this would be limited to identical twins. The tissue is syngeneic or congeneic. Syngraft replaces the misleading term "isograft," misleading because the prefix *iso-* has been used so extensively in immunology to mean same species and not same antigen. An autograft occurs when the donor and the recipient are the same individual. Syngrafts and autografts are always successful, since there are no novel antigens presented by the donor to the recipient. Xenografts, grafts between individuals from different species, can always be expected to fail for the opposite reason.

These judgments of graft success or failure and the discussion of hyperacute, first, and second set rejection are based on the premise that the surgical technique has been adequate, that sepsis was prevented, and that no further immunologic or chemotherapeutic interventions were permitted to alter the natural outcome of the tissue transplant. Unequivocal evidence is now available that when these restrictions are met and the graft still fails, it is due to an immune response of the recipient directed against antigens of the donor.

Table 11-1. Relationships of immunologic, surgical, and genetic terms used in transplantation

Genetic term	*Immunologic term*	*Surgical term*	*Tissue*	*Application*
Autograft	Autograft	Autograft	Autogeneic	Donor and recipient are same person
Syngraft	Isograft	Homograft or isograft	Syngeneic or congeneic	Donor and recipient are genetically identical
Allograft	Isograft	Homograft	Allogeneic	Donor and recipient are antigenically nonidentical but in same species
Xenograft	Heterograft	Heterograft	Xenogeneic	Donor and recipient of different species

Histocompatibility antigens

Although antibodies directed against the ABO(H) or other erythrocyte antigens can contribute to graft rejection, as a matter of practice grafts across the blood group barriers are not attempted. Even so, the usual allograft is rejected, and this rejection is based on immunologic phenomena. The antigens responsible for the failure of grafts are known as histocompatibility or transplantation antigens, although other organ or tissue-specific antigens may also contribute to graft rejection. All of the histocompatibility antigens are not of equal potency in inducing tissue rejection and have accordingly been divided into the major and minor antigens. It is believed that leukocytes contain all or nearly all of the major antigens, and this accounts for their designation as HL (human leukocyte) antigens.

The formation of histocompatibility antigens is genetically regulated by two associated loci consisting of a number of alleles. These are designated as the A loci, and this accounts for the abbreviation HL-A (human leukocyte—series A) for the human histocompatibility antigens. The first series locus regulates the synthesis of antigens HL-A1, A2, A3, A9, and A11 plus additional antigens Ba, Li, W19, etc. not yet assigned numbers. Antigens HL-A5, A7, A8, A12, A13, etc. are controlled by the second series locus (Table 11-2). Since these antigens are controlled by paired genes, the antigens are transmitted in pairs. Consequently, the HL-A composition of any individual can be considered in respect to the two antigens (or genes) inherited from each parent, and this is known as the haplotype (half-type). For example, a person with antigens 1 and 5 (from the first and second series, respectively) and 2 and 7 (again from the first and second series) would possess the haplotypes 1,5 and 2,7.

The transplantation or histocompatibility antigens are located on the external surface of nucleated cells. A vast number of purification methods, beginning with the cell membranes as the starting material, have been attempted. Extraction with detergents, salts, lipid solvents, freeze-thaw cell rupture, sonic oscillation, or similar treatments served as a usual first step. HL-A antigens are also present in the cell cytoplasm and even in blood. These may prove to be superior sources of these antigens and are certainly more convenient sources, since the antigens are already in soluble form. Crude preparations of the HL-A antigens contain lipid, carbohydrate, and protein. The lipid is nonessential and can be removed without losses in HL-A activity. The carbohydrate (1% to 10%) is intimately associated with the protein that exists as a glycoprotein, but it too appears noncontributory to antigenicity. The HL-A antigens are destroyed by protein denaturants or proteolysis and consist of glycoproteins with molecular weights of 31,000 to 35,000. The biochemistry of the transplantation antigens is very similar in all mammalian species examined so far.

Table 11-2. Genetic distribution of human histocompatibility antigens

First series (locus)	*Second series (locus)*	*Third series (locus)*	*Mixed lymphocyte culture*
A1	A5	Numbers not yet assigned	Numbering system now being developed
A2	A7		
A3	A8		
A9	A12		
A10	A13		
A11	A14		
A28	A17		
Plus at least 6 unassigned numbers	A27		
	Plus perhaps 10 unassigned numbers		

Histocompatibility testing

The assessment of graft success relies on a determination of the antigenic similarity between the donor and the recipient. This can be determined by analyzing tissues of each participant for the coincidence of their major histocompatibility antigens or, alternatively, one can assay for an antagonistic reaction between tissues of the donor and recipient in vitro, which is presumed to reflect the future reaction in vivo if the graft was actually made.

Cytotoxicity assay. A basic premise in cytotoxicity testing for HL-A antigens is that an antiserum exists that will detect each antigen. This is probably not true; all of the HL-A antigens themselves have probably not yet been recognized. The cytotoxicity test is a good predictor of transplant success, because antisera do exist for most of the important antigens. The test is also relatively inexpensive and simple to perform compared to its alternative, the mixed lymphocyte culture.

To conduct the cytotoxicity test, lymphocyte preparations from the donor and recipient are harvested from blood and incubated separately with antiserum to each of the HL-A antigens in the presence of serum complement. The incubation, usually for 1 hour at room temperature or 37° C in multiple concavity microtrays, is sufficient to inaugurate the complement-dependent killing of any cell-bearing antigens that correspond with the antiserum placed in that concavity. The dead cells are stained with trypan blue or eosin. Microscopic examination then reveals which antisera were toxic to the lymphocytes, and this identifies the antigens corresponding to the specificity of these antisera. With this information the antigenic composition of both donor and recipient tissues is determined. Modification of the method includes the use of dyes that stain only living cells or the release of radioisotopes from labeled cells as evidence of damaged membranes. The cells are not lysed by the serologic reaction.

Regardless of the modification used, the interpretations are the same. When the donor cells contain an antigen not present on cells of the recipient, the graft is not attempted. Such a graft would only immunize the recipient against the foreign HL-A antigen and induce the transplant rejection process.

Mixed lymphocyte culture. When lymphocytes from unrelated donors are placed in culture, lymphocyte transformation observed as a stimulation of DNA synthesis, enlargement of the cell nucleus, increase in mitotic figures, and cell enlargement and division can be detected (Fig. 11-2). These changes can be detected microscopically, but this is time-consuming and subject to interpretative error as to what constitutes a transformed cell. To hasten the process and to increase the sensitivity of the test, tritiated thymidine is added to the cultures, and isotope incorporation is used as an index of DNA synthesis and cell proliferation.

Mixed lymphocyte reactions appear to reflect disparities only in the major histocompatibility antigens, and differences in the minor antigens apparently go undetected. Since some grafts matched by cytotoxicity testing are nevertheless rejected, the mixed lymphocyte culture (MLC) reaction may be measuring antigens more critical to graft success. These MLC antigens are regulated by MLC genes. The nomenclature and classification of MLC antigens are yet to be constructed but are under study.

One obvious drawback to the MLC test as described is the potential for donor lymphocytes to respond to recipient lymphocytes in the absence of any recipient response to donor lymphocytes and yet be interpreted as a histocompatibility mismatch. In the MLC reaction the only important determination for routine grafting is to determine if the recipient is reacting against donor cells. This can be done if the donor lymphocytes are poisoned with mitomycin C or irradiation before adding them to the culture. Mitomycin C blocks DNA metabolism in the donor cells so that any lymphocyte transformation becomes an index

Normal mixed lymphocyte culture

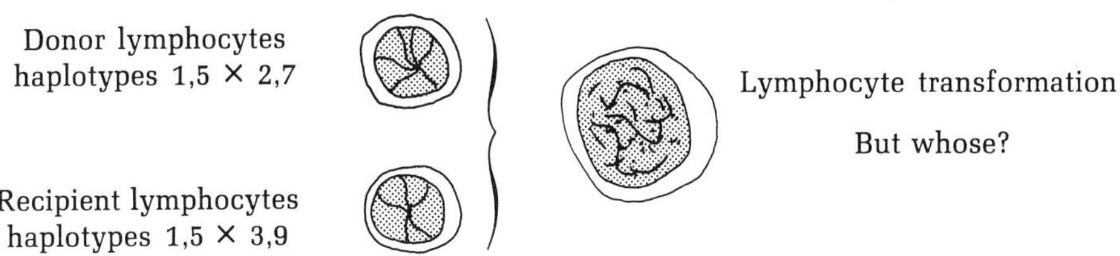

One-way mixed lymphocyte culture

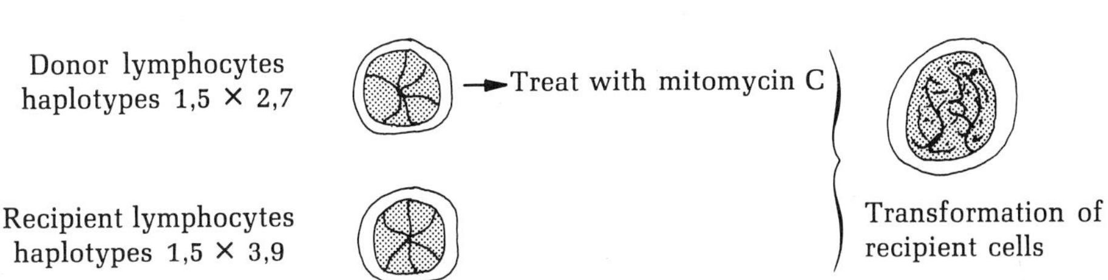

Fig. 11-2. Poisoning donor lymphocytes assures that a positive mixed lymphocyte culture is result of recipient lymphocyte transformation.

only of the recipient's response, and the test is thus a one-way MLC.

Graft-versus-host reaction

If the one-way MLC were conducted in the opposite fashion so that only the recipient's cells were poisoned, then the test would be an index of the graft-versus-host reaction. Graft-versus-host reactions can occur when immunocompetent tissues are transferred into an immunologically penalized host. This situation has been observed to occur naturally in a few neonates who received maternal lymphocytes during the pregnancy. These cells mount their immune attack on the indefensible fetus and runt disease results. Runt disease may be characterized as an underweight offspring that fails to grow, has a distinct splenomegaly, erythematous skin, anemia, and diarrhea. Human victims of runt disease have been observed, and their symptomatology mimics very closely that seen in experimental runt disease where lymphocytes are given to fetal animals by injection. Fortunately graft-versus-host reactions do not necessarily terminate fatally, especially when the graft and the host share a number of the major HL-A antigens. It was this fact that encouraged bone marrow transplantation in children devoid of B and T lymphocytes to repair their immunologic deficit and into patients with aplastic anemia to repair their red blood cell deficit.

Graft-versus-host disease is rarely a consequence of the lymphoid population of organs that are grafted to patients who are then treated with immunosuppressants to minimize the usual host-versus-graft reaction, since the transferred cells are also immunosuppressed. Graft-versus-host reactions can also be prevented by pretreating the lymphoid tissue to be transferred with immunosuppressant chemicals or irradiation before the graft is effected. There is no need for this when heart, skin, or other lymphocyte-poor tissues are transferred, even though the defense system of the host may be compromised by immunosuppressant treatments.

Immunosuppression

It is a rare transplant that is not accompanied by immunosuppression of the recipient to modify the graft rejection process even in instances of apparently suitable matching of HL-A or MLC antigens. Virtually all forms of immunosuppression have been tested—irradiation, most chemical inhibitors of the immune response, and antilymphocyte serum or its globulin fraction (ALS or ALG). These have been applied singly and in combination. Naturally the selection of these inhibitors varies from one situation to another and from one transplant team to another. ALG is included in most regimens despite obvious handicaps in assessing its potency before use, its tendency to produce erythema and pain on injection, and the hazard of producing serum sickness or anaphylaxis. Even though the grafted patient is usually receiving other immunosuppressants that would tend to reduce the allergic response to ALG, the fact remains that most do develop an allergic reaction to ALG, which demands its removal from the therapeutic program.

Among the chemical immunosuppressants the steroids, cyclophosphamide, the purine analogs, and methotrexate have all been used. A significant danger in the use of these agents is that they are general depressants that ease the infectiousness of bacteria, viruses, and other pathogens of all sorts. Even more serious is the observation of an increased incidence of cancer in immunosuppressed patients. It appears that depression of the immune system to prevent its elimination of foreign cells also handicaps the elimination of oncogenic host cells as well. This heightened incidence of cancer in immunosuppressed graft recipients has been used as evidence that cell mutation to the cancerous state occurs regularly, but that the cancer growth is easily destroyed in the healthy patient.

Privileged sites and tissues

Circumstances do exist in which allograft acceptance can be accomplished without the need for immunosuppression. Corneal transplants, now practiced for decades in human medicine, are a classic example. The cornea is physiologically rather inert, and it apparently releases antigens very slowly when transferred to a new host. Moreover, the cornea is placed in a relatively avascular bed distant from the lymphatic drainage system. These features of corneal transplants combine to protect the transferred tissue from the lymphocyte-dependent rejection process of the host and ensure success of the graft. When ideal surgical conditions are not met and vessel damage or bleeding develops at the relocation site, then corneas are rejected in the same fashion as other tissues.

The developing fetus is a prime example of an immunologically protected tissue. Except in the breeding of syngeneic laboratory animals, all fertilizations require that the fetus contain antigens derived from its father that are foreign to the mother. In utero these antigens stimulate no graft rejection response. The exact reason for this is uncertain but may be related to the thick trophoblastic layer that separates the uterine wall from the fetus. It has been speculated that this tissue layer is impermeable to lymphocytes. The feeble role of antibodies in allograft rejection is demonstrated by the observation that immunization of the mother with tissues from the father is noncontributory to fetal abortion.

Other experiments have also demonstrated that prior immunization with tissue antigens has no detrimental effect on graft rejection and indeed prior immunization may prolong the acceptance of the graft. This has been termed immunologic enhancement and is presumed to operate much like blocking antibodies produced in allergic individuals. The enhancing antibodies apparently attach to the tissue antigens but in themselves are not cytotoxic. Their presence blocks the approach of T lymphoctyes or a combination of T lymphocytes and cytotoxic antibodies so that the graft is spared.

TUMOR IMMUNOLOGY

Tumor-specific antigens

When a neoplastic cell develops, it expresses a large set of new properties not possessed by the surrounding cells; among these is the formation of new antigens. Some of these antigens are restricted to the intracellular portion of the cells, but others are located on the cell surface. The former are anatomically protected from the defense system of the host, whereas those on the cell surface, like the histocompatibility antigens of any foreign cell, are situated in physically vulnerable positions in terms of the immune activities of the host. Despite this, these cells all too often escape these host resistance forces, proliferate, interrupt the physiologic and structural pattern of surrounding tissues, and may cause the death of the host.

Virus-induced antigens. Two interesting observations have been made about these antigens, the first of which led to the use of the term "tumor-specific transplantation antigen" (TSTA) or simply "tumor-specific antigen" (TSA). Tumors provoked in experimental animals by a carcinogenic chemical, with few exceptions, are antigenically unrelated, even when multiple tumors are induced in different locations on the same animal. Virus-induced tumors, on the other hand, are antigenically the same from animal to animal or between tumors located on the same animal. The latter are identified as TSTA, and both DNA and RNA viruses have been recognized to induce their formation in experimental animals (Table 11-3). As yet there is no final proof that this transpires in man because of the difficulty in establishing the viral etiology of human cancer. However, Burkitt's lymphoma may be caused by the Epstein-Barr virus and may be the first accepted instance. There is already proof that human adenoviruses are carcinogenic for laboratory animals, but again, there is no final proof of their oncogenic behavior in man. The fact that these viruses induce TSTA suggests several possibilities, one of which is that an immune response directed only against the TSTA antigens would destroy the tumor with no effect on other host cells. It is also obvious that detection of the antigen would assist in the diagnosis of cancer, and quantitation of TSTA levels in blood or other tissues of a patient would serve as a prognosticator of therapeutic efficacy.

Table 11-3. Carcinogenic agents and tumor antigens

Chemically induced	*Viral induced*
Antigenically variable	Antigenically constant for any one virus
Inducers include benzpyrene, methylcholanthrene, and many unidentified compounds	Viral inducers
	RNA viruses
	Leukemia-sarcoma group of mice, cat, rat, guinea pig, hamster, etc.
	Mouse mammary tumor
	DNA viruses
	Herpesvirus*
	Adenovirus*
	Polyomavirus
	Papillomavirus*

*Includes viruses of human origin that cause cancer in experimental animals.

Embryonic antigens. The second observation regards an interesting group of antigens identified in human tumors that have been termed oncofetal antigens, maturation antigens, regression antigens, carcinoembryonic antigens, etc. These antigens although not viral induced, are antigenically constant from one example to the next and constitute a second class of TSTA; they have been identified in tumors of specific organs or organ systems and in embryonic tissue from these same organs, and this distribution accounts for their many synonyms. The first recognized of these is the carcinoembryonic antigen (CEA) associated with cancerous tissue from the human digestive system. This includes cancers of the small intestine, colon, stomach, liver, and pancreas. CEA is found in these same normal tissues in the human fetus, but it is not restricted to these solid tissues. It is also found in the blood of individuals with digestive system tumors, and from this arose the hope that recognition of this antigen in blood would serve to diagnose these conditions. For two reasons the results have not met this expectation. The first of these is that all such patients do not have CEA in their blood—perhaps only 60% to 80% will be positive. And as more and more sensitive serologic methods have been used in an effort to increase these percentages, the incidence of CEA in cancer-free persons has climbed. This has not discouraged interest in CEA, however, for in those patients with proved digestive tract tumors and CEA, a decrease in CEA titer may be a very useful index to the efficacy of therapy. The present opinion is that fetal antigens may be more useful in prognosis than in diagnosis (Table 11-4).

Two other fetal antigens associated with oncogenesis, are α-fetoprotein, present in normal fetal liver and in hepatomas, and a sulfoglycoprotein, isolated from stomach cancers and the fetal stomach. After birth the infant gradually halts its synthesis of these antigens, and only when tissues of the involved organ regress to the oncogenic state is their synthesis regenerated.

Table 11-4. Characteristics of embryonic tumor-specific antigens

Synthesis	By embryonic organ systems and tumors of the same organ in adults; fetal synthesis ceases near birth
Source	Embryonic organs; cancerous organs; or blood
Specificity	For organ system producing them
Chemistry	Protein or glycoproteins; 25,000-150,000 mol wt
Identification	Immunoassay with antisera rendered specific by adsorption with normal tissues
Importance	As prognostic aid; possibly also in diagnosis

Immunotherapy

It is obvious that prophylactic immunization against cancer is impossible, since there is no method to predict which persons will develop cancer or which cancer they will develop. Moreover, all cancers do not possess TSTA. Although the possibility of immunoprophylaxis is quite remote, the hope for a successful immunotherapy remains high, because this type of therapy would have no effect on normal tissues, an inescapable complication of cytotoxic drug therapy.

Immunotherapy with specific antisera directed against tumor antigens of experimental animals has been an outright failure. Indeed, the tumors were as often enhanced as destroyed, a discovery that leads to the prospect of immunologic enhancement to improve allograft survival. Since foreign cells are more susceptible to T cell than B cell activities, modification of tumor antigens with haptens to encourage a T cell response that would then involve the whole hapten-tumor cell complex has been attempted, but with only partial success. The alternative, to improve the immune response of tumor-bearing patients, appears to offer a greater chance for success. One thought is that cancer patients may be naturally tolerant to tumor antigens or at least to the tumor antigens that are of fetal origin. In this case it would be difficult to cause the host to muster an immune response against the tumor cells. It is also possible that cancer patients do not reject their tumors, because the antigenic load of the tumor is sufficient to create a specific immune tolerance. The attraction of this hypothesis is the observation that animals can reject tumor transplants of small size but not when they exceed a critical amount. Another hypothesis for which some evidence has been presented is that the T lymphocytes of cancer patients are essentially anergic in their response to all antigens, and a recovery of these cells from this condition would be therapeutic.

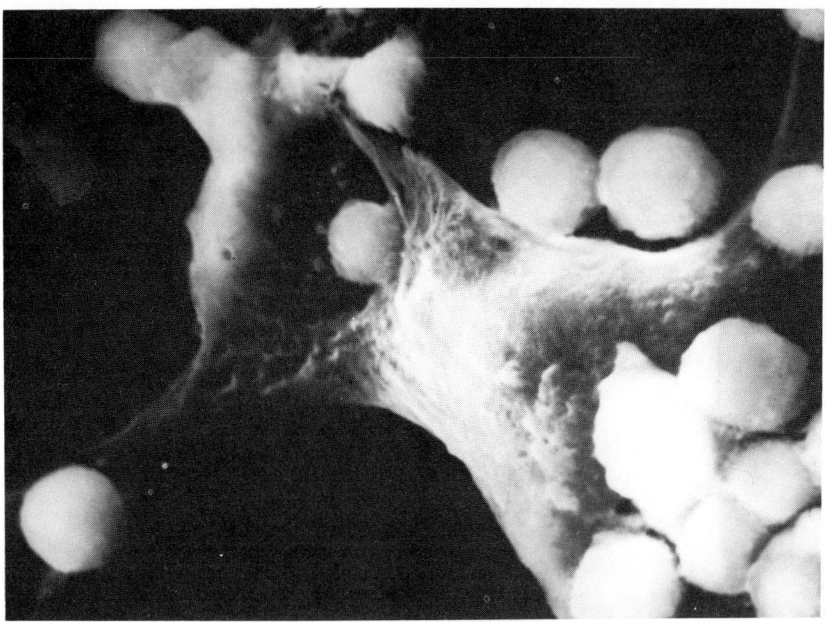

Fig. 11-3. White balls seen in scanning electron microscope view are T lymphocytes attacking a much larger Walker carcinoma cell. T lymphocytes are a significant part of our defense against foreign, including cancer, cells. (Courtesy Dr. E. Adelstein.)

One method of magnifying the nonspecific immune system of the cancer patient relies on the injection of bacille Calmette Guérin (BCG) into the area of the tumor. BCG, it will be recalled, is the living but attenuated *Mycobacterium tuberculosis* var. *bovis* used to immunize against tuberculosis. It is well known that BCG produces a potent allergy of infection that activates the T lymphocytes and macrophages. Lymphokine activity is nonspecific, and lymphotoxin elaborated from the sensitized T cells would attack the BCG organisms and any other foreign cells (Fig. 11-3). Macrophages would assist in this process and be aided by macrophage inhibition factor and chemotaxins. BCG treatment of tumors in laboratory animals has been surprisingly effective, and the hope is that this method can be applied to human beings. Modifications will undoubtedly be required to meet this prospect, and it may be possible to isolate the active compounds from the microorganisms and use them in a purified state. Adjuvants for T cells and macrophages that are superior to BCG may eventually be recognized.

BIBLIOGRAPHY

Alexander, P.: Immunological reactions of the host against primary tumors: their possible role in therapy. In Irvine, W. T., ed.: Scientific basis of surgery, Baltimore, 1972, The Williams & Wilkins Co.

Bach, F. H., and Bach, M. L.: Fundamental immunogenetics—their application to histocompatibility, Clin. Immunobiol. **1**:157, 1972.

Baker, M. A., and Taub, R. N.: Immunotherapy of human cancer, Prog. Allergy **17**:227, 1973.

Billingham, R. E., and Silvers, W. K.: The immunobiology of transplantation, Englewood Cliffs, N.J., 1971, Prentice-Hall, Inc.

Burnet, F. M.: Immunological surveillance in neoplasia, Transplant. Rev. **7**:3, 1971.

Calne, R. Y., ed.: Clinical organ transplantation, Oxford, 1971, Blackwell Scientific Publications, Ltd.

Calne, R. Y., ed.: Immunological aspects of

transplantation surgery, New York, 1973, John Wiley & Sons, Inc.

Cerottini, J.-C., and Brunner, K. T.: Cell-mediated cytotoxicity, allograft rejection, and tumor immunity, Adv. Immunol. **18**:67, 1974.

Congdon, C. C.: Bone marrow transplantation, Science **171**:1161, 1971.

Feldman, J. D.: Immunological enhancement: a study of blocking antibodies, Adv. Immunol. **15**:167, 1972.

Fortner, J. G., and Shiu, M. H.: Organ transplantation and cancer, Surg. Clin. North Am. **54**:871, 1974.

Gold, P.: Antigenic reversion in human cancer, Annu. Rev. Med. **22**:85, 1971.

Hellström, K. E., and Hellström, I.: Lymphocyte-mediated cytotoxicity and blocking serum activity to tumor antigens, Adv. Immunol. **18**:209, 1974.

Klein, G.: Tumor immunology, Clin. Immunobiol. **1**:219, 1972.

Lance, E. M., Medawar, P. B., and Taub, R. N.: Antilymphocyte serum, Adv. Immunol. **17**:1, 1973.

McKhann, C. F., and Jagarlamoody, S. M.: Evidence for immune reactivity against neoplasms, Transplant. Rev. **7**:57, 1971.

Monaco, A. P.: Progress in clinical organ transplantation, Surg. Annu. **3**:97, 1971.

Najarian, J. S., and Simmons, R. L., eds.: Transplantation, Philadelphia, 1972, Lea & Febiger.

Starzl, T. E., and Putnam, C. W.: Transplantation immunology, Clin. Immunobiol. **1**:76, 1972.

chapter 12

Immunodeficiency and immunoproliferation

Good health is the expression of the body's natural and acquired defense forces to cope with internal and external antigenic threats to it's well-being. Just as cuts and scratches of the skin can create a breach in the natural defense system and open the body to infection, so also can fissures in other parts of the defense system—in phagocytosis, in immunoglobulin synthesis, in T cell activities, and in the complement system—render the body susceptible to otherwise easily repelled organisms. Immunodeficiencies may arise from a genetic inability to produce a required cell or cell product, or they may be acquired, in which case the true etiology of the condition rarely becomes known. Excessive proliferation of one kind of immunocompetent cell may likewise result in an increased susceptibility to disease, presumably by crowding out other required cells and creating an imbalance in the defense system.

In the following discussion, immunodeficiencies related to B lymphocytes, T lymphocytes, the phagocytic cell system, and the complement system will be considered separately, and in the case of the B and T cells as combined immunodeficiency (Table 12-1). This is not meant to minimize the interaction of these cell systems, which is necessary for a complete immune response. The participation of a healthy phagocytic system and T cell population for the perfect functioning of B cells, at least to certain antigens, is well recognized and was discussed in Chapter 2.

IMMUNODEFICIENCIES INVOLVING LYMPHOCYTES

Immunodeficiencies involving B lymphocytes

The critical product of the B lymphocyte is ultimately immunoglobulin, even though the immunoglobulins arise directly from plasma cells and only indirectly (or rarely) from B lymphocytes. Any break in the differential pathway leading from the stem cells of the bone marrow to mature functioning plasma cells will depress or totally prevent immunoglobulin synthesis. Points of interruption in the sequence presented in Fig. 12-1 are stated for each immunoglobulin deficiency.

Although the term "agammaglobulinemia" is well entrenched in the immunologic literature, traces of gamma globulin, perhaps only 5 to 500 μg/ml, can be found in sera of agammaglobulinemic patients. Thus hypogammaglobulinemia is a more exact term, but the two will be used interchangeably here.

Transient neonatal agammaglobulinemia. Transient hypogammaglobulinemia of the newborn infant is the summation of the infant's inability to synthesize significant amounts of immunoglobulin until it has been challenged with antigen and the inability of IgA and IgM to pass the placental barrier from mother to fetus. The total amount of gamma globulin in the serum of the newborn infant is 1044 ± 201 mg/100 ml or approximately two thirds of the normal adult level of 1457 ± 353 mg/

Table 12-1. Classification of immunodeficiencies

Condition	*Characteristics*
B lymphocyte deficiencies	
Transient neonatal agammaglobulinemia	Does not involve IgG
Congenital agammaglobulinemia	
Bruton type	Sex linked, involves all immunoglobulin classes
Dysgammaglobulinemia	Involves one or more immunoglobulin classes
Acquired immunoglobulin deficiency	Often associated with reticuloendothelial system malignancy
T lymphocyte deficiencies	
Nezelof's syndrome	True congenital failure in thymic embryogenesis
Acquired T cell defects	
DiGeorge's syndrome	Nongenetic failure in thymic embryogenesis
Episodic lymphopenia	Due to lymphocytotoxin, an antibody against T cells
Partial T cell loss	Leprosy, chronic mucocutaneous candidiasis, other infections
Combined B and T lymphocyte deficiencies	
Sex-linked agammaglobulinemia	Not Bruton type!
Swiss-type agammaglobulinemia	Not sex linked
Wiskott-Aldrich syndrome	Depressed IgM
Ataxia-telangiectasia	Lowered IgA and IgE
Phagocytic system deficiencies	
Chronic granulomatous disease	Failure to form singlet oxygen
Job's syndrome	Etiology uncertain
Glucose-6-phosphate dehydrogenase deficiency	Failure of phagocyte to oxidize
Myeloperoxidase deficiency	Failure to utilize H_2O_2
Chédiak-Higashi disease	Abnormal lysosomes
Complement system deficiencies	
C1 deficiency	C1q, C1r, and C1s forms noted
C2 deficiency	More common
C3 deficiency	Few examples
C5, 6, and 7 deficiencies	Few examples of each
$C\bar{1}$ INH deficiency	Well known, associated with hereditary angioneurotic edema

100 ml (Fig. 12-2). Since maternal IgG can pass the placenta, the IgG level in newborn sera (1031 ± 200 mg/100 ml of serum) compares favorably with the adult level of 1158 ± 305 mg/100 ml. Neonatal levels of IgM and IgA average 11% and 1%, repectively, of the adult levels of 99 ± 27 mg/100 ml and 200 ± 61 mg/100 ml. IgD is difficult to detect in the sera of newborn infants, and IgE is found at approximately 15% of the adult level of 225 μg/ml.

After birth the infant's IgG level falls steadily for approximately 3 months. Between 3 and 6 months of age, when IgG is at its low ebb (300 to 600 mg/100 ml), the infant displays its greatest sensitivity to infectious disease. After the third month of life the IgG level increases steadily so that about 75% of the adult level is achieved by 3 years of age. IgM is synthesized earlier in infancy than IgG and increases in concentration so rapidly after birth that 50% of the adult level is reached within the first 6 months, whereas IgA does not achieve 50% of the adult level until the child is 1 year of age. At 5 years of age the IgD levels are still one-third that of adults, and IgE reaches approximately two-thirds that of the adult level.

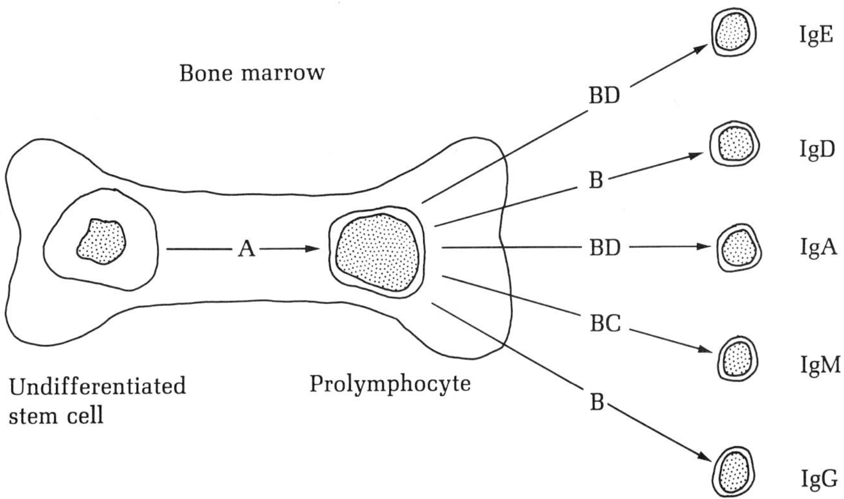

Fig. 12-1. Schematic representation indicating origin of immunoglobulins from bone marrow. Intermediate stages include prolymphocyte, B lymphocyte, and plasma cell. Prolymphocyte is probably source of T lymphocytes as well.

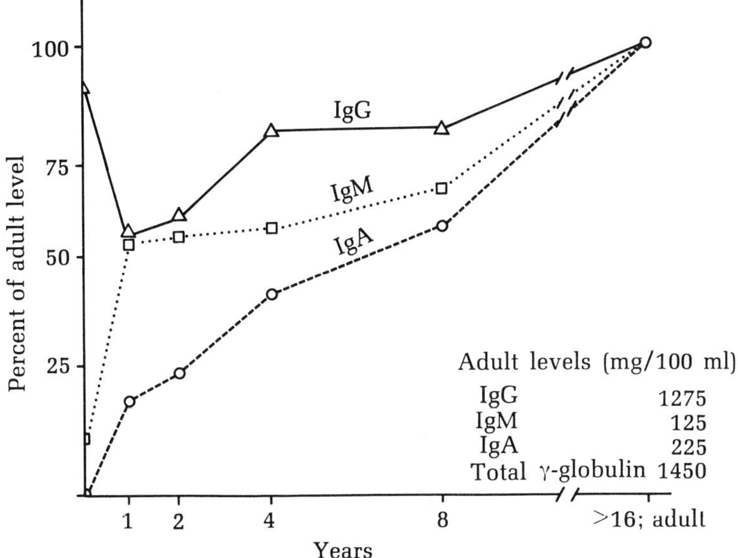

Fig. 12-2. At birth, the human infant has 80% to 90% of the adult level of IgG but is deficient in other immunoglobulins.

Congenital agammaglobulinemia. Congenital or genetic hypogammaglobulinemia results from a permanent inability to synthesize gamma globulins. The afflicted children suffer from repeated bouts of infectious disease, often caused by feeble pathogens. If no accompanying penalty of the T cell system is involved, hypogammaglobulinemic children will contract and recover normally from the usual viral and fungal diseases of childhood. In the preantibiotic era these children died of bacterial septicemia before it could be recognized that they were hypogammaglobulinemic. In the 1950s the development and use of broad-spectrum antibiotics kept these children alive long enough for their congenital condition to be diagnosed. Now antibiotics and passive immunization with pooled human gamma globulin allow these individuals to lead a relatively normal life.

Bruton-type agammaglobulinemia. A World Health Organization committee has recommended that infantile sex-linked agammaglobulinemia be used as the official name of the disease commonly known as Bruton's agammaglobulinemia or Bruton's sex-linked agammaglobulinemia. As the new name indicates, this is a disease transmitted by the mother only to her male children. The disease does not become apparent until about 6 months of age, at which time the immunity the child derived from maternal IgG has waned. These young boys then begin what will invariably develop into a series of bacterial infections involving the usual pathogens of childhood, *Hemophilus, Streptococcus, Staphylococcus, Pseudomonas,* and other less pathogenic gram-negative bacilli. These primary bacterial infections do not result in immunity and the synthesis of immunoglobulins; instead, they signal the fact that recurrences of otitis media, conjunctivitis, pneumonia, meningitis, pyoderma, and septicemia will follow. The gamma globulin concentration of these children may fall below 25 mg/100 ml of serum. All classes of immunoglobulins are absent or extremely low. Lymphocyte counts in peripheral blood are within the normal range, but these are T cells not B cells.

These children respond normally to most viral diseases of childhood (measles, mumps, chickenpox, etc.) and they develop a lasting immunity. Their response to chemicals that provoke contact dermatitis is normal, also indicating that their T cell system is functioning suitably. Even after intensive stimulation with antigens, plasma cells are rarely found in lymphoid tissues. All the evidence suggests that infantile sex-linked agammaglobulinemia is a total incapacity to synthesize immunoglobulins concurrent with a normal T cell responsiveness. Since all the immunoglobulin classes are involved in the deficiency, the cellular fault lies early, possibly at the point labeled *A* in Fig. 12-1, in the pathway to mature B lymphocytes.

Dysgammaglobulinemia. Far more common than generalized hypogammaglobulinemia is selective or variable hypogammaglobulinemia, in which only one or a combination of immunoglobulins is missing or present in a much lower than normal concentration. This condition is also known as dysgammaglobulinemia. Individuals with selective hypogammaglobulinemia cannot always be identified by a decrease in total gamma globulin levels, since a decrease in one class of immunoglobulin may be compensated by a disproportionate hypergammaglobulinemia of another class of immunoglobulin. For example, several patients deficient in IgG and IgA have been described but they had sufficiently increased IgM to have a normal gamma globulin level. Diagnosis of selective immunoglobulinemia is best made by quantitative radial immunodiffusion analyses for the separate immunoglobulin classes, although a first clue to the diagnosis is often an abnormal immunoelectrophoretic serum profile. An increased incidence of infectious diseases is an unreliable diagnostic criterion, since single deficiencies, except where IgG is the deficient immunoglobulin, do not always lead to an increased incidence of infectious disease. Patients with dysgammaglobulinemia often display a malabsorption syndrome with a noninfectious diarrhea of variable severity. When IgG is involved, it is usually low, often below 500 mg/100 ml but not as low as in sex-linked agammaglobulinemia. IgG levels over 250 mg/100 ml are usually adequate for protection against most bacterial infections.

Virtually all mathematically possible forms of dysgammaglobulinemia have been detected, that is, those in which only one of the immunoglobulins is missing, all the possible combinations where two are missing, where three are missing, etc. Of the selective hypogammaglobulinemias the most frequently recognized is that involving a familial loss of IgA. The incidence of single IgA dysgammaglobulinemia has been estimated at 1 in 500 to 1 in 3500 persons. Both serum and secretory IgA are diminished or absent, although secretory piece is produced. There is frequently a corresponding increase in IgM. Patients with an isolated IgA loss commonly seek medical assistance because of an associated autoimmune disease. Diseases involved here include rheumatoid arthritis, lupus erythematosus, and thyroiditis. IgA losses are also associated with sinopulmonary disease, a feature of the deficiency that indicates that secretory IgA is important in protecting mucous membranes. A noninfectious diarrhea is also a common feature of IgA deficiency. The locus of dysgammaglobulinemic defects is indicated in Fig. 12-1 at the several points labeled *B*.

Acquired immunoglobulin deficiency. Immunoglobulin deficiency associated with malignancies of the reticuloendothelial system—thymoma, chronic lymphocytic leukemia, lymphoma, and lymphosarcoma—probably result from a combined loss of a lymphoid cell's capacity to synthesize a gamma globulin and its conversion to a neoplastic state. These conditions develop during the person's lifetime and are not genetic, at least in terms of the immunoglobulin loss. Multiple myeloma is the best known example of a neoplastic malignancy in which a hypogammaglobulinemia of one class of globulin develops. These diseases will be discussed further in the section on immunoproliferative disease in this chapter.

Immunodeficiencies involving T lymphocytes

The contemporary interest in the T lymphocyte and its contribution to immunity is best delineated by those human illnesses associated with a loss only of the T lymphocyte. Until recently it was believed there were only two such examples—Nezelof's and DiGeorge's syndrome. More recently a series of acquired T cell defects has been encountered, including leprosy, sarcoid disease, and others that lack the proliferative aspects of Hodgkin's disease and the leukemias. A synthesis of the results from all of these conditions has contributed much to our understanding of the biologic role of the T lymphocytes.

Nezelof's syndrome. Infants with Nezelof's syndrome are athymic by virtue of an autosomal recessive trait whose inheritance prevents normal lymphoid development of the gland. Since the connective tissue of the gland is reasonably intact, the defect does not reside in embryogenesis of the thymus gland per se from the third and fourth pharyngeal pouches but in its fulfillment as a lymphoid organ. Consequently, the block in cellular development resides in or near the stem cell level and its inability to generate the lymphocytes destined to become T cells (Fig. 12-1). Children with Nezelof's syndrome generate typical germinal centers in the far cortical or B cell regions of their lymph nodes, produce plasma cells, and have a reasonably normal immunoglobulin response. However, the lymphoid development of the paracortical and medullary regions of lymph nodes, the T cell regions, is markedly restricted. This is demonstrated early in infancy by the development of infectious diseases that are resisted primarily by a suitable T cell activity—*Candida albicans* infections and those by other yeasts or fungi and severe, even fatal, chickenpox or a fatal outcome from smallpox vaccination. Respiratory disease due to the feebly pathogenic *Pneumocystis carinii* and to bacteria is also prominent. A high incidence of malignancy is also noted in these unfortunate children.

Acquired T cell defects. Although Nezelof's syndrome is the sole example of an isolated T cell defect with a direct genetic origin, several forms of acquired T cell defects are known. One of these, the DiGeorge syndrome, in some ways mimics Nezelof's disease. Both are detectable in the very young infant; both are the result of aplasia of the lymphoid elements of the thymus and the effects that this has on the secondary lymphoid tissues. Infants with either disease respond normally to immunization with toxoids or killed bacterial vaccines and yet fail to resist viruses and fungi.

DiGeorge's syndrome. DiGeorge's syndrome is the result of an accidental failure in embryogenesis of the third and fourth branchial pouches and is not a familial, inherited disease like Nezelof's syndrome. In the DiGeorge form of congenital thymic hypoplasia, abnormalities of the aortic arch, the mandible, the ear, and the parathyroid may accompany those of the thymus gland, since all of these tissues have a common embryonic origin. Of these accessory deficits that of the parathyroid gland is the most important from a diagnostic viewpoint. The parathyroid gland is the regulatory organ for blood calcium. During fetal life the level of this mineral in fetal blood is regulated in part by the maternal parathyroid hormone. After birth, when this is no longer possible, the infant progresses toward a condition of hypocalcemia that is soon expressed as an involuntary rigid muscular contraction (tetany). Restoration of the blood calcium level by calcium or parathyroid hormone relieves this condition but, of course, can do nothing to restore thymic functioning. DiGeorge's syndrome is not a genetic disease, but its etiology is unknown. It may arise from an intrauterine infection. Presumably this infection would occur before the fourteenth week of gestation when the development of the involved tissues ordinarily begins.

Episodic lymphopenia. A third condition that involves only the T cell system is episodic lymphopenia with lymphocytotoxin. This toxin is actually an antibody directed against lymphocytes, so this could be classified as an autoimmune disease. Destruction of T lymphocytes by the antibody is complement dependent. Only a few instances of this disease are known, but they share common chromosome abnormalities and have a familial distribution.

Partial T cell loss. There exist several conditions that involve only a partial T cell loss.

Sarcoidosis is a granulomatous disease that involves the lung, liver, spleen, and other deep-seated organs plus the superficially situated peripheral lymph nodes. Histologically, the granulomas are difficult to distinguish from the granulomas caused by the tubercle bacillus. Each contains many mononuclear cells and giant cells, but the tuberculoid granuloma has a tendency toward central, caseous necrosis. Although sarcoidosis, sometimes known as Boeck's sarcoid, might be confused histologically with tuberculosis, the sarcoid patient does not usually display a delayed-type hypersensitivity skin reaction to tuberculin. Bacille Calmette Guérin (BCG) vaccination generally fails to convert the sarcoid patient to a tuberculin-positive status. Passive acquisition of tuberculin sensitivity by sarcoid patients is possible, but this is not expressed systemically—only near the site where the sensitized lymphocytes were injected. Only 50% to 60% of sarcoid patients display a dermal sensitivity to yeast and fungal allergens that evoke positive reactions in a much larger percentage of normal adults. These findings plus the knowledge that chemical sensitizers of the contact type such as a halogenated nitrobenzene are inert in sarcoid patients indicates that the sarcoid patient has an impaired T cell responsiveness. This is further demonstrated by in vitro experiments that reveal the general inactivity of T cells from the sarcoid patient to stimulation by a variety of antigens. The etiology of sarcoid disease is still a mystery. Its diagnosis is aided by the Kveim reaction, a skin reaction of the granulomatous type in response to an intradermal injection of tissue from a sarcoid donor.

Unlike sarcoidosis the etiology of leprosy is clearly established as due to *Mycobacterium leprae*. Leprosy divides itself into two easily recognized clinical forms, lepromatous and tuberculoid leprosy. In the former the disease is progressive; the bacterial population is high and increases steadily with an associated increase in the necrotic destruction of tissue, and when untreated, it offers a bleak prognosis. On the other hand, tuberculoid leprosy has a better prognosis; there is less tissue destruction and a lower bacillary load. Diagnostic skin testing of lepers with lepromin, an extract of human tissue containing *M. leprae,* has revealed that those with the tuberculoid form of the disease give the typical delayed type of skin reaction, whereas those with lepromatous leprosy are more often than not unreactive to lepromin. Since bacteriologic and histologic evidence can confirm that both types of patients have leprosy, the unresponsiveness of those with the lepromatous type of disease demands an explanation.

The explanation, although not the mechanism for this situation, has recently been revealed. Patients with lepromatous leprosy have depleted paracortical and medullary regions in their lymph nodes; their lymphocytes are unresponsive to mitogens such as phytohemagglutinin or *M. leprae* antigens in vitro and fail to produce lymphokines in culture. A recent study has revealed that the T cell population in the peripheral circulation of persons with lepromatous leprosy (but not those with tuberculoid leprosy) is depressed. The degree of this T cell loss is directly correlated with the bacillary load. It is tempting to conclude that the bacteria or products of the leprosy bacillus specifically destroy the T cells that might protect the patient against the disease. Considerably more experimentation is needed before such a sweeping suggestion can be confirmed. It is interesting that patients with lepromatous leprosy have about twice the B cell population of those with tuberculoid disease, but since immunoglobulins contribute so little to protection and recovery from leprosy, this is of little benefit to them.

One of the first infectious diseases recognized to have an attendant defect in the T cell system was chronic mucocutaneous candidiasis. The etiologic agent of this disease, a yeast, is a relatively feeble pathogen and is a common part of the normal flora of the female birth canal. As a consequence, neonates not infrequently develop mild infections with this yeast. Candidiasis, also known as moniliasis, can also present itself as an extensive and severe disease in those persons with a thymus defect. Recurrent serious infections with *Candida albicans* have been noted in patients with DiGeorge's or Nezelof's syndrome and in patients with thymoma. Patients with chronic mucocutaneous candidiasis exhibit extensive destruction of the nail beds and persistent infections of the mucous membranes and the skin. The normal features of the skin may be almost totally obliterated by the serous exudate, crust, and granuloma formation of the affected regions. Patients with this disease do not respond to dermal injections of

Candida, and in vitro tests of lymphocytes from these patients reveal their inability to produce lymphokines. The cellular defect is probably not identical in all of these patients—some may have a generalized T cell defect and others a specific *Candida* defect.

Coccidioidomycosis and generalized vaccinia are two other instances where T cell defects may result in serious infectious disease, and it is almost certain that more examples will be recognized as our understanding of T cells increases.

Combined immunodeficiency disease

Combined immunodeficiency diseases are those in which there is a decided loss in both B and T lymphocyte functions. As a consequence of this superimposed loss of humoral and cellular immunity, survival beyond infancy, until recently, was rare. Persons with combined immunodeficiency disease have an extraordinarily high incidence of infectious disease and malignancy and an abbreviated life expectancy.

Sex-linked agammaglobulinemia. Sex-linked agammaglobulinemia, in which there is a defect in cellular immune mechanisms associated with the agammaglobulinemia, must not be confused with infantile sex-linked agammaglobulinemia of the Bruton type in which no generalized loss of cellular immunity has ever been noted. In sex-linked agammaglobulinemia there is considerable variation in the immunoglobulin class that is deficient, and not all classes (as in Bruton's disease) may be involved. Likewise, the extent of the immunoglobulin loss may not be as severe as in Bruton's disease. Points *A* or *B* of Fig. 12-1 may be affected plus T cell development. Losses in cellular immunity may not be absolute, but the thymus is small, weighing only about 1 gm as compared to an expected weight of 4 gm for the normal infant. The combination of B cell and T cell losses results in a life expectancy of only 2 years. The condition is seen only in male children and is inherited as a recessive characteristic.

Swiss-type agammaglobulinemia. A second disease embodying losses in both cellular and humoral immunity is Swiss-type agammaglobulinemia. Several dozen cases have been described since the original description of this disease in 1950 by Glanzmann and Riniker, two Swiss pediatricians. The afflicted children, either male or female since this disease is transmitted as an autosomal recessive disease, are vulnerable to severe diarrheas and severe pyogenic infections caused by the usual bacterial pathogens of childhood. More reflective of their severe immunologic handicap is the inability of these children to resist even feeble pathogens such as *Escherichia coli, Pseudomonas aeruginosa,* and *Pneumocystis carinii.* Childhood viral and fungal diseases—measles, chickenpox, smallpox vaccination, and *Candida* infections—can all be fatal or contribute to fatality.

Autopsied tissues do not reveal plasma cells or germinal centers, and little if any immunoglobulin is present in the blood. This is characteristic of a blockade at point *A* in Fig. 12-1. The thymus exists as an epithelial structure without lymphoid elements. This is the key to the inability of these patients to resist viral or fungal pathogens or to respond to other stimuli for T cells such as the contact sensitizers dinitrochlorobenzene or dinitrofluorobenzene.

Wiskott-Aldrich syndrome. The Wiskott-Aldrich syndrome is a sex-linked recessive disease whose victims suffer innumerable bacterial, viral, fungal, and protozoan infections as a result of their failure to generate a typical immunoglobulin or T cell response. In terms of the immunoglobulin aspect of their disease it has been noted that the total immunoglobulin level may be normal. This is due to an elevated IgA and depressed IgM level in the presence of essentially normal or elevated levels of IgG. The restriction of the immunoglobulin loss to IgM suggests that the B cell deficit is related primarily to polysaccharide antigens. The true locus of the defect may not be in the lymphocyte cell system at all but in the macrophages that process the polysaccharide antigens for the B cells. (The specific site *C* is indicated in Fig. 12-1.) Further studies are needed to confirm the site of the metabolic error, but it is well known that patients with Wiskott-Aldrich syndrome respond poorly to *Salmonella* vaccines and have only low levels of hemagglutinins for red blood cells, both of which depend on polysaccharide antigens. The location of the defect in the T cell system is also obscure. The thymus itself is relatively normal; only peripheral lymphoid organs demonstrate losses in T cells. This appears to be a progressive condition associated with thrombocytopenia and eczema.

Ataxia-telangiectasia. Ataxia-telangiectasia, the term for the disease in which a progressive loss in muscle coordination is associated with small blood vessel dilation most obvious in the conjunctivae, is also an important disease because of its combined cellular deficiency and lowered IgA and IgE levels. Although the depressed IgE may have little to do with the immune status of these persons, the loss of IgA (in the presence of normal or increased total immunoglobulin level) has been associated with a heightened incidence of sinopulmonary disease. Abnormalities in the cell-mediated arm of the immune response include an abnormal thymus, lymphopenia, and failure to display or develop the expected delayed dermal hypersensitivities. It is believed that the disease is inherited as an autosomal recessive characteristic. The developmental block would occur at the positions in Fig. 12-1 marked *D*.

DEFICIENCIES IN THE PHAGOCYTIC SYSTEM

Chronic granulomatous disease

Chronic granulomatous disease (CGD) is a sex-linked recessive disease of male infants that is usually recognized within the first few months of birth. A second, less severe form of the disease is found in females and is probably transmitted as an autosomal recessive trait. Immunologic examination of infants with CGD has confirmed that they have a normal or even elevated immunoglobulin level, that they respond normally to vaccines, and that they have normal B and T lymphocyte functions and complement levels. Nevertheless, victims of CGD develop a series of infections early in infancy due to bacterial pathogens such as *Klebsiella* species, *Proteus vulgaris, Staphylococcus epidermidis, Escherichia coli, Aerobacter aerogenes, Serratia marcescens,* and the more virulent *Staphylococcus aureus.* Feebly virulent yeasts and fungi such as *Candida albicans* and *Aspergillus* may also be involved in infections of far more serious proportions in these children than in the usual child. Suprisingly the pathogenic bacteria that cause the most serious diseases of childhood—*Neisseria meningitidis, Hemophilus influenzae, Streptococcus pyogenes,* and *Streptococcus (Diplococcus) pneumoniae*—are combatted effectively.

As a result of these repeated infections, CGD patients typically have elevated immunoglobulin levels. A leukocytosis and granulomatous lymphadenitis are also hallmarks of the disease. Tissue biopsies will reveal granuloma formation in virtually every organ. Granulomas typically include tissue macrophages in various stages of digestion of bacterial cells, giant cells containing several nuclei, monocytes, and epithelioid cells. All parameters in the immune defense system function normally in these patients except for their intraphagocytic destruction of certain bacteria (Fig. 12-3). Even the phagocytic cells of patients with CGD have normal chemotactic responses and are as active in engulfment as other phagocytes. Neutrophils of CGD patients kill engulfed bacteria at a reduced rate, and the recovery of 50% to 100% of ingested bacteria at a time when only 1% to 10% of bacteria can be recovered from normal leukocytes is typical (Fig. 12-4).

The biochemical lesion in neutrophils of

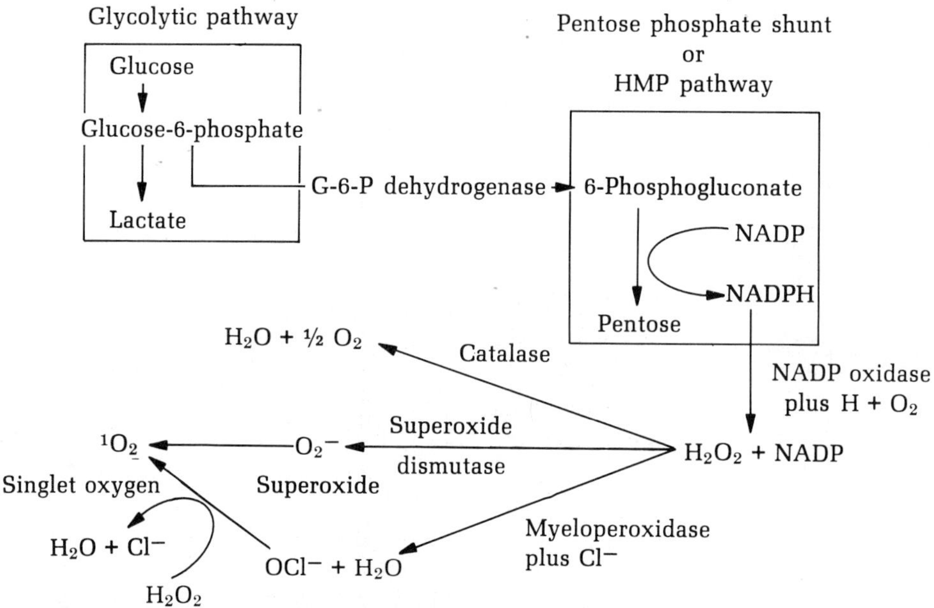

Fig. 12-3. Diagram indicating the many steps necessary to reach singlet oxygen. Failure at any level will result in phagocytic deficiency.

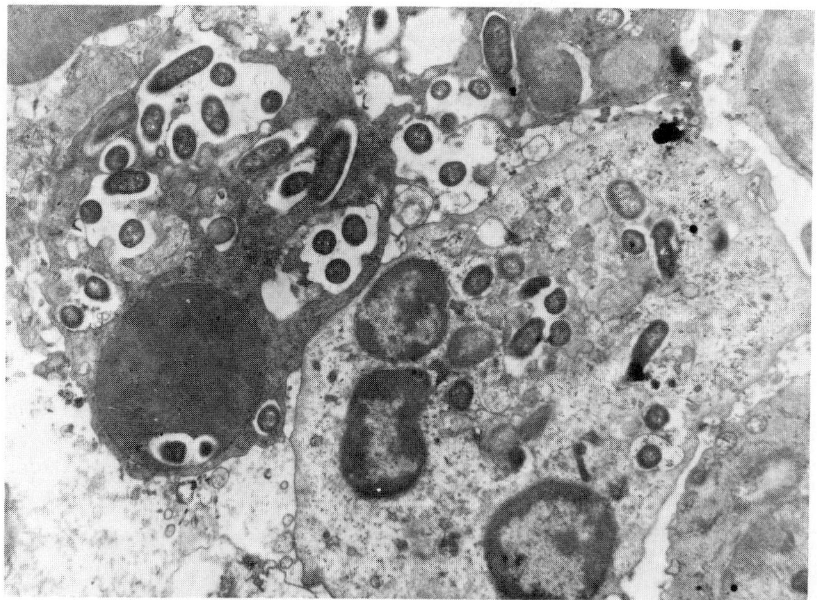

Fig. 12-4. Granulocytes from young boy with chronic granulomatous disease are literally filled with bacteria, but bacteria are not in process of dissolution. In fact, bacterium superimposed over nucleus of left phagocyte seems to be dividing.

CGD patients has been identified as a failure to accumulate H_2O_2 during phagocytosis. Prior to phagocytosis these cells utilize anaerobic glycolysis as their source of energy. During and after phagocytosis these cells demonstrate a burst in respiratory activity as they shift to the hexose monophosphate (HMP) shunt as their energy source. Utilization of the HMP pathway typically results in the formation of H_2O_2 as hydrogen is transferred by the nicotinamide adenine dinucleotide phosphate (NADP) system to oxygen.

The resultant hydrogen peroxide appears to function in cooperation with lysosomal myeloperoxidase to iodinate and kill intracellular bacteria. This may be mediated by singlet oxygen derived from the hydrogen peroxide (Fig. 12-3). Neutrophils of CGD patients do not make the shift to aerobic metabolism and hence fail to accumulate H_2O_2 and to kill intracellular bacteria. The role of H_2O_2 is clearly related to the type of pathogen that causes the most trouble for the CGD patient. Organisms such as *Hemophilus, Neisseria,* and *Streptococcus* produce H_2O_2 but lack a catalase that can destroy it. Consequently, these bacteria develop a microenvironment just like that created in normal phagocytes, and this is suicidal. The feebler pathogens that are so often involved in CGD infections have a high level of catalase, an enzyme that converts H_2O_2 to water and oxygen. Neutrophils of the CGD patient simply do not produce enough H_2O_2 to overcome the bacterial catalase. Bacteria-causing infections in CGD patients are typically those that do produce catalase, whereas bacteria that lack catalase but produce their own H_2O_2 are resisted by these patients.

The metabolic shift of normal phagocytes to oxidative metabolism can be determined easily by the nitroblue tetrazolium (NBT) reductase test. In this test neutrophils in the act of phagocytosing latex spherules are incubated in a solution of NBT dye that serves as a hydrogen acceptor instead of oxygen as oxidative metabolism ensues. This reduces the dye to its insoluble formazan, which is seen as distinct blue intracytoplasmic granules. Leukocytes of the CGD patient are not engaged in active oxidative metabolism and thus cannot reduce NBT. Female carriers of CGD have approximately a 50% loss in their ability to reduce NBT.

Job's syndrome

A specific phagocytic defect that permits *Staphylococcus aureus* to produce abscesses of the skin and subcutaneous tissue in the absence of any significant inflammatory response is known as Job's syndrome. Phagocytes from these individuals are normally active in endocytosis but are unable to kill the staphylococci, and the NBT test is negative. The location of the cellular defect has yet to be determined.

Glucose-6-phosphate dehydrogenase deficiency

An inability of neutrophils to destroy engulfed bacteria has also been associated with a deficiency in the enzyme glucose-6-phosphate dehydrogenase (G-6-PD) (Fig. 12-3). This enzyme must be considered as the first in the hexose monophosphate shunt, where it diverts G-6-PD from the glycolytic pathway. Accordingly, individuals who are devoid of this enzyme have a penalized ability to generate H_2O_2; in fact, it is estimated that their phagocytes produce only 25% of the normal level of hydrogen peroxide. *Staphylococcus, Escherichia,* and *Serratia* survive inside these phagocytes, but H_2O_2-producing microbes do not.

Myeloperoxidase deficiency

Benzidine staining of granulocytes for myeloperoxidase activity has exposed a deficiency of this enzyme in certain patients with severe acute infections. During phagocytosis the shift of phagocytic metabolism to the oxygen-consuming pentose pathway occurs normally in these patients, which suggests that normal amounts of H_2O_2 are formed. Cell studies have revealed that little or no iodination of intracellular microbes occurs and that the killing rate is depressed. The similarity of myeloperoxidase deficiency to CGD is obvious; patients with the latter disease have myeloperoxidase but little H_2O_2, whereas patients with the former disease have H_2O_2 but no myeloperoxidase. Both are required for protection against many pyogenic bacteria (Fig. 12-3).

Chédiak-Higashi disease

Chédiak-Higashi disease (CHD) is characterized by a pigmentary dilution of the eyes and skin (oculocutaneous albinism), extreme sensitivity to light (photophobia), rapid involuntary eye movements (nystagmus), and frequent pyogenic infections. The primary cellular defect noticed in victims of CHD is the presence of abnormally large granules in all phagocytic cells. Due to the recurrent infections, these persons have fever, lymphadenopathy, and hepatosplenomegaly and a mean survival age of 6 years. In only 13 of 56 reported cases have the patients lived beyond 10 years of age.

The giant granules found in phagocytic cells of patients with CHD are found in the highly active phagocytic cells of the tissue and blood such as the tissue macrophages, alveolar macrophages and neutrophils, and other cells of the myeloid series. An analysis of host defenses in CHD patients has revealed that immunoglobulin synthesis, cell-mediated immunity, and phagocytic endocytosis are all normal. The central defect is an inability to form normal primary granules in cells of the granulocytic series. Primary granules are the typical lysosomal granules that contain β-glucuronidase, peroxidase, lysozyme, several hydrolases, etc. and can be compared to the secondary granules that contain alkaline phosphatase. Victims of CHD have enlarged pleomorphic granules in their granulocytes. Even though the phagocytic activity of these cells is normal, their bactericidal activity against *Staphylococcus aureus,* streptococci, pneumococci, and lesser pathogenic bacteria proved to be deficient. Retarded intraphagocyte killing is not the result of depressed H_2O_2 formation nor any associated iodination of engulfed bacteria, but it is related to an inability of cells to degranulate normally. In CHD there is also a generalized neutropenia and an impaired chemotactic response, both of which would favor bacterial pathogens.

DEFICIENCIES OF THE COMPLEMENT SYSTEM

A deficiency in the C1q molecule of the first component of complement has been detected in several patients with hypogammaglobulinemia. Some of these patients had a pure B cell and others a combined immunodeficiency disease. Since persons with only T cell deficits have nearly normal C1q levels, the loss of C1q must be related to B cell rather than T cell activities, if indeed it can be related to either B or T lymphocytes. The lowered levels of C1q in these patients may be related to hypercatabolism rather than depressed synthesis. A C1r deficiency has been described in at least three patients, and supplements of this component to the patients' sera completely restored the hemolytic capacity of the sera even though C1s was present at a level of only 50% of normal. These persons had the usual concentration of C1q. A single instance of C1s loss has also been recorded.

At least 24 instances of deficiency of C2 in humans have been discovered. Both the homozygous and heterozygous state have been described. Homozygotes have 0.5% to 4% of the expected C2, and heterozygotes have 30% to 60% of the normal values. The characteristic is transmitted as an autosomal recessive trait. The depressed hemolytic activity of the sera of these patients is restored by purified C2. The alternate pathway of complement activation is normal in these individuals. Immune adherence, which unlike hemolysis requires only traces of C2, can be demonstrated in these patients.

Three examples of C3 loss in humans have been detected in which the persons had approximately half the standard amount of C3. This suggests that the individuals were heterozygous. Other members of the same family also had depressed C3 levels. Further studies of this family may unravel the genetic basis of C3 defects.

Dysfunctional C5 has been discovered in at least two families. On immunochemical analysis they appear to have the normal level of C5, and yet hemolytic assays for C5 indicate its presence at about 10% in these sera; this biologically inactive molecule cross-reacts with the antibody to native C5.

C6 deficiency has been described in two individuals, as has C7 deficiency. Lack of C8 or 9 in humans has not yet been recognized.

Deficiencies of these molecules of the complement cascade are not always associated with an increased incidence of infectious disease, although this appears to be the situation with C5 dysfunction. Some patients with a C2 loss are also more susceptible to infectious diseases.

A genetic deficiency of the inhibitor of the first component of complement, $C\bar{1}$ inhibitor ($C\bar{1}$ INH), has a direct relationship with the disease hereditary angioneurotic edema. $C\bar{1}$ INH has been identified as an α_2-neuraminoglycoprotein found in the α_2-globulin fraction of the serum proteins at a level of 180 μg/ml. It is a relatively large protein (mol wt 90,000) with a high content of neuraminic acid (17%) and total carbohydrate (31%). $C\bar{1}$ INH is an inhibitor of a number of esteroproteases, including plasmin, Hageman factor, kininogenase, and $C\bar{1}$ esterase, by virtue of its stoichiometric combination with C1r. Two forms of $C\bar{1}$ INH deficiency exist: one in which a dysfunctional molecule identical serologically with $C\bar{1}$ INH exists in serum but does not neutralize $C\bar{1}$ and a second in which levels of about one-sixth the normal blood level of $C\bar{1}$ INH are obtained. Genetic analysis indicates the second form of the deficiency is transmitted as an autosomal dominant trait.

Patients with $C\bar{1}$ INH deficiency were described in 1963, and amply confirmed since, to suffer from hereditary angioneurotic edema. This is an episodic edematous condition that affects the tissues around the eyes, lips, and other tissue associated with the respiratory and digestive systems. The edema usually lasts no longer than 3 days. The primary mediator of the disease is apparently the C2-associated kinin, liberated by the activity of $C\bar{1}$ and C4 on C2. Whether this occurs as a result of an antigen-antibody activation of complement or is an effect of the coagulation (alternate) pathway on complement activation is uncertain. In any event normal levels of $C\bar{1}$ INH prevent activation of complement and hereditary angioneurotic edema. But when the already depressed $C\bar{1}$ INH levels of the deficient person are further exhausted, $C\bar{1}$ catalysis of C2 and formation of the C2 kinin occurs. The disease is preventable by ϵ-aminocaproic acid, which inhibits plasma proteases, or by the transfusion of $C\bar{1}$ INH present in normal blood into the victims.

IMMUNOLOGIC RECONSTITUTION

Restoration of a suitable immune status to persons with uncomplicated agammaglobulinemia presents no novel problems; it is only necessary to provide them passive immunity by periodic injections of pooled human gamma globulin (Table 12-2). Indeed, this has been practiced from the first recognition of these individuals, as Bruton's index case of a patient with sex-linked agammaglobulinemia, diagnosed as a young child and now a married man living an outwardly normal life, will attest.

Selective deficits in T cell responses are also subject to correction by a simple technical procedure (Fig. 3-10 and Table 12-2). Nonviable T cell extracts or transfer factor (TF) prepared from T cells of donors with a normal status of cell-mediated immunity can be injected into the T cell–deficient person to convert him to the immune condition of the donor. It is notable that this procedure is peculiar to man—T cell extracts of lower animals do not transfer cell-mediated immunity to others of the same species, although their concentrated RNA may. In human studies, T cell extracts are not injected in their crude form. The lymphocytes of a donor with good T cell responses are subjected to several freeze-thaw cycles. Cell fragments are removed by centrifugation, and high molecular weight molecules are trapped inside a dialysis membrane. The low molecular weight dialysate, the fraction originally described by Lawrence as TF, is used. Human TF is probably an antigen-specific low molecular weight oligonucleotide or peptide. Its mode of action in the recipient is unknown, but the recipient's lymphocytes are converted to a condition in which they will respond to foreign antigens in the typical way. This is generally determined externally by a skin test of the recipient with purified protein derivative (PPD), dermatophytin, coccidioidin, or some other preparation known to provoke a delayed skin reaction in the donor.

TF injections have been applied in the treatment of chronic mucocutaneous candidiasis, coccidioidomycosis, Swiss-type agammaglobulinemia, sex-linked agammaglobulinemia, ataxia-telangiectasia, Wiskott-Aldrich syndrome, sarcoidosis, vaccinia gangrenosa, leprosy, and several forms of cancer. The results have been quite encouraging. Of seven patients with mucocutaneous candidiasis, four showed definite improvement; of 11 patients with Wiskott-Aldrich syndrome, six responded with a change in skin test results, five no longer have the eczema, and four became free of infection; and some patients with coccidioidomycosis showed improvement after treatment with TF.

Successful reconstitution of the immune status with TF demands that the individual have a reasonably normal population of lymphocytes. TF merely triggers existing lymphocytes into activity; it does not generate lymphocytes. When these lymphocytes are not present or are present in extremely low numbers, TF injections can be

Table 12-2. Immunologic reconstitution of immunodeficiency diseases

Condition	*Method*
B lymphocyte deficiencies	
Transient agammaglobulinemia	None needed
Bruton-type agammaglobulinemia	Pooled human gamma globulin
Dysgammaglobulinemia	Pooled human gamma globulin if IgG missing
T lymphocyte deficiencies	
Nezelof's syndrome	Bone marrow or thymus grafts
DiGeorge's syndrome	Bone marrow or thymus grafts
Sarcoidosis, leprosy, chronic mucocutaneous candidiasis	Transfer factor
Combined B and T lymphocyte deficiencies	
Sex-linked agammaglobulinemia	Transfer factor plus pooled human gamma globulin or bone marrow and thymus depending on extent of T cell loss
Swiss-type agammaglobulinemia	
Wiskott-Aldrich syndrome	
Ataxia-telangiectasia	
Phagocytic system deficiencies	Granulocyte transfusions (temporary value only)
Complement and complement-inhibitor deficiencies	Human plasma

expected to fail. In these instances (Nezelof's and DiGeorge's syndrome and some cases of combined immune deficiency disease) transplantation of bone marrow or thymus may be required to provide the needed T lymphocytes. Bone marrow transplants would also provide the B lymphocytes, but this is usually not the primary purpose of bone marrow transplants, since B cell products (immunoglobulins) are readily available. Bone marrow transplantation suffers the innate hazard of creating graft-versus-host reactions, since immunoresponsive cells are being transferred to an immunodeficient host. This problem is not met when the transplantation is between identical twins or between a histocompatible donor and recipient.

Since DiGeorge's and Nezelof's syndrome are characterized by the loss of only the cell-mediated arm of the immune response, marrow grafts to supply B cells are unnecessary, and thymus grafting alone is sufficient. Fetal thymus that has not yet reached immunologic maturity is the preferred tissue and has successfully reconstituted patients with Nezelof's and DiGeorge's syndrome.

IMMUNOPROLIFERATIVE DISEASE

Just as immunodeficiencies may center on either the B or T lymphocyte–dependent portions of the immune response, so also may B or T cells serve as neoplastic cells that lead to an immunoproliferative disease. As in the section on immunodeficiency, immunoproliferative diseases involving B lymphocytes will be considered before T cell neoplasms are discussed.

Immunoproliferative diseases involving B lymphocytes

Multiple myeloma and Waldenström's macroglobulinemia. The simplest definition of multiple myeloma is that it is the result of the neoplastic growth of plasma cells and is thus a plasmacytoma (Table 12-3). This dyscrasia of plasma cells may encompass several histologic or anatomic forms, but multiple myeloma is usually expressed as a proliferation of plasma cells in bone marrow with a concomitant erosion of the surrounding bone. Bone destruction is observable on roentgenographic examination as discrete holes in the osseous tissue and can be so extensive as to cause the fracture of long bones under moderate weight stress. Bone marrow aspirates may reveal that 10% to 20% of the cells are plasma cells compared to about 3% or less in normal marrow. These plasma cells will differ slightly in morphology from one case to another but are often classified as one of two types. The most easily recognized is the classic pyroninophilic plasma cell with a spokelike arrangement of its nuclear chromatin. The

Table 12-3. Classification of immunoproliferative diseases as B or T cell disorders

Diseases	*Comment*
B cell disorders	
Multiple myeloma	IgG, IgA, IgD, or IgE mono- or polyclonal globulin; Bence Jones protein often present
Waldenström's macroglobulinemia	IgM; Bence Jones protein often present
Heavy chain disease	Gamma, mu, and alpha types recognized; chain incomplete
Amyloidosis	Some forms are light chain diseases
Chronic lymphocytic leukemia	Arrested B cell maturation
Acute lymphocyte leukemia	Some are T cell diseases
Burkitt's lymphoma	May be virus-altered B cells
T cell disorders	
Hodgkin's disease	Generalized T cell inadequacy
Sézary syndrome	T cell lymphoma

other cell will contain numerous acidophilic structures, disklike or globular in appearance, that are known as Russell's bodies. Russell's bodies are intracellular concretions of immunoglobulin. Since plasma cells normally produce the immunoglobulins and multiple myeloma is a malignant plasmacytoma, it is not unexpected that patients with multiple myeloma should have unusual concentrations of immunoglobulins and also quite often of light chains in their tissues, blood, and urine. Multiple myeloma is often diagnosed by recognizing these excessive gamma globulins in the blood or light chains, known as Bence Jones proteins, in urine.

Ordinary serum electrophoresis on paper or cellulose is very helpful in establishing the diagnosis of multiple myeloma, which characteristically produces a sharp, abnormal peak in the tracing of the gamma globulin portion of the serum profile (Fig. 12-5). This peak, which appears in about 75% of sera from myeloma patients, represents the excess immunoglobulin produced by the neoplastic cells. This supplementary protein is known as the myeloma (M) protein or M component. A single, sharp peak, which represents an electrophoretically homogeneous protein, indicates that a single clone of aberrant plasma cells has developed, and the protein is described as a monoclonal M component. Less frequent is the appearance of several new proteins representing an aberration in several clones of plasma cells. This situation is aptly termed "polyclonal gammopathy." In certain instances the electrophoretic positioning of the M component may suggest that the excess immunoglobulin is of the IgG, IgA, or other immunoglobulin class. Especially if the M component has a slow gamma mobility, myeloma of the IgG class can be anticipated. However, identification of the M protein class is best confirmed by the use of specific antisera for IgG, A, etc. in immunoelectrophoretic or radial immunodiffusion tests.

It should be noted that immunoproliferative disease involving IgM is generally described as Waldenström's macroglobulinemia. Waldenström's macroglobulinemia is distinguishable from multiple myeloma by the fact that the proliferative cell is more lymphocytic than plasmacytic in appearance, and the punched-out bone lesions are more rare than in multiple myeloma. Due to the hyperviscosity of blood in Waldenström's macroglobulinemia, vascular disease is more prominent than in the other myelomas. Of the myelomas, 60% are of the IgG class, 16% of the IgA class, and less

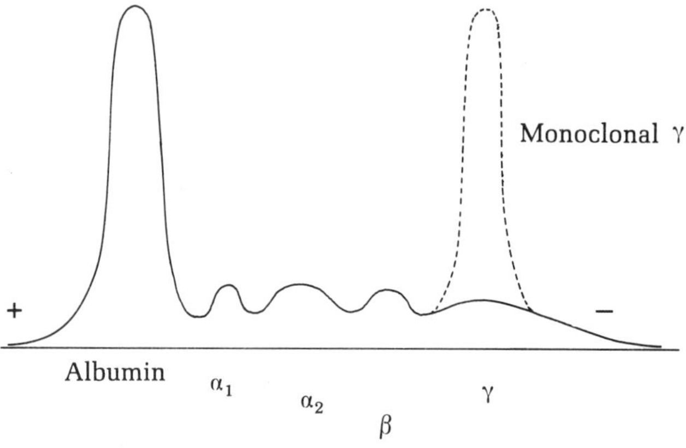

Fig. 12-5. Example of serum electrophoretic profile of patient with pronounced monoclonal gammopathy.

than 1% each of the IgD and IgE classes. Waldenström's macroglobulinemia represents about 14% of the total.

Although myeloma proteins were once considered paraproteins (structural but nonfunctional counterparts of normal proteins), it is now accepted that they are immunoglobulins with normal serologic activity. The original problem was simply to identify the antigen, a search that has now been completed for many human myeloma proteins. Ten IgG myeloma proteins have been recognized to neutralize streptolysin O; others have been identified that react with staphylolysin, transferrin, dinitrophenyl hapten, *Leptospira*, and *Brucella*. Serum albumin, human blood group antigens A_1 and I, cardiolipin, *Klebsiella*, and dinitrophenyl groups are among the antigens known to react with different IgM myeloma proteins. Fewer antigens have been identified to correspond with IgA myelomas because the IgA myelomas are more rare, but these include human blood group I and dinitrophenyl groups. In many instances the Fab fragment of the myeloma protein has been demonstrated to combine with the antigen. As yet no certain antigenic stimulus can account for the serologic activities of myeloma proteins, but the knowledge that they have serologic activity strengthens the clonal selection concept of antibody formation.

In addition to being characterized by large quantities of a circulating immunoglobulin, many patients with multiple myeloma or macroglobulinemia have in their blood or excrete in their urine a protein described as Bence Jones protein. Bence Jones proteins have a molecular weight of 20,000 to 22,000, although dimeric forms are also known. In about 10% of all myelomas the only aberrant protein detectable is the Bence Jones protein, and none of the complete immunoglobulins can be found. Serologic study of human Bence Jones proteins has revealed that they are identical to the light chains of the immunoglobulins; that is, some are κ-type and some are λ-type chains. When a patient has hyperimmunoglobulinemia with Bence Jones protein, the light chain of the gamma globulin is usually of the same type as the Bence Jones protein. This indicates that the neoplastic cell is synthesizing light chains faster than heavy chains and cannot complete the formation of the full immunoglobulin molecule under these conditions. The amino acid sequence and other structural aspects of human κ- and λ-chains was actually determined by study of purified Bence Jones proteins (Chapter 3).

Although patients with multiple myeloma or Waldenström's macroglobulinemia may be hypergammaglobulinemic, these diseases are genuine immunodeficiency diseases. A majority of these patients have low antistreptolysin titers and lower levels of antibodies to influenza, poliomyelitis, and measles virus than the general population. Their response to vaccines is subpar. They may have recurrent pneumonia or pyelonephritis. No special relationship to mycotic infections has been established.

Heavy chain disease. Heavy chain disease refers to any condition in which all or part of an immunoglobulin heavy chain is found in the serum and/or urine. It is rare to recover the entire heavy chain; usually structural rearrangements, internal deletions, and proteolysis significantly alter the heavy chain from the structure of the protein normally produced. Patients with heavy chain disease have a proliferative disease of cells (Table 12-3) that fail to synthesize the requisite amount of light chain to bind with the heavy chain, resulting in overproduction and excretion of the latter.

From its first description in 1968 until the middle of 1973, 59 patients have been described who had alpha chain disease. These patients generally display the clinical features of malabsorption syndrome, weight loss, diarrhea, steatorrhea, and abdominal pain. Other lymphoid tissues may be normal, but an infiltration of plasma cells into the lamina propria with accompanying medium-sized lymphocytes and reticulum cells is a typical cellular finding. Mesenteric nodes present a similar histologic pattern.

Diagnosis of alpha chain disease, the most common of the heavy chain diseases, is difficult since the needed tissues are seldom available for diagnosis until late in the study of the patient. Serum electrophoresis may not reveal more than a broadening of the β- and γ-globulin region and that in only 50% of the cases. Sharp monoclonal peaks of the α-chain are rarely seen.

The α-chain excreted by the aberrant plasma cells exists as a dimer of 3S to 4S, but larger polymeric forms are also known. The molecular weight of the protein varies from patient to patient and usually consists of the entire Fc and hinge region, amounting to one-half to three-fourths the size of the α-chain. A segment is missing in the Fd portion that includes the V_H and C_H1 regions. In addition, proteolysis at the amino terminal end shortens the protein from different individuals to different degrees. Cells making the faulty H chain do not make light chains, and the cells involved are disproportionately of the A1 subclass. As yet, not a single α-chain disease has been associated with the A2 subclass, whereas 41 have been identified as A1.

Gamma heavy chain disease has been described in over 30 patients who have a disease ordinarily labeled as a malignant lymphoma rather than multiple myeloma. The gradual onset of the disease ultimately causes lymphadenopathy, fever, malaise, hepatosplenomegaly, lymphocyte and plasma cell accumulation in bone marrow. Serum immunoelectrophoresis is often the key to the diagnosis and typically reveals a protein in the β- and γ-region that will not react with antiserum to light chains. The serum spike is broad and represents the formation of an aberrant protein whose molecular weight may vary from 45,000 to 55,000. Of 26 proteins listed, 20 were classified as γ_1, one as γ_2, four as γ_3, and one as γ_4. Some of the proteins were obviously deletion mutants in the hinge region or Fd portions alone or in combination. Some are of uncertain structure and so large as to suggest an origin from unusually large γ-chains.

Mu chain disease is more rarely observed than either alpha or gamma chain disease. A molecular weight of 55,000 for one isolate suggests it was an Fc rather than complete heavy chain disease.

Delta and epsilon chain variants of heavy chain diseases have not yet appeared in the immunologic literature.

Amyloidosis. A disease that may take several forms but is characterized by the deposition of a protein with a high content of carbohydrate (amyloid) in the tissues is called amyloidosis. The amyloid deposits appear hyaline in tissues because they are refractory to the usual stains, but special dyes will stain them. Electron microscopy has revealed that certain amyloid deposits have a fibrillar structure. Fluorescent antibody microscopy has identified gamma globulin in these deposits. Purification of amyloid protein from different patients indicates that they differ in molecular weight and in amino acid composition and sequence. Amyloid purified from two patients was found to consist of portions of κ-type light chains. The larger of these had a molecular weight of 18,500 and the smaller 7500. The suggestion that amyloidosis is the result of faulty synthesis or partial digestion of light chains has been made, but this does not exclude the possibility that other forms of amyloidosis may exist.

Leukemias. The leukemias are proliferative diseases in which a surplus of some type of white blood cell is seen in blood smears. Leukemias may involve cells of the granulocytic series or of the agranulocytic series such as the lymphocytes.

In chronic lymphocytic leukemia the predominant cell is a well-differentiated small lymphoid cell; this is not the case in acute lymphocytic leukemia, where the distinction between lymphocytic and other forms of leukemia is sometimes difficult. Patients with the chronic form of the disease have decreased gamma globulin levels and a depressed antibody response to routine vaccines. The vast majority of these patients can be described as having an arrested maturation of the B-type lymphocyte (Table 12-3), and these cells regularly exceed 70% of the circulating lymphocytes. It must be remembered that the normal B cell population of peripheral blood is approximately 15%. Immunoglobulin can be detected on the surface of these cells but is not being excreted into the blood, hence the tendency toward hypogammaglobulinemia in these patients. Analysis of the immunoglobulin class of the membrane-bound globulin has revealed that about half are pure IgM, a quarter are IgG, and many are mixed IgM and IgG with a rare case of IgA.

Immunoproliferative diseases involving T or B lymphocytes

In acute lymphocytic leukemia the affected cell may be either a B or T lymphocyte (Table 12-3). In an early French study only five of 35 cases were classifiable as T cell disorders, and a group of six patients studied in Norway all had B-type leukemias. Other Scandinavian studies have reported a separation of acute lymphocytic leukemia into B and T cell types.

Lymphomas. The lymphomas may be considered a neoplasm of any type of cell found in lymphoid tissue. Under this banner a leukemia can be considered a lymphoma, although traditionally the two are considered separately. The most outstanding example of lymphoma is Hodgkin's disease, although lymphocytic lymphoma (lymphosarcoma) and Burkitt's lymphoma are two other well-known examples.

In the examination of nine patients with lymphosarcoma, membrane-bound immunoglobulin on lymph node and peripheral blood cells was identified in eight instances. Of these, six were of the IgM class and two were IgG.

Human B cells have receptors for Epstein-Barr virus, which is the presumed etiologic agent of Burkitt's lymphoma. Burkitt cells are pyroninophilic, and established culture lines of these cells synthesize and excrete a monoclonal immunoglobulin.

Immunoproliferative diseases involving T lymphocytes

A T cell disturbance has been identified in each of three patients with Sézary syndrome, a form of lymphoma. The abnormally large lymphocytes that invade the skin in this disease were destroyed by antiserum to T-type lymphocytes. These cells were devoid of cell membrane–bound immunoglobulin.

Hodgkin's disease (Table 12-3) is a neoplastic lymphoma characterized by progressive granuloma formation and enlargement of lymphoid tissue. Multinucleate giant cells in lymphoid tissue with concurrent depletion of tissue lymphocytes and a developing lymphopenia are the cytologic hallmarks of Hodgkin's disease. Intensive studies of these patients with an extensive battery of immunologic tests has accumulated considerable evidence to support the contention that these patients are undergoing a progressive loss of T cell function. Patients who were previously positive to tuberculin or fungal allergens develop a gradual anergy and may remain tuberculin negative even after BCG vaccination. The induction of contact dermatitis with dinitrochlorobenzene, which is successful in 95% of all normal subjects, fails in most victims of Hodgkin's disease. Transplant rejection is slowed, and in vitro tests for T cell functions are negative or depressed; among these, the response to allogeneic cells and the production of lymphokines such as lymphotoxin and migration inhibition factor can be mentioned. Since patients with Hodgkin's disease respond typically to bacterial vaccines and toxoids, no deficit in B cell function is suspected, only in T cells. The mechanism and etiology of the disease is unknown. Recovery from the anergic state during chemotherapy is a good prognostic sign for recovery from the disease.

CLINICAL APPLICATION

The student who is sharply oriented toward medical practice may question the clinical relevance of some of the material presented in this chapter on the basis that the immunologic disorders discussed are exotic and unlikely to be encountered in general medical practice. To some extent this criticism is justified. After all, no more than a few hundred cases of agammaglobulinemia have been described. Except for the deficiency of $C\bar{1}$ INH, persons with a deficiency in any component of the complement system total less than 200. The risk of developing acute lymphocytic leukemia in the age group at highest risk (under 10 years of age) is only 1 in 2500. Deaths due to Hodgkin's disease probably do not exceed 4000 in the United States annually. Thus there is no refuting that the incidence of the immune deficiency and immune proliferative diseases is low. What, then, is the basis for the extensive discussion they have received?

There are several answers to this question. One, and probably the least satisfying to critics, is that the examination of persons with these semiesoteric diseases has definitely improved our knowledge of human physiology. Chronic granulomatous disease is a good example. Now, approximately 90 years after Metchnikoff's discovery that adequate phagocytosis of yeast cells in the water flea would protect it against disease, we are close to defining the mechanism of the bactericidal activity of phagocytic cells. With this information we can perhaps uncover the basis of other phagocytic defects, and once this is known the next discovery will inevitably be the cure.

A second answer is simply an exercise in mathematics. Statistics compiled from 1972 indicated that approximately 5% of physicians had a pediatric practice, 13.5% were internists, and 15.5% were in general practice. If it is assumed that a physician can examine 30 patients a day or conduct 10,000 examinations per year, then the low incidence of some of these diseases takes on another connotation, namely, that roughly 30% of all physicians have the chance to see approximately four patients with leukemia a year. The mortality rates in both immunoproliferative and immunodeficiency diseases is high. An understanding of all aspects of these diseases can go a long way toward sparing those lives. Almost certainly every pediatrician has at one time or another seen a child diagnosed as having "failure to thrive" syndrome or had patients who developed unexpected fatalities that might have had an immunodeficient undercurrent.

What should a physician do to evaluate the immunologic competence of a patient? Immunologic assessment must include a determination of the patient's previous immunologic status and his present responsiveness if at all possible. These determinations should include tests of humoral and cellular immunity in all cases and for phagocytic and complement activities if the clinical situation so indicates.

Tests for evaluating potential B or T cell immunodeficiency diseases

- Detection of preexisting B cell function
  - Total gamma globulin (for agammaglobulinemias)
  - Serum electrophoresis (for dysgammaglobulinemia)
  - History of successful immunization with toxoids or certain bacterial vaccines
  - Presence of antistreptolysin O or other common antibodies
- Detection of preexisting T cell function
  - History of natural course of viral infections
  - Positive delayed-type skin tests to OT or PPD, vaccinia virus, mumps, oidiomycin, histoplasmin, etc.
- Assay of current B cell status
  - Assay response to bacterial toxoid or bacterial vaccine by following antibody titers
- Assay of current T cell status
  - Determine T cell population by rosette or other tests
  - Assay delayed-type skin response to 0.1% or 0.05% dinitrochlorobenzene 2 weeks after sensitization with a 10% to 30% solution of the compound
  - Measure in vitro response of T cells to transformation by concanavalin A or other mitogens

Analysis for the A and B blood group isohemagglutinins in persons more than a few months of age is useful in evaluating the patient's past antibody-synthesizing ability. If an immunization record is available, this would also be helpful since it would permit an evaluation of the response to specific antigens. In the absence of such a record the level of immunoglobulins to widely prevalent antigens such as streptolysin O should be determined. An estimation of total serum immunoglobulins by immunoelectrophoresis may be followed by quantitative determinations of specific immunoglobulin classes if deemed necessary. Current immunoglobulin responsiveness is tested by measuring the antibody response to standard vaccines and toxoids. Only killed vaccines such as DPT or inactivated poliomyelitis vaccine are used!

A past history of T cell function can be estimated by dermal tests with PPD or OT, trichophytin, oidiomycin, and *Candida* or in certain geographic areas with histoplasmin and coccidioidin. The present status is easiest determined by exposing the individual to 0.05 ml of a 30% solution of dinitrochlorobenzene. This will evoke a contact dermatitis in more than 95% of normal persons. This sensitivity is determined by the dermal application of 0.05 ml of a 0.1% solution 14 days after the sensitizing exposure.

Tissue biopsy of lymph nodes and bone marrow may also be important in assessing the current status of T and B cells.

Complement levels can be determined by simple hemolytic assays or serologic tests for C3 or 4. Phagocytic function is usually measured by the NBT test or bactericidal test.

BIBLIOGRAPHY

Alper, C. A., and Rosen, F. S.: Genetic aspects of the complement system, Adv. Immunol. **14**:251, 1971.

Alper, C. A., and Rosen, F. S.: Clinical applications of complement assays, Adv. Intern. Med. **20**:61, 1975.

Azar, H. A., and Potter, M., eds.: Multiple myeloma and related disorders, Hagerstown, Md., 1973, Medical Department, Harper & Row, Publishers, Inc.

Baehner, R. L.: Disorders of leukocyte function, Adv. Pediatr. **20**:323, 1973.

Bergsma, D., ed.: Immunological deficiency diseases in man, New York, 1968, National Foundation.

Bernier, G. M.: Structure of human immunoglobulins: myeloma proteins as analogues of antibody, Prog. Allergy **14**:1, 1970.

Biggar, W. D., Park, B. H., and Good, R. A.: Immunologic reconstitution, Annu. Rev. Med. **24**:135, 1973.

Braylan, R. C., Jaffe, E. S., and Berard, C. W.: Malignant lymphomas: current classification and new observations, Pathol. Annu. **10**:213, 1975.

Gelfand, E. W., Biggar, W. D., and Orange, R. P.: Immune deficiency: evaluation, diagnosis, and therapy, Pediatr. Clin. North Am. **21**:745, 1974.

Higby, D. J., and Henderson, E. S.: Granulocyte transfusion therapy, Annu. Rev. Med. **26**:289, 1975.

Kagan, B. M., and Stiehm, E. R., eds.: Immunologic incompetence, Chicago, 1971, Year Book Medical Publishers, Inc.

Kaplan, H. S.: Hodgkin's disease, Cambridge, Mass., 1972, Harvard University Press.

Klein, G.: Immunological aspects of Burkitt's lymphoma, Adv. Immunol. **14**:187, 1971.

Levin, A. S., Spitler, L. E., and Fudenberg, H. H.: Transfer factor therapy in immune deficiency states, Annu. Rev. Med. **24**:175, 1973.

Padgett, G. A., Holland, J. M., Davis, W. C., and Henson, J. B.: The Chédiak-Higashi syndrome—a comparative review, Curr. Top. Pathol. **51**:175, 1970.

Pruzanski, W., and Ogryzlo, M. A.: Abnormal proteinuria in the malignant diseases, Adv. Clin. Chem. **13**:335, 1970.

Rosen, F. S.: Immunological deficiency disease, Clin. Immunobiol. **1**:271, 1972.

Rosen, F. S.: Primary immunodeficiency, Pediatr. Clin. North Am. **21**:533, 1974.

Samter, M., ed.: Immunological diseases, ed. 2, Boston, 1971, Little, Brown & Co.

Stiehm, E. R., and Fulginiti, V. A., eds.: Immunologic disorders in infants and children, Philadelphia, 1973, W. B. Saunders Co.

Turk, J. L.: Immunology in clinical medicine,

ed. 2, New York, 1972, Appleton-Century-Crofts.
Uhr, J. W., and Landy, M., eds.: Immunological intervention, New York, 1971, Academic Press, Inc.
Williams, R. C., Jr., and Messner, R. P.: Alterations in T- and B-cells in human disease states, Annu. Rev. Med. **26**:181, 1975.
Windhorst, D. B.: Functional defects of neutrophils, Adv. Intern. Med. **16**:329, 1970.

Case histories

CASE 1. HODGKIN'S DISEASE

J. D., a 47-year-old postal delivery man, was first seen in February, 1972, for evaluation of a fever of undetermined origin. At this time the patient had no cough or sign of upper respiratory disease, although he had a positive PPD skin test. He weighed 178 pounds. The fever subsided spontaneously, and no diagnosis was established. All cultures were negative for tubercle bacilli. In September, 1972, the patient returned with complaints of cervical lymphadenopathy, fever, night sweats, and occasional chills. His weight at this time was 164 pounds; he appeared pale and acutely ill. His blood pressure was 112/88 and his temperature 103.2° F (39.6° C); the white blood cell differential count showed 67 polymorphonuclear leukocytes, 19 lymphocytes, and 14 monocytes and the total white blood cell count was 4740/mm^3. A lymph node biopsy, sternal bone marrow aspiration, and serum protein electrophoresis was ordered. An immunologic assessment of the patient was indicated, and he was skin tested with PPD as the first step in that direction.

Questions

1. What cells of the immune system are involved in Hodgkin's disease?
2. What further immunologic tests are suggested to assist in the diagnosis of Hodgkin's disease?
3. In what way is the chemotherapy of Hodgkin's disease related to its immunocytology?

Discussion

Lymph node biopsy and bone marrow aspirations are recommended aids to the diagnosis of most immunoproliferative diseases. Peripheral white blood cell counts and differential counts are also useful. Hodgkin's disease is separable from the other lymphoproliferative diseases on the basis of two cytopathologic criteria: (1) the relative pleomorphism of the cellular constituents involved and (2) the near constant appearance of Reed-Sternberg cells. In Hodgkin's granuloma, neoplastic elements are variable in appearance. A mixture of plasma cells, eosinophils, Reed-Sternberg cells, and fibrous elements are detectable. Variable foci of necrosis appear in the lymph nodes. The Reed-Sternberg cell ranges from 12 to 40 μ, has a prominent lobulated nucleus, and may contain a pair of nuclei. The cytoplasm does not stain intensely, and it may be either acidophilic or basophilic. Its presence establishes the diagnosis.

The position of the Reed-Sternberg cell in any maturation sequence of the T cell series is uncertain, but it probably arises from a primitive, relatively undifferentiated cell. Hodgkin's disease is a form of T cell lymphoma, but the cellular defect escapes unequivocal positioning.

Serum protein electrophoresis and PPD testing were included as part of the immunologic evaluation of this patient. It is rare to find any significant change in the immunoglobulin pattern of patients with Hodgkin's disease, since B lymphocyte functions are not particularly disturbed in this disease. The knowledge that this patient had a recent positive skin test to PPD challenge is very helpful in assessing his immunologic status. Other tests should include mumps virus and *Candida* skin testing plus sensitization to dinitrochlorobenzene. The incidence of delayed-type skin reactions in healthy adults and patients with Hodgkin's disease to these tests is tabulated as follows.

	Controls (%)	*Hodgkin's* (%)
PPD (intermediate)	24	14
Mumps	88	63
Candida	52	36
Dinitrochlorobenzene	95	70

Retesting of J. D. revealed a loss of PPD sensitivity. No tests for B cell functioning were deemed necessary.

Combined radiotherapy and chemotherapy are suggested for Hodgkin's disease; both are indicated for their destructive effect on lymphoid tissue. Nitrogen mustard, cyclophosphamide, and chlorambucil are among the drugs used. Purine and pyrimidine analogs (5-fluorouracil) and methotrexate have proved surprisingly ineffectual. Prolonged maintenance on corticosteroids is difficult. The therapeutic success can be evaluated by retesting for the emergence of positive skin tests to PPD, mumps, etc.

REFERENCES

Brown, R. S., Haynes, H. A., Foley, H. T., Godwin, H. A., Berard, C. W., and Carbone, P. P.: Hodgkin's disease. Immunologic, clinical and histologic features of 50 untreated patients, Ann. Intern. Med. **69:** 291, 1967.

Smithers, D., ed.: Hodgkin's disease, Edinburgh, 1973, Churchill Livingstone.

Kaplan, H. S.: Hodgkin's disease, Cambridge, Mass., 1972, Harvard University Press.

CASE 2. MULTIPLE MYELOMA

B. C., a 60-year-old white male, was admitted to the hospital with pains in his back and legs. Enlarged lymph nodes were noted in the cervical, axillary, and groin areas. His hemoglobin was 12.4 gm/100 ml, white blood cell count was 9200/mm^3, and the serum bilirubin level was increased. Urinalysis was 1+ for protein. Serum protein electrophoresis indicated a possible polyclonal gammopathy of the A and G classes. Total serum protein levels were normal. Skeletal x-ray films, bone marrow aspiration, and quantitative immunoglobulin determinations were ordered.

Questions

1. What is the probable nature of the proteinuria?
2. How does the total serum level remain normal with a concurrent polyclonal gammopathy?
3. How can a polyclonal gammopathy be suggested only from serum electrophoresis?
4. What is the preferred procedure for immunoglobulin quantitation?

Discussion

The proteinuria is undoubtedly due to Bence Jones protein. To test for Bence Jones protein it may be necessary to acidify the urine to pH 4.5 with dilute acetic acid. The exact temperatures at which precipitation and dissolution will occur vary from patient to patient; some Bence Jones proteins do not dissolve at 100° C. The frequency of Bence Jones protein in urine has varied from as low as 30% to as high as 88% of myeloma cases. This wide range is undoubtedly due to differences in technique (acidity of urine), protein concentration, and temperature criterion. The electrophoresis of 5- to 10-fold concentrated urine has done much to improve the urinary identification of Bence Jones protein. Systematic investigation indicates an incidence in urine in excess of 50%. The Bence Jones protein is frequently the only protein in the urine, where it is situated in the electrophoretic position occupied by the gamma globulins. It is the light chain of the immunoglobulins or dimeric or polymeric forms of the molecule.

As an aside it is interesting that Sir Henry Bence Jones has had his name perpetuated by this protein. He was a clinical pathologist who recognized the protein in a urine sample supplied by Dr. Dalrymple, and another physician, Dr. Watson, later cared for the patient. The names of the patient and the two attending physicians have fallen into obscurity!

Polyclonal and monoclonal M components do not necessarily disturb the total gamma globulin concentration of the serum; in fact, hypogammaglobulinemia is seen in 12% of all patients with myeloma. This has been interpreted as an elimination of normal plasma cells by cells of the plasmacytoma. Serum electrophoresis may identify the class of the hypo- as well as the hypergammaglobulinemic protein. Simple serum electrophoresis will often distinguish an IgG myeloma from the others. Mixed IgA and IgM proteins will appear in nearly the same electrophoretic position and obscure the identification of the condition as a polyclonal disease. IgG with either IgA or IgM is more easily identified, although whether the second protein is A or M is often difficult to decide. In the recent past this distinction has been made via immunoelectrophoretic determinations of a crude quantitative nature with specific antisera against IgG, IgA, and IgM with normal strength and diluted serum. If the serum IgG and IgA are no longer detectable with specific antisera tested against diluted serum but the IgM is, then the indication is that the myeloma is of the IgM class. Radial immunodiffusion tests are now preferred because they are more sensitive and quantitative. In the patient described the Mancini test recovered 3.2 gm/100 ml of IgG and 0.6 gm of IgA. Normal values should approximate 1.3 gm for IgG and 0.3 gm for IgA; thus the patient had a combined IgG and IgA myeloma.

REFERENCES

Engle, R. L., and Wallis, L. A.: Immunoglobulinopathies, Springfield, Ill., 1969, Charles C Thomas, Publisher.

Osserman, E. F.: Plasma-cell myeloma. II. Clinical aspects, N. Engl. J. Med. **261**:1006, 1959.

Waldenström, J.: Diagnosis and treatment of multiple myeloma, New York, 1970, Grune & Stratton, Inc.

CASE 3. SELECTIVE IgA DEFICIENCY

L. H., a 3-year-old female, was referred to a regional hospital by her local physician in a small farming community because of recurrent respiratory infections. On admission she weighed 29 pounds, appeared thin and pale, had a temperature of 37.5° C, had a reddened throat, and had small white foci on her tonsils. The child's history indicated that she has had recurrent tonsillitis since 1½ years of age. Rarely were any significant pathogens isolated, but on one occasion *Streptococcus pyogenes* group A was recovered. Her present white blood cell count was moderately elevated, with a shift to the left. Throat cultures were taken, and blood was drawn for serum electrophoretic analysis.

Questions

1. Why is this child not considered to have agammaglobulinemia?
2. What is the status of secretory IgA in the serum IgA–deficient person?
3. What diseases are associated with IgA dysgammaglobulinemia?
4. Is IgA antigenic for the patient with IgA dysgammaglobulinemia?

Discussion

It is the general experience that even though many IgA-deficient individuals are asymptomatic, recurrent infections are also common. Recognized infectious diseases include tonsillitis, otitis media, febrile disease with cough and nasal discharge, and other upper respiratory diseases not further identified. In older children and adults, asthmatic episodes are triggered by these infections, which suggests an allergic disposition toward the pathogens. This is not the case in hereditary telangiectasia, where an IgE deficiency accompanies the IgA loss. Since this child had not had a life-threatening illness in the first years of her life, combined immunodeficiency disease was not considered. Because the child was female, Bruton's agammaglobulinemia was discounted.

Individuals deficient in serum IgA are likewise deficient in secretory IgA. Since the patient with IgA dysgammaglobulinemia has never experienced any self-contact with IgA, it is recognized as a foreign antigen. The immune response to external IgA in plasma or blood transfusions could result in anaphylaxis if a prior exposure induced sufficient antibody formation.

REFERENCES

Rockey, J. H., Hanson, L. Å., Heremans, J. F., and Kunkel, H. G.: Beta-2A aglobulinemia in two healthy men, J. Lab. Clin. Med. **63:** 205, 1964.

Tomasi, T. B., and Grey, H. M.: Structure and function of immunoglobulin A, Prog. Allergy **16:**81, 1972.

West, C. D., Hong, R., and Holland, N. H.: Immunoglobulin levels from the newborn period to adulthood and in immunoglobulin deficiency states, J. Clin. Invest. **41:**2054, 1962.

Glossary

This glossary is not intended to be a complete listing of all immunologic terms. Students desiring fuller definitions or definitions of additional words, phrases, or abbreviations are advised to consult the following sources.

Halliday, W. J.: Glossary of immunological terms, New York, 1971, Appleton-Century-Crofts.

Herbert, W. J., and Wilkinson, P. C., eds.: A dictionary of immunology, Oxford, 1971, Blackwell Scientific Publications, Ltd.

ABO antigens Antigens of the major human blood group system.

acquired immunity Immunity developed after birth as compared to inherited immunity.

activated macrophage Macrophages from antigen-sensitized or otherwise stimulated animals.

adjuvant Substance, usually injected with an antigen, that improves the immune response, either humoral or cellular, to the antigen.

adrenergic drugs Drugs such as adrenaline that constrict blood vessels, relax smooth muscle, and inhibit histamine release from mast cells.

agammaglobulinemia Condition in which all of the immunoglobulins are absent from the serum. See also *Hypogammaglobulinemia.*

agglutination Aggregation of cellular or particulate antigens by an antiserum containing antibodies to one or more surface antigens.

agglutinin Antibody directed toward surface antigens and capable of causing agglutination.

agglutinin adsorption Removal of agglutinins by allowing them to combine with the cellular antigen. The antigen and attached antibodies are then removed by filtration, centrifugation, etc.

ALG See *Antilymphocyte globulin.*

alkylating agent Agent that reacts with electronegative centers in another compound and forms covalent bonds with it during the reaction. Such compounds are often immunosuppressants.

allergen Substance (antigen or hapten) that causes an allergy, that is, stimulates IgE synthesis and/or T lymphocytes.

allergy Altered state of reactivity to an antigen or hapten; used synonymously with hypersensitivity.

allogeneic Of different genetic and hence antigenic type, but usually applied to antigens possessed by another member of one's own species.

allograft Graft that contains antigens different from those in the graft recipient, as considered within a single species. Replaces the term "homograft."

allotype Existence within a single species of molecules differing in antigenicity but sharing similar or identical functions.

alpha chain Heavy peptide chain of IgA.

ALS See *Antilymphocyte serum.*

alternate pathway Mechanism to activate complement at the level of C3 in which antibodies are not absolutely required.

anamnestic response The rapid rise in the immunoglobulin content of blood following a second or subsequent exposure to antigen; synonymous with booster or secondary response.

anaphylactoid reaction Pseudoanaphylactic reaction that is similar to it in most respects except that it is not created by an antigen-antibody reaction.

anaphylatoxin Originally a substance that caused histamine release; now specific peptides from complement fractions 3 and 5, C3a and C5a, that release histamine from mast cells and basophils.

anaphylaxis Unexpected, detrimental reaction to a second exposure to antigen in which histamine, SRS-A, etc. are released by a reaction of antigen with IgE on the surface of mast cells (*ana,* meaning without; *phylaxis,* meaning protection).

anergy Inability to respond to an antigen in the expected way.

angioneurotic edema Sporadic edematous condition related to a genetic deficiency in $C\bar{1}$ esterase inhibitor.

antibody Proteins of the gamma globulin fraction of serum that are induced by and react with antigens; synonymous with immunoglobulin.

antibody fragments Portion of an antibody molecule as created by enzymatic hydrolysis or chemical dissociation.

antigen Macromolecule that will induce the formation of immunoglobulins or sensitized lymphocytes that will react specifically with the antigen.

antigen determinant sites Unique portions of an antigen that are responsible for its activity.

antiglobulin test Test to determine the presence of a globulin with an antibody to that globulin, as in the Coombs' test.

antihistamine Drug that is an inhibitor, usually a competitive inhibitor, of histamine.

antilymphocyte globulin Globulin fraction of an antilymphocyte serum.

antilymphocyte serum Antiserum prepared against lymphocytes of either the B, T, or usually a mixture of the B and T types.

antiserum Serum that contains antibodies.

antitoxin Antibody (or antiserum) prepared in response to a toxin or toxoid.

Arthus reaction Necrotic, dermal reaction due to antigen-antibody precipitation, complement fixation, and neutrophilic inflammation in tissues of an animal inoculated intracutaneously with antigen.

ataxia-telangiectasia Loss of muscle coordination and blood vessel dilation combined with deficits in IgA production and T lymphocyte activities.

atopy IgE-dependent allergy often arising from an unknown exposure to an antigen or autocoupling hapten.

attenuation Weakening of the virulence of a pathogenic organism while retaining its viability.

autoallergic disease Disease in which a self-directed immune response is detectable; synonymous with autoimmune disease.

autoantibody Antibody that is reactive with antigens of the animal producing the antibody.

autograft Graft of tissue in which the donor and recipient are the same individual.

autoimmune disease Synonym of autoallergic disease.

autoimmunization Immunization with self-antigens.

avidity Firmness of the combination of antigen or hapten with antibody.

B cell Lymphocyte from the bursa of Fabricius or one that is of the immunoglobulin-forming type.

bacteriolysis Dissolution of the bacterial cell wall by specific antibody and serum complement.

bacteriotropin Immune opsonin that stimulates phagocytosis of a bacterium, other cell type, or particle.

Bence Jones protein Immunoglobulin light chain often found in urine or blood of patients with a myeloma.

blocking antibody Antibody that prevents the action of another antibody, that is, antibodies formed during desensitization aganst atopic allergies. Also an antibody that blocks the activity of a T lymphocyte.

blood group antigen Antigens that are genetically determined and present on the surface of red blood cells.

booster response See *Anamnestic response.*

Boivin antigen Heat-stable antigen extractable from gram-negative bacteria; essentially synonymous with endotoxin.

Boyden technique Procedure for attaching protein antigens to erythrocytes by first treating the cells with tannic acid.

bradykinin Specific peptide of nine amino acids formed during anaphylaxis that produces pain, vasodilation, edema, and smooth muscle contraction. See also *Vasoactive amine.*

Bruton-type agammaglobulinemia Sex-linked

congenital inability to form B cells and hence immunoglobulins.

bursa of Fabricius Cloacal organ in fowl from which the immunoglobulin-synthesizing B lymphocytes originate.

C1 to C9 Components of serum complement numbered sequentially.

C1 esterase Esterase formed during activation of the C1s component of complement.

C3 INAC C3 inactivator, KAF, conglutinogen activating factor.

C3 PA C3 proactivator.

C3 PAse Enzyme that converts C3 PA to C3 activator; also known as C3 PA convertase.

capsular swelling Apparent enlargement of the capsule of a microorganism on its reaction with specific antibody; synonymous with quellung reaction.

Cell-mediated immunity Immunity dependent on T-type lymphocytes and phagocytic cells; also known as cellular immunity.

CGD See *Chronic granulomatous disease.*

C_H1, C_H2, and C_H3 Portions of γ-chains and other heavy chains that have nearly constant amino acid sequences.

Chédiak-Higashi syndrome Disease based on faulty phagocytic destruction of parasites and related to lysosomal abnormalities.

chemotaxis Attraction of leukocytes or other cells by chemicals; synonymous with leukotaxin in reference to white blood cells.

chimera Animal possessing antigens, which are not its own antigens in a genetic sense, from its twin or acquired by experimental procedures.

chronic granulomatous disease Sex-linked hereditary disease resulting in faulty phagocytic destruction of ingested parasites.

C_L Portions of κ- and λ-chains with constant amino acid sequences.

classic pathway Activation of complement by antigen-antibody combination; involving all nine components of complement.

clonal selection theory Theory of immunoglobulin formation that suggests that an antigen causes the replication of a cell to form a clone of cells producing antibody to that antigen.

complement System of nine major serum proteins that interact with antigen and antibody to produce cytolytic, chemotaxic, anaphylactic, and other effects.

complement fixation Binding or utilization of serum complement in a reaction with antigen and antibody.

concanavalin A Phytohemagglutinin that is specific for T lymphocytes.

constant region That region of an immunoglobulin chain with a close sequence homology to other chains of that class or subclass.

contact dermatitis Delayed or cell-mediated hypersensitive response to cutaneously applied allergens.

Coombs' test Form of antiglobulin test in which the globulin antigen is a nonhemagglutinating antibody.

corticosteroids Natural (or synthetic) compounds from the adrenal cortex that are anti-inflammatory and immunosuppressive.

counterimmunoelectrophoresis Electrophoretic movement of antigen and antibody toward each other to promote their precipitation.

C-reactive protein An albumin excreted by liver cells only during an inflammatory disease.

cross-reaction Reaction of an antibody with an antigen closely related in structure to the antibody-inducing antigen.

crossed immunoelectrophoresis Electrophoretic migration of antigen(s) into a gel containing antibody.

cytophilic antibody Antibodies that attach nonspecifically to macrophages.

cytotropic antibody Antibodies that attach nonspecifically to mast cells and basophils.

delayed hypersensitivity Synonym of cell-mediated hypersensitivity. A form of allergy expressed by T lymphocytes, not involving immunoglobulins, and developing slowly when provoked dermally.

delta chain Heavy chain of immunoglobulin D.

desensitization Elimination or reduction of allergic sensitivity, usually through a programmed course of antigen treatment.

DiGeorge's syndrome Birth defects in embryonic development of the thymus resulting in losses of immune competence related to T lymphocytes.

double-antibody procedure Serologic test in which an antibody to an antigen serves also as an antigen for a second antibody.

dysgammaglobulinemia Imbalance in the normal concentration of the immunoglobulins or a malfunction of one or more immunoglobulins.

ECF-A See *Eosinophilic chemotactic factor of anaphylaxis.*

endotoxin Toxins present as a structural part of the cell wall of gram-negative bacteria and essentially synonymous with O antigen.

Eosinophilic chemotactic factor of anaphylaxis Product of mast cells that is chemotactic for eosinophils.

epsilon chain Heavy chain of IgE.

erythroblastosis fetalis Disease of the newborn caused by maternal antibodies that pass the placenta and destroy fetal erythrocytes.

Fab fragment Fragment of an immunoglobulin consisting of one light chain and approximately one half of the heavy chain. The heavy chain class may be designated Fabγ, Fab_{α}, etc.

$F(ab)_2$ fragment Two Fab fragments plus an additional portion of the heavy chain of the immunoglobulin joined by disulfide bonds, as after papain treatment of IgG. The heavy chain class may also be designated $F(ab)_{2\gamma}$, etc.

Fc fragment Carboxyl terminal portion of an immunoglobulin heavy chain. The heavy chain class may also be designated as Fc_{γ}, etc.

ferritin-labeled antibody Immunoglobulin conjugated to ferritin for use in electron microscopy.

flocculation 1. Specific type of precipitation that occurs over a narrow range of antigen concentration. 2. Aggregation of colloidal particles in a serologic reaction, as in syphilis serology.

fluorescent antibody Immunoglobulin conjugated to a fluorescent dye for use in ultraviolet microscopy.

folic acid antagonist Structural analogs of folic acid that function as immunosuppressants (aminopterin, methotrexate, etc.).

Forssman antigen Hapten (not an antigen) distributed widely through both the plant and animal kingdoms.

Freund's adjuvant Adjuvant consisting of an oil and emulsifying agent (incomplete Freund's adjuvant) with which antigen solutions are emulsified. For the complete adjuvant, mycobacteria are also incorporated into the mixture.

gamma chain Heavy chain of IgG.

gamma globulin Portion of the serum proteins in which the immunoglobulins are found; characterized by low electrophoretic mobility at pH 8.3.

germinal center Discrete cellular structure in lymphoid organs of antigenically stimulated animals containing macrophages, T or B lymphocytes, and/or plasma cells.

Gm group Allotypic group based on antigenic changes in heavy chain antigens of IgG.

graft-versus-host reaction Reaction resulting from the attack of immunocompetent tissue in a graft against an immunologically compromised host.

H antigen Flagellar antigen(s) of bacteria.

H chain disease Condition characterized by the presence of heavy chains of an immunoglobulin or portions thereof in serum.

H substance Antigen on the human erythrocyte that is a precursor substance for the A and B antigens.

Hageman factor Plasma protein that can activate prokininogenase; also known as PF/dil.

hapten Nonantigenic material that, when combined with an antigen, conveys a new antigenic specificity on the antigen.

heavy chain Large polypeptide chain, of which two exist, in the basic tetrapeptide structure of immunoglobulins.

helper function Capacity of T cells to assist B cells in immunoglobulin formation.

hemagglutination Agglutination of erythrocytes, especially by antiserum.

hemolysin Antibody with a specificity for erythrocytes that, in cooperation with serum complement, will lyse the red blood cells.

hemolysis Lysis of erythrocytes by specific antibody and serum complement.

heterocytotropic antibody Antibody from one species that will attach to mast cells of another species.

heterograft Graft of a different antigenic composition than the host. Replaced by allograft and xenograft as appropriate.

heterotopic graft Graft placed in an abnormal anatomic position.

histamine Specific chemical compound released from mast cells and producing vasodilation, smooth muscle contraction, and edema during anaphylaxis.

histamine releasers Synthetic compounds, often polyamines, that will release histamine from mast cells.

histocompatibility antigen Antigen on the surface of a cell that, when the cell is transplanted to a different host, induces the response leading to graft rejection; synonymous with transplantation antigen.

HL-A antigen Human histocompatibility antigen, originally identified as human leukocyte A antigen.

Hodgkin's disease Neoplastic, lymphoproliferative disorder characterized by a progressive loss of T cell function.

homocytotropic antibody Antibody that will attach to the mast cells of the species producing it.

horror autotoxicus Fear of self-poisoning, as related to the usual inability of an antigen to serve as an autoantigen.

host-versus-graft rejection Usual etiology of graft rejection; the loss of grafted tissue by immunologic responses of the grafted individual toward foreign antigens of the graft.

humoral immunity Immunity due to immunoglobulins.

hypogammaglobulinemia Opposite of hypergammaglobulinemia, or decreased levels of gamma globulin in plasma.

hyposensitization Desensitization to an allergic condition.

idiotype An antigen, unique to an individual or small group of individuals, as opposed to allotype.

immediate hypersensitivities Allergies related to IgE or similar immunoglobulins in lower species, such as hay fever, food allergies, and certain drug allergies.

immune adherence Adhesive nature of antigen-antibody complexes to inert surfaces when complement is bound into the complex.

immune-complex disease Disease caused by or associated with the formation of antigen-antibody complexes, for example, glomerulonephritis and serum sickness.

immune enhancement Improved transplantability or survival of tissue in hosts with antibodies to the antigens of the tissue.

immune paralysis Failure to produce an antibody following proper exposure to antigens, especially massive doses; often used interchangeably with immunologic tolerance.

immunity Condition of being resistant to an infection.

immunoblast Cell intermediate between the lymphocyte and plasma cell.

immunodiffusion Diffusion of soluble antigens and/or antibodies toward each other leading to their precipitation in gel.

immunoelectrophoresis Electrophoretic displacement of antigen(s) or antibodies followed by immunodiffusion.

immunoglobulin A Immunoglobulin possessing α-heavy chains. Exists in serum and secretory forms.

immunoglobulin D Immunoglobulin in lowest concentration in serum and possessing δ-heavy chains.

immunoglobulin E Serum immunoglobulin with a potent homocytotropic tendency for mast cells and possessing ϵ-heavy chains; synonymous with allergic reagin.

immunoglobulin G Serum globulin in greatest concentration (75% to 95% of the total) and possessing γ-heavy chains.

immunoglobulin M Serum immunoglobulin of greatest molecular weight (about 900,000) formed earliest after antigen exposure and possessing μ-heavy chains.

immunologic tolerance Failure or depression in the immune response on proper exposure to antigen, especially massive doses.

immunosuppression The suppression of an immunologic response by chemical, physical, or biologic means.

incomplete antibody Antibody that does not continue into the aggregative phase of the reaction with antigen.

inherited immunity Immunity conferred by one's genetic constitution, not acquired by exposure to infectious agents; synonymous with innate immunity.

innate immunity See *Inherited immunity.*

interferon Protein(s) released from a cell that is infected by an intracellular parasite and which protects neighboring cells from invasion by the same or other intracellular parasites.

Inv groups Antigenic groups on κ-chains that create allotypic subclasses.

Ir gene Gene that permits an immune response to an antigen.

isogeneic Of the same genetic and hence antigenic constitution; synonym of syngeneic.

isograft Graft from another individual within the same species. Allograft or syngraft is now the preferred terminology as appropriate.

isohemagglutinin Antibody of an animal that will agglutinate erythrocytes from another animal of the same species.

isoimmunization Immunization of an individual with antigens of another individual of the same species.

isologous Referring to the same species. Preferred usage is now allogeneic or syngeneic as appropriate.

J chain Polypeptide chain found attached to secretory IgA and IgM that may function as a joining chain.

Jones-Mote reaction Hypersensitive reaction that appears to be mixed immediate and delayed reaction.

kallidin Lysylbradykinin or kinin 10.

kallikrein Protease(s) that releases kinins from kininogen; synonymous with kininogenase.

kappa chain Antigenic form of light chain of the immunoglobulins.

kininogenase See *Kallikrein.*

kininogens Alpha globulin proteins of serum that are precursors to kinins.

kinins Peptides or polyamines released during anaphylaxis that possess vasodilating and muscle-contracting activity.

Koch's phenomenon Rejection of subcutaneously placed tubercle bacilli by tuberculous animals as an expression of cell-mediated immunity.

Kveim reaction Specific reaction in the skin of sarcoid patients provoked by tissue from others with sarcoidosis.

lambda chain Antigenic form of light chain of the immunoglobulins.

LE cell Polymorphonuclear cell that has engulfed the enlarged nucleus of another white blood cell distorted by antinuclear antibody.

light chain Smallest of the two types of polypeptide chains (light and heavy) of immunoglobulins, of which two exist in the tetrapeptide unit.

lymph node permeability factor High molecular weight substance extractable from lymph node cells that will mimic the delayed hypersensitive skin reaction when injected into normal persons.

lymphocyte Agranular leukocyte with sparse cytoplasm and round nucleus derived from bone marrow and found in lymph nodes, blood, spleen, etc. Exists as B or T types.

lymphocyte transfer reaction Reaction in the skin of a normal recipient of lymphocytes from a donor, the extent of which is believed to indicate their histocompatibility difference.

lymphocyte transformation Active nucleic acid metabolism and nuclear enlargement of a lymphocyte on contact with antigen.

lymphokines Low molecular weight peptides elaborated by antigen-exposed T lymphocytes.

lymphotoxin Cell-destroying toxin excreted by T lymphocytes sensitized to a cellular antigen.

lysosome Intracellular structure serving as a condensed source of hydrolytic enzymes.

MAF Macrophage aggregation factor produced by T lymphocytes.

M component Serum protein produced in excessive concentration in cases of myeloma or macroglobulinemia.

macrophage Tissue or blood phagocytes, 20 to 80 μ in diameter, containing lysosomes, vacuoles, and partially digested debris in their cytoplasm.

Mancini test Radial immunodiffusion test, usually based on diffusion of antigen through a gel containing antibody.

mast cell Cell found in connective tissue in which heparin and histamine are stored in numerous intracytoplasmic granules.

mast cell degranulation Loss of mast cell granules during a serologic reaction on the cell surface or produced by certain chemicals.

Masugi nephritis Form of glomerulonephritis produced by passive immunization with antikidney serum.

memory cell Cell that responds more quickly to the second exposure to antigen than the primary exposure and is responsible for the anamnestic response.

MIF See *Migration inhibition factor.*

migration inhibition factor Protein (mol wt 23,000 to 55,000) produced by antigen-sensitized T lymphocytes when in the presence of antigen; prevents macrophage migration.

mixed leukocyte reaction Transformation of leukocytes in cultures with foreign leukocytes;

believed to indicate the histoincompatibility of their donors.

MLR See *Mixed leukocyte reaction.*

monovalent antibody Antibody that does not complete the aggregative phase of the serologic reaction.

mu chain Heavy chain of IgM.

multiple myeloma See *Myeloma.*

myeloma Plasma cell neoplasm resulting in excessive production of one or more immunoglobulins.

natural antibody Antibody formed in the absence of a known antigenic exposure.

natural immunity Inherited, not acquired, immunity.

neoantigen A "new" antigen formed by modification of an "old" antigen by haptenic addition or other means.

Nezelof's syndrome Genetic failure of T lymphocyte development and hence cell-mediated hypersensitivity.

nitroblue tetrazolium reduction test Test to measure the oxidizing and thus bactericidal activity of leukocytes.

O antigen Surface somatic antigens of bacteria; not to be confused with ABO antigens of human erythrocytes.

opsonin Antibody that attaches to a cellular or particulate antigen and "prepares" it for phagocytosis.

orthotopic graft graft placed in its usual anatomic position.

Ouchterlony test Immunodiffusion test based on diffusion of both antigen and antibody through gels; named for the scientist who designed it.

O_z group Antigenic unit responsible for different allotypic forms of λ-light chains.

paraproteinemia Presence of protein molecules in plasma that are antigenically similar to but originally believed lacking the biologic activity of normal molecules, especially as regards immunoglobulins.

passive cutaneous anaphylaxis Form of anaphylaxis caused by dermal injection of cytotropic antibodies followed by systemic injection of antigen.

passive hemagglutination Hemagglutination resulting from antibodies directed toward antigens adsorbed to the erythrocyte surface.

passive immunization Acquisition of immunity through injection of antibodies or antiserum produced in another animal.

PF/dil Permeability factor present in serum only after its dilution; synonymous with activated Hageman factor.

Pfeiffer's phenomenon Bacteriolysis with antiserum and complement.

phagocytic index

$$\frac{\text{Log conc. of particles at } T_1 - \text{Log conc. of particles at } T_2}{T_2 - T_1}$$

where T = time.

phagocytosis Engulfment of cells or particulate matter by leukocytes, macrophages, or other cells.

phytohemagglutinin Extract of a plant, usually *Phaseolus,* that will agglutinate erythrocytes.

PK test See *Prausnitz-Küstner test.*

Plasma cell Cell 10 to 20 μ in diameter that can actively synthesize immunoglobulins and be distinguished morphologically from similar cells.

plasmacytoma Neoplasm consisting of plasma cells.

polymorphonuclear leukocyte White blood cell with a granular cytoplasm and multilobed nucleus that is very active in phagocytosis.

postzone Failure of a serologic reaction to occur in extreme dilutions of antibody.

Prausnitz-Küstner Test for immediate hypersensitivity performed in a normal subject who has been passively sensitized by immunoglobulin from the allergic individual.

precipitation Formation of an insoluble complex of antibody with soluble antigen.

prekallikrein Prokininogenase.

prokininogenase Proenzyme of kininogenase.

properdin Complex serum protein capable of activating complement.

prozone Failure of a serologic reaction to occur in a high concentration of antibody.

quellung reaction Precipitation of specific antibody on the capsule of an organism producing the appearance of capsular swelling.

radioimmunoassay test Immunologic test utilizing radiolabeled antigen, antibody, complement, or other reactants. May be adapted to radioimmunodiffusion, radioprecipitation, etc.

RAST Radioallergosorbent test. See also *Radioimmunoassay.*

reagin 1. IgE, with specificity for allergens. 2. Syphilitic reagin, with specificity for cardiolipin antigens.

reticuloendothelial blockade Malfunction of

phagocytic cells caused by prior exposure to phagocytosable particles.

reticuloendothelial system Collective term for cells of varying morphology and tissue residence with the common feature of being actively phagocytic.

Rh antigens System of human blood group antigens shared by the rhesus monkey.

rheumatoid factor IgM associated with arthritis with a specificity toward IgG.

rosette technique 1. Test involving antibody-producing or antibody-binding cells mixed with a cellular antigen and forming a rosette. 2. Test for T lymphocytes from nonimmunized animals based on their ability to form rosettes with sheep red blood cells.

Schultz-Dale reaction In vitro anaphylactic response of sensitized uterus or gut when exposed to antigen.

secretory IgA Form of IgA found on mucosal surfaces consisting of two IgA units, secretory piece and J chain.

secretory piece Portion of secretory IgA not present in serum IgA and not produced in plasma cells.

serotonin Chemical mediator of anaphylaxis; 5-hydroxytryptamine.

serum sickness Protracted anaphylactic reaction due to the presence of antigen at the time that antibody is being formed.

Shwartzman reaction Necrotic reaction in tissue produced by endotoxins.

slow-reacting substance A Material that causes a slow or prolonged contraction of smooth muscle; believed to be released during anaphylaxis.

somatic antigen Antigen that is part of the body of a cell as opposed to flagellar or capsular antigen.

SRS-A See *Slow-reacting substance A.*

suppressor activity Ability of T cells to suppress immunoglobulin formation.

Swiss-type agammaglobulinemia Genetic disease resulting in deficiencies in both T and B lymphocyte functions.

syngeneic Of identical genetic and hence antigenic constitution.

T lymphocytes Lymphocyte modified in the thymus that is responsible for cell-mediated hypersensitivity and cell-mediated immunity.

target cell destruction Destruction of tumor or other cells by T lymphocytes previously exposed to these cells.

TF See *Transfer factor.*

thymic aplasia See *DiGeorge's syndrome.*

thymosin Hormonelike substance from thymus believed to be the active component of T lymphocytes.

thymus Gland located near the parathyroid and thyroid whose lymphocytes (T type) regulate cell-mediated hypersensitivity and interact with B cells for immunoglobulin formation.

titer Greatest dilution of a substance used in a serologic reaction that will produce the desired result.

toxoid Toxin treated to preserve its native antigenicity but to eliminate its toxicity.

transfer factor Ribonucleotide (mol wt 700 to 4000) that can transfer (in human species) the cell-mediated hypersensitivities of the lymphocytes from which it is extracted.

translation inhibitory protein Protein believed to be the mechanism by which interferon interrupts replication of intracellular parasites.

transplantation antigen Antigen on tissue that, when grafted, induces the immune responses critical to tissue rejection. Histocompatibility antigen.

TSTA See *Tumor-specific transplantation antigen.*

tumor-specific transplantation antigen Transplantation antigen(s) acquired by tumor cells.

vaccine Suspension of living or dead organisms used as an antigen.

valence Number of antigenic determinant sites available on an antigen (or antibody) to which an antibody (antigen) can combine.

vasoactive amine Amine or peptide that produces vasodilation.

V_H region Region of heavy chains that have a variable sequence.

V_L region Same as V_H but involving light chains.

Waldenström's macroglobulinemia Myeloma involving IgM or IgM-like molecules.

Wiskott-Aldrich syndrome Sex-linked genetic disease with combined losses of B and T lymphocytes, especially of IgM production.

xenograft Graft of tissue between different species.

Index

G

H

I

O

P

Q

R